NCLEX-RN® Notes

Core Review & Exam Prep Third Edition

Barbara A. Vitale, RN, MA

A Davis's Notes Book

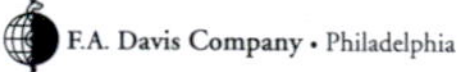

F. A. Davis Company
1915 Arch Street
Philadelphia, PA 19103
www.fadavis.com

Printed in China

Last digit indicates print number: 10 9 8 7 6 5 4 3 2 1

Publisher, Nursing: Terri Wood Allen
Content Project Manager: Julia L. Curcio
Electronic Project Editor: Sandra A. Glennie
Cover Design: Carolyn O'Brien
Contributors: Jane Brody RN, PhD; Mary Ann Hellmer-Saul RN, PhD, CNE; Michael Mangino Jr., RN, NP-P; Patricia Nugent RN, EdD.
Medical Consultant: Joanne Vitale, RPA-C.
Consultants: Joan Carnosso RN, MS, EdS; Doreen DeAngelis MSN, RN; Patricia Delmoe RN, MN; Melissa Garno EdD, RN; Jan Hartig MSN, RN; Elizabeth A. Kassel MSN; Pamela D. Korte RN, MS; Dara Lanman MSN, RN, CNE; K. Shea Mobley FNP; Emily Dawn Orr RN, BSN, CCRN; Cindy Parsons DNP, PMHNP-BC, FAANP; Jean M. Schroeder PhD, RN; Brenda Sloan RN, MA, ACNS; Kim Stevens MSN, RN; Virginia E. Tufano EdD, MSN, RN

↑	Increase
↓	Decrease
→	Cause, contribute to
>	Greater than
≥	Equal to or greater than
<	Less than
≤	Equal to or less than
ABG	Arterial blood gas
ADH	Antidiuretic hormone
ADL	Activities of daily living
ADHD	Attention deficit hyperactivity disorder
BM	Bowel movement
bpm	Beats per minute, breaths per minute
BR	Bed rest
BUN	Blood urea nitrogen
Ca	Cancer
C&S	Culture and sensitivity
CHO	Carbohydrate
cm	Centimeter
CNS	Central nervous system
CO_2	Carbon dioxide
CSF	Cerebrospinal fluid
CT	Computed tomography
DBP	Diastolic blood pressure
D&C	Dilation and curettage
D/C	Discontinue
DFV	Deficient fluid volume
DM	Diabetes mellitus
DVT	Deep vein thrombosis
ECG	Electrocardiogram
EFV	Excess fluid volume
EPS	Extrapyramidal side effects
FDA	Food and Drug Administration
F&E	Fluid and electrolytes
FHR	Fetal heart rate
g	Gram(s)
Hb	Hemoglobin
Hct	Hematocrit
HDL	High-density lipoprotein
HF	Heart failure
HOB	Head of bed
HR	Heart rate
hr	Hour(s)
HTN	Hypertension
IBD	Irritable bowel disease
I&O	Intake and output

ICP	Increased intracranial pressure
ICU	Intensive care unit
IVF	Intravenous fluids
K	Potassium
L	Liter
lb	Pound(s)
LDL	Low-density lipoprotein
LLQ	Left lower quadrant
LOC	Level of consciousness
LUQ	Left upper quadrant
MAOI	Monoamine oxidase inhibitor
mcg	Microgram
Med(s)	Medication(s)
mg	Milligram(s)
MI	Myocardial infarction
min	Minute(s)
mL	Milliliter(s)
mL/kg	Milliliter per kilogram
mo	Month(s)
MRI	Magnetic resonance imaging
N&V	Nausea and vomiting
Na	Sodium
NGT	Nasogastric tube
NPO	Nothing by mouth
NS	Normal saline
NSAID	Nonsteroidal anti-inflammatory drug
OT	Occupational therapy
OTC	Over the counter
PE	Pulmonary embolism
pH	Degree of acidity or alkalinity of a substance
PN	Parenteral nutrition
PROM	Premature rupture of membranes, passive range of motion
PT	Prothrombin time, physical therapy
PTT	Partial thromboplastin time
QI	Quality improvement
RDA	Recommended daily allowance
Rh	Rh blood group system
RLQ	Right lower quadrant
RUQ	Right upper quadrant
RT	Respiratory therapy
SBP	Systolic blood pressure
sec	Second(s)
SNS	Sympathetic nervous system
SOB	Shortness of breath

ST	Speech therapy
STI	Sexually transmitted infection
TB	Tuberculosis
TPN	Total parenteral nutrition
UTI	Urinary tract infection
wk	Week(s)
yr	Year(s)

NCLEX-RN® Overview

The National Council Licensure Examination for Registered Nurses (NCLEX-RN) measures the knowledge and abilities necessary for entry-level nurses.

- It is administered by computer-adaptive testing (CAT), which individualizes tests to match the unique competencies of each test taker.
- Each exam adheres to the NCLEX-RN Test Plan, which describes the content and scope of RN competencies.
- Practices basic to nursing (nursing process, caring, teaching, learning, communication, documentation, culture, and spirituality) are integrated throughout, and most questions require application and analysis of information.

NCLEX-RN Test Plan: Distribution of Content

Client Needs and Percentage of Items

Client Needs	Percentage of Items
Safe and Effective Care Environment	
• Management of Care	17%–23%
• Safety/Infection Control	9%–15%
Health Promotion and Maintenance	6%–12%
Psychosocial Integrity	6%–12%
Physiological Integrity	
• Basic Care/Comfort	6%–12%
• Pharmacological/Parenteral Therapies	12%–18%
• Reduction of Risk Potential	9%–15%
• Physiological Adaptation	11%–17%

Taking the NCLEX-RN Test on a Computer

- You will receive general information about the exam and the testing center. Your time spent on this will not count.
- You will take a tutorial on how to use the computer to answer the questions on the NCLEX-RN. Your answers will not count toward your score, but the time you take will be subtracted from the total 6 hr you have for the exam.
- You will then be presented with NCLEX-RN items; there will be between 75 and 265 items. The test ends when it is 95% certain your ability is ↑ or ↓ the passing standard.

- Answers may be selected or deleted several times if desired before confirming a final answer. You must answer every question. You cannot return to a previous question.
- A time-remaining clock is in the screen's upper right-hand corner.
- A calculator on the computer is available for calculations.

Go to www.NCSBN.org to access an NCLEX tutorial to practice multiple-choice and alternate format items on the computer.

Content in Davis*Plus*.FADavis.com

To maximize your test-taking performance you should begin by focusing on your critical thinking abilities, use of general and specific study skills, and use of test-taking techniques. See Davis*Plus*.FADavis.com for a detailed presentation of the topics in the outline below along with over 850 practice test items. The practice test items encompass the following clinical disciplines: Basic Information, Childbearing, Pediatrics, Mental Health, Medical-Surgical, and Medication and Medication Administration. These questions include Multiple-Choice items as well as all types of Alternate Format Items.

Critical Thinking

Definition, Influences, and Uses
Maximize Your Critical-Thinking Abilities: Actions and Benefits

General Study Skills

Use Techniques Appropriate for Learning Domains: Cognitive, Affective, Psychomotor

Specific Study Skills

How to Remember and Recall Information: Commit Facts to Memory
How to Manipulate Information: Apply, Solve, Modify, and Use Information
How to Analyze Information: Examine the Organization, Structure, and Interrelationship of Information
Test-Taking and Study Tips
Alternate Format Questions and Test-Taking Tips

Practice Test Items

Basic Life Support by Health-Care Providers (Cardiopulmonary Resuscitation, CPR) (American Heart Association)

Definition: External cardiac compression and ventilation to ↑ blood flow to heart and brain.

1. Assess breathing and pulse simultaneously. No breathing or only gasping and no pulse within 5–10 seconds, then proceed with procedure. Palpate carotid pulse for adult or brachial/femoral pulse for infant/child.
2. If no response: If alone, for an adult, activate emergency system and get AED before CPR; for child or infant, follow steps for adult if collapse is witnessed or if unwitnessed give 2 minutes of CPR then activate the emergency system, get AED, and then resume CPR.
3. Ensure victim is on hard surface in supine position before cardiac compressions.

CPR	Infant (<1 yr)	Child (>1 yr–adolescent)	Adult
Rate of compressions.	100–120 compressions per min. Rotate health-care provider every 2 min; interruptions less than 10 sec.		
Hand placement.	2 fingers in center of chest just below nipple line (1 rescuer). 2 thumbs with hands encircling center of chest, just below nipple line (2 rescuers).	2 hands or 1 hand for small child on lower half of sternum.	Heel of one hand with fingers interlocked with the other on lower half of sternum.
Depth of compressions; allow full recoil after each compression.	⅓ of anteroposterior (AP) diameter. About 1.5 inches.	⅓ of AP diameter. About 2 inches.	At least 2 inches. No more than 2.4 inches.
Ratio of compressions to ventilations.	30 to 2 (1 rescuer). 15 to 2 (2 rescuers).		30 to 2 (1 or 2 rescuers).

4. Assess and establish airway; open airway (head-tilt, chin-lift maneuver or jaw thrust without neck hyperextension if cervical injury suspected).
5. If not breathing, instill air into lungs at the rate indicated in the fourth row of the chart "Ratio of compressions to ventilations" (maintain head-tilt or jaw thrust maneuver while pinching victim's nostrils).
6. Maintain ratio of compressions to ventilations for five cycles and then reassess pulse; allow for full recoil after each compression; do not lean on chest between compressions.
7. Defibrillate; minimize length of interruptions to ↓ than 10 seconds.
8. If successful, discontinue CPR and position victim in recovery position.
9. If unsuccessful, resume compressions and ventilations according to appropriate age and number of rescuers; terminate CPR when ordered by primary health-care provider or rescuer exhaustion.

Foreign Body Airway Obstruction (American Heart Association)

	Infant (<1 yr)	Child (≥1 yr–Adolescent) and Adult
Assess Extent of Obstruction	**Partial:** Can cough and make sounds, stridor. **Total:** Cannot cough, make sounds, speak; difficulty breathing; cyanosis.	**Partial:** Can cough and make sounds. **Total:** Cannot cough, make sounds, speak; difficulty breathing; cyanosis; hands may encircle throat (universal choking sign).
Victim Is Conscious	**Partial:** Monitor; allow victim's efforts to dislodge object.	
	Total • Sit with infant face down on your forearm, head angled down. • Give 5 back blows; turn infant face upward; deliver 5 chest thrusts. • Alternate back blows with chest thrusts until object is expelled, victim can breathe, or victim is unconscious.	**Total** • Initiate abdominal thrust maneuver: Encircle victim's waist and with intertwined clenched fists, thrust upward and inward against diaphragm. • Deliver abdominal thrusts until object is expelled, victim can breathe, or victim is unconscious.

Foreign Body Airway Obstruction (American Heart Association)—cont'd

	Infant (<1 yr)	Child (≥1 yr–Adolescent) and Adult
Victim Is Unconscious	• Implement head-tilt, chin-lift maneuver to open airway; inspect mouth; remove object if present; start CPR as per guidelines in previous chart; inspect mouth before each 2 rescue breaths.	

Ethical and Legal Foundations

Basics of Ethical Decision Making

- **Patient Care Partnership** (American Hospital Association): Information about what clients should expect about their rights and responsibilities when hospitalized, including high-quality hospital care, clean and safe environment, involvement in care, protection of privacy, and help when leaving the hospital and with billing. www.aha.org/aha/issues/Communicating-With-Patients/pt-care-partnership.html.
- **Autonomy**: Support personal freedom and decision making.
- **Beneficence**: Promote good.
- **Fidelity**: Keep promises and commitments.
- **Justice**: Treat people fairly and equally.
- **Nonmaleficence**: Do no harm.
- **Paternalism**: Make or allow a person to make a decision for another.
- **Respect**: Acknowledge rights of others.
- **Veracity**: Tell the truth.

Legal Terms

- **Advance directive**: Written document that addresses treatment desires in the future if unable to make decisions.
  - **Living will**: Specifically identifies treatment desires.
  - **Health-care proxy** (durable power of attorney): Assigns decision making to another.

  - **Do not resuscitate:** Order stating that a client should not be revived; at request of client when able; health-care proxy, family member, or legal guardian when client is unable to give consent.
- **Assault:** Threat of unlawful touching of another.
- **Battery:** Unlawful touching of another without consent, such as procedures performed without consent.
- **False imprisonment:** Restriction/retention of client without consent; use restraints in compliance with policy and procedure; have client sign release if desiring to leave facility against medical advice.
- **Good Samaritan law:** Legal protection for those who render care in an emergency without expectation of remuneration.
- **Libel:** Written statement causing harm to client.
- **Malpractice:** Professional negligence; for example, when the nurse owed a duty to the client but did not carry out that duty, and it resulted in injury to the client.
- **Negligence:** Failing to perform an act that a reasonable prudent nurse would do under similar circumstances; may be an act of omission or commission. Examples: Failure to ensure client safety (falls); improper performance of a treatment (burns from warm soak); med errors; inappropriate use of equipment (excessive IVF via pump); and failure to assess, report, or document a client's status.
- **Organ donation:** Donor card, living will, or family consent if client is unable to participate in decision is necessary to donate organs.
- **Respondeat superior:** Latin term meaning "let the master answer"; employer is responsible for acts of employees causing harm during employment activities.
- **Slander:** Oral statement resulting in damage to a client; for example, nurse incorrectly tells others that a client has AIDS and it affects the client's business.
- **Uniform Determination of Death Act:**
  - **Cardiopulmonary criteria:** Irreversible cessation of circulatory and respiratory function.
  - **Whole-brain criteria:** Irreversible cessation of all functions of the entire brain and brain stem; organs may be healthy for donation even though meeting whole-brain criteria.

Disease and Treatment Mnemonics

CAUTION: Early Signs of Cancer	INFECT: S&S of Infection
Change in bowel or bladder habits. **A** sore that does not heal. **U**nusual bleeding or discharge. **T**hickening or lump. **I**ndigestion; dysphagia. **O**bvious change in a wart or mole. **N**agging cough or hoarseness.	**I**ncreased pulse, respirations, white blood cells (WBCs). **N**odes are enlarged. **F**unction is impaired. **E**rythema, edema, exudate. **C**omplains of discomfort or pain. **T**emperature—local or systemic.

Treatment for Acute Injury

Rest: Decreases stress/strain on injury.
Ice: Vasoconstriction decreases edema and pain.
Compression: External pressure decreases edema and pain.
Elevate: Gravity decreases edema.

Phases of the Therapeutic Nurse-Client Relationship

Phase	Nurse	Client
Preinteraction: Begins before client contact.	• Explore personal feelings, values, attitudes. • Collect data about client. • Plan for first interaction.	• Has no role in this phase.
Orientation: Introductory phase; begins at first meeting.	• Listen; be empathetic. • Identify boundaries of relationship (termination begins here). • Clarify expectations. • Establish rapport.	• Recognize need for help. • Commit to a therapeutic relationship. • Begin to test relationship.
Working: Begins when client identifies problems to be worked on.	• Assist with exploration of issues. • Support healthy problem solving.	• Develop trust in nurse. • Examine personal issues. • Develop strategies to resolve issues.

Continued

Phases of the Therapeutic Nurse-Client Relationship—cont'd

Phase	Nurse	Client
	• Assist with strategy development. • Identify own reactions to client based on own needs, conflicts, relationships (**counter-transference**).	• May superimpose feelings from another relationship onto the nurse-client relationship (**transference**).
Resolution: Termination phase; begins when problems are resolved and ends when relationship is terminated.	• Review goals and objectives achieved. • Reinforce adaptive behaviors. • Share feelings about termination. • Avoid discussing previous or new issues. • Encourage independence; focus on future. • Promote positive family interactions. • Refer to community resources.	• Share feelings about termination (anger, rejection, regression; negative feelings may be expressed to deal with loss). • May attempt to discuss previous or new issues. • Assume responsibility for use of community resources.

Interviewing

Interviewing Skills

- **Active listening**: Absorbs content and client's feelings; uses all senses. *Nurse:* Verbal/nonverbal attending, appropriate gestures (head nodding), eye contact, sitting, open posture, vocal cues ("mmm").
- **Clarification**: Asks for more information; checks accuracy; ↓ ambiguity. *Nurse:* "I am not sure I know what you mean by that."
- **Confrontation**: Presents reality; identifies inconsistencies; ↑ self-awareness; use gently after trust is developed. *Client:* "I never have any visitors." *Nurse:* "I was here yesterday when you had three visitors."
- **Direct**: Collects specific information quickly. *Nurse:* "Where is your pain?"

- **Focusing**: Lets client finish thoughts; centers on key elements to ↓ rambling. *Nurse:* "When talking about your house, you mentioned scatter rugs. Let's talk more about being safe in your home."
- **Nonverbal**: Promotes verbalization. *Nurse:* Lean forward, nod head, smile, use gestures.
- **Open-ended**: Invites elaboration; nonthreatening; avoids yes and no answers. *Nurse:* "Tell me about what a typical day is like for you."
- **Paraphrasing**: Restates message in similar words; focuses on content; encourages discussion. *Client:* "I may not make it." *Nurse:* "You think you are going to die?"
- **Reflection**: Describes or interprets feelings or mood. *Nurse:* "You sound upset."
- **Silence**: Allows for reflection and client response; prompts talking; useful when client is sad or remaining quiet.
- **Summarizing**: Reviews key elements; brings closure; clarifies expectations. *Nurse:* "Today we talked about . . ."
- **Touch**: Conveys caring; is reassuring; may invade personal space. *Nurse*: Hold client's hand, gently pat client's shoulder, avoid touching suspicious, paranoiac, or angry clients.
- **Validation**: Confirms what the nurse heard or observed. *Nurse:* "I understand that you just said . . ."

Barriers to Communication

- Pain
- Advising
- Changing topic
- Failing to listen
- Trite, common expressions (clichés)
- Judgmental or minimizing comments
- Direct probing and "how" and "why" questions
- Overly optimistic statements (false reassurance)
- Challenging, defensive, or disapproving responses
- Interruptions, environmental noise, or extremes in temperature

Basic Theories

Maslow's Hierarchy of Needs

- Needs are ranked in hierarchy of importance.
- Physiologic: First level; need for air, food, water, shelter, elimination, rest, sleep, activity, sex, temperature.

- Safety and security: Second level; physically and emotionally protected from injury.
- Love and belonging: Third level; give and receive love and acceptance and connection to others.
- Self-esteem: Fourth level; positive self-regard; independent, confident.
- Self-actualization: Fifth level; achieve highest potential within abilities.

Erikson's Stages of Psychosocial Development

- Consists of 8 stages; each requires specific tasks to achieve growth.
- Inability to achieve a task affects ability to achieve later tasks.
- Tasks: Infant—trust/mistrust; toddler—autonomy/shame and doubt; preschooler—initiative/guilt; school-age child—industry/inferiority; adolescent—identity/role confusion; young adult—intimacy/isolation; middle-age adult—generativity/self-absorption; older adult—integrity/despair.

Leadership and Management

Leadership and Management Terms

- **Accountability**: Answerable for actions and judgments regarding care.
- **Autonomy**: Nurse can make independent decision to act.
- **Case management**: Coordination of interdisciplinary care for client.
- **Decentralized management**: Staff participates in decision making.
- **Performance appraisal**: Evaluation of a nurse's compliance (quality and quantity) with standards and roles within job description.
- **Professional standards:** Actions consistent with minimum safe professional conduct. Description of responsibilities (American Nurses Association, Joint Commission, agency policy and procedure).
- **Quality improvement**: Activities to ↑ achievement of ideal care.
- **Responsibility**: Duties and activities the nurse is hired to perform.

Leadership Styles

- **Autocratic**: Complete control over decisions, goals, plans, and evaluation of outcomes; firm, insistent; often used in emergencies or when staff is inexperienced or new.
- **Democratic**: Participative; shares responsibilities; uses role to motivate staff to achieve communal goals **(shared governance)**; encourages intercommunication and contributions; used to help staff grow in abilities; ↑ motivation; ↑ staff satisfaction.

- **Laissez-faire:** Nondirective; relinquishes control and direction to staff; best used with experienced, expert, mature staff who know roles.
- **Transformational:** Presents vision for the future, provides supportive climate, acts as coach or mentor, inspires commitment to the good of the group, promotes creativity; best used in self-governing situations.

Leader Qualities

Effective leaders and managers need to:

Understand human behavior.

- Have insight into its relationship to beliefs, values, feelings.
- Be sensitive to others' feelings and problems.

Use effective communication skills.

- Be clear, concise, avoid ambiguity.
- Use appropriate format (verbal, written, formal, informal).
- Be aware of own nonverbal behavior.

Use power appropriately.

- Power of authority—use of position attained through place in table of organization.
- Power of coercion—use of a threat or unfavorable outcome.
- Power of expertise—use knowledge, expertise, or experience.
- Power of reward—use an incentive or positive outcome.
- Do not abuse power.

Respond to staff needs.

- Listen attentively; attend to needs; provide positive feedback; avoid favoritism; set realistic expectations; avoid mixed messages.
- Treat staff with respect; counsel privately; keep promises; avoid threats, superior attitude, criticism, or aggressive confrontation.

Delegate appropriately (leader retains accountability).

- Right person (competent subordinate).
- Right task (within scope of practice).
- Right situation (appropriate to abilities and client acuity).
- Right communication (clear instructions, validate understanding).
- Right supervision (assess actions, evaluate outcomes).

Provide opportunities for personal growth.

- Help less-experienced nurse to ↑ knowledge, experience, responsibility (mentor/preceptor, continuing education, staff education).

Use critical thinking and problem solving.

- Encourage staff to engage in critical thinking by involving in assessing, planning, and evaluating outcomes.

Recognize and address conditions conducive to change.

- Refer to Lewin's Force-Field Model of change theory: Unfreezing stage—problem awareness; moving stage—planning/implementing change; refreezing stage—integrating/stabilizing change.
- Ensure that all staff have a stake in the outcome; include all creatively in the process; focus on benefits; provide positive feedback; offer incentives.
- Ensure change is planned, introduced gradually, and initiated in a calm rather than chaotic atmosphere; best after a prior successful change.
- Recognize and address resistance; identify causes of resistance: threatening; lack of understanding; disagreeing with purpose/approach, beliefs, values; ↑ in responsibility; content with status quo; fear of failure.

Levels of Management

First level: Supervises nonmanagerial staff; oversees day-to-day activities of a group (team leader, charge nurse).
Middle level: Supervises a group of first-level managers (supervisor, coordinator).
Upper level: Organizational executives; sets goals and strategic planning (VP for nursing, associate director of nursing).

Nurse Manager Role

- Functions as a role model regarding professional conduct.
- Sets standards of performance; establishes goals for the unit with the staff; mobilizes staff and agency resources to attain goals.
- Supports mutual trust; treats staff with respect; counsels privately.
- Empowers staff; supports innovation; seeks staff members' opinions; promotes professional environment and growth; rewards growth.
- Performs client rounds with multidisciplinary team.
- Evaluates nursing practice and achievement of standards.
- Designs and implements a QI program for the unit; engages staff in QI activities.
- Assists in staff development plan and orientation of new employees.
- Schedules staffing for unit; conducts staff meetings with all shifts.
- Evaluates performance of subordinates (performance appraisal).
- Participates in intradepartmental and interdepartmental meetings.
- Manages conflict; involves all concerned; explores solutions; and negotiates resolution.

Staff Nurse Role

- Functions as role model regarding professional conduct.
- Communicates and collaborates with other nurses and health team members responsible for the client's care.
- Assesses, analyzes, and interprets data; identifies client problems or needs; formulates a plan of care; evaluates client responses to care and extent of outcome achievement.
- Sets priorities regarding client needs; progresses from those who have an immediate threat to survival (problems with breathing, VS, ↓ LOC); to requests for help (mobility, toileting); to important but not immediate needs (teaching).
- Coordinates and/or performs care for assigned clients; uses time-management skills; completes all care assigned.
- Performs professional procedures such as sterile irrigations, insertion of a urinary catheter, colostomy irrigation, tracheal suctioning, administering meds and parenteral therapies, client teaching.
- Delegates care to subordinates that is within their job description.
- Evaluates care delegated; establishes clear expectations; encourages communication; evaluates client outcomes related to delegated tasks (nurse retains accountability for delegated tasks).
- Engages in QI activities.
- Participates in intradepartmental and interdepartmental meetings.

Unlicensed Assistive Personnel Role

- Works within scope of practice determined by agency policy; performs activities with established sequence of steps with little or no modification and reasonably predictable results; provides direct care for only stable clients.
- Cannot engage in activities outside their role; pervasive functions of assessment, planning, evaluation, and nursing judgment cannot be delegated (NCSBN 2005); examples: performing a physical assessment, formulating plans of care, teaching, implementing complex tasks, caring for unstable clients.
- Obtains VS.
- Performs hygiene and comfort activities (bathing, backrub).
- Assists clients with ADLs such as eating, drinking, toileting (bedpan, commode), ambulation (walking, transfer).
- Changes linens.
- Empties urinary retention collection device.
- Transports clients.

Community Nursing

- **Community health nursing (public health nursing):** Nursing care for a specific population living in the same geographical area, or groups having similar values, interests, needs; aims to develop a healthy environment.
- **Public health functions:** Community assessment, policy development, facilitating access to resources; cohesiveness is promoted by engaging community members in the problem-solving process and promoting empowerment through education, opportunities, resources; successful public health programs are congruent with that of the interests and goals of the community.
- **Assessment of a community:**
  - **Structure (milieu):** Geographical area, environment, housing, economy, water, sanitation.
  - **Population:** Age and sex distribution, density, growth trends, educational level, cultures and subcultures, religious groups.
  - **Social systems:** Education, communication, transportation, welfare, health-care delivery systems (governmental, voluntary agencies).
- **Community-based nursing:** Nursing care delivered in the community while focused on a specific individual's or family's health-care needs; individual viewed within the larger systems of family, community, culture, society.
- **Vulnerable populations:** Homeless, living in poverty, migrant workers, living in rural communities, pregnant adolescents, suicidal individuals, frail older adults.
- **Stigmatized groups:** People viewed with disdain because of a disease or behavior (HIV, substance misuse, mental illness).
- **Settings in which nurses work:** Homes, community health centers, clinics, industry, rehabilitation centers, schools, crisis intervention centers and phone lines, shelters, halfway houses, sheltered workshops, day-care centers, forensic settings.
- **Roles of nurses:** Discharge planner, case manager, counselor, health promoter, case finder, caregiver, educator, researcher, consultant, advocate, role model, change agent.
- **Hospice care:** Supportive care **(palliative)** for dying persons and their caregivers usually during last 6 mo of life; experts in pain and symptom management; focuses on preserving dignity and quality over quantity of life; supports bereavement; Medicare Care Choices Model is studying the option of allowing curative care.
- **Respite care:** Temporary care for the homebound so caregivers have relief from day-to-day responsibilities.

Client Education

Learning Domains

Cognitive

- Thinking, acquiring, comprehending, synthesizing, evaluating, storing, recalling information.
- Builds on what client knows; presents essential information first; adds information as client asks questions.
- Teaching strategies: Lecture, discussion, audiovisuals, printed material, computer-assisted instruction, Web-based instruction.
- Evaluation: Assesses knowledge by verbal and written means.

Affective

- Addresses attitudes, feelings, beliefs, values.
- Recognizes that it takes client time to internalize need-to-change behavior.
- Understands own value system; respects uniqueness of each client; helps client explore feelings.
- Teaching strategies: Discussion, play, role-modeling, panel discussion, groups, role-playing.
- Evaluation: Evidence of behavior incorporated into lifestyle.

Psychomotor

- Addresses physical and motor skills; requires dexterity and coordination to manipulate equipment; ultimately performs a task with skill.
- Ensures mastery of each step before moving to next step.
- Teaching strategies: Audiovisuals, pictures, demonstrations, models.
- Evaluation: Observation of performance of skill (return demonstration).

Teaching and Learning: General Concepts

- Education can prevent illness; promote or restore health; ↓ complications; ↑ independence and coping; ↑ individual and family growth; incorporate throughout health-care delivery.
- Environment should be conducive to learning: Private, quiet, well lit, comfortable, lacking distractions (close doors and curtains; shut off TV).
- Teaching process should follow format of the nursing process (assessment, analysis, planning, implementation, and evaluation).
- Both short- and long-term goals should be set to ↑ motivation and allow for evaluation; goals must be client centered, specific, measurable, realistic, and have a time frame; point out goal achievement.
- A variety of teaching strategies that use different senses should be used (written materials, videos, discussion, demonstration).

- Teaching can be formal or informal, and individualized or within a group.
- Information should move from simple to complex, from known to unknown, and be appropriate for client's cognitive and developmental levels.
- Shorter, more frequent sessions are most effective (15–30 min).
- Learning is ↑ with repetition, consistency, and practice.
- Evaluation and documentation are essential elements of teaching.

Client Factors That Influence Learning

Culture, Religion, Ethnicity, Language

Commonalities and differences exist among cultures and among people from within the same culture.

Nursing Care

- Be culturally sensitive and nonjudgmental.
- Avoid assumptions, biases, stereotypes; seek help from multicultural team.
- Provide teaching in client's language; use professional translator.

Knowledge and Experience

Can promote or deter learning.

Nursing Care

- Identify what client already knows; build on this foundation.
- Explore concerns related to experiences; correct misconceptions.

Literacy

Years in school may not accurately reflect reading ability.

Nursing Care

- Assess ability to read, comprehend material (confusion, nervousness, excuses may indicate ↓ ability to read).
- Use illustrations, models, videos, discussion.
- Provide privacy.

Developmental Level

Children

The younger the child, the shorter the attention span; may regress developmentally when ill; imagination can ↑ fear and misconceptions; toddlers and preschoolers are concrete thinkers; school-age children are capable of logical thinking.

Nursing Care

- Identify developmental age to determine appropriate strategies (dolls, puppets, role-playing, drawing, games, books).
- Use direct, simple approach.
- Include parents.

Adolescents
Need to be similar to peers; seek autonomy; focus on the present.

Nursing Care
- Be open and honest about the illness.
- Respect opinions and need to be like peers.
- Support need for control.
- Ensure learning has immediate results.

Adults
Need to be self-sufficient and in control; learning most effective when self-directed.

Nursing Care
- Assess for readiness; explore perceived benefit.
- Build on prior knowledge and experience.

Older Adults
Needs are highly variable; functional changes, stress, fatigue, chronic illness can ↓ learning; changes may include slower cognition and reaction time, becoming overwhelmed with too much detail, ↓ ability to recall new information.

Nursing Care
- Do not underestimate learning ability.
- Plan shorter, more frequent teaching sessions.
- Decrease pace of teaching to allow more time to process information, make decisions.
- Teach main points and avoid irrelevant details.

Readiness to Learn: Receptiveness to Learning
Client has to recognize need to learn and be physically and emotionally able to participate.

Nursing Care
- Identify readiness: Client states misconceptions, asks questions, demonstrates health-seeking behaviors, is physically comfortable, and anxiety is less than moderate.
- Identify physical adaptations that may interfere with learning: Pain, acute or chronic illness, O_2 deprivation, fatigue, weakness, and sensory impairment.
- Identify emotional and mental adaptations that interfere with learning: Depression, anxiety, anger, denial, and impaired cognition.
- Select teaching aids appropriate for client's sensory limitations (↓ sight, ↓ hearing).
- Postpone teaching until client is able to focus on learning; address factors that interfere with learning.

Motivation

Motivation is the drive that causes action; essential to learning.

Nursing Care

- Identify the client's personal desire to learn (intrinsic motivation, internal locus of control).
- Identify the client's desire to learn because of an external reward (extrinsic motivation, external locus of control).
- Be sincere and nonjudgmental.
- Ensure material is meaningful; make contractual agreement; set short-term goals to ensure success.
- Identify and praise progress (positive reinforcement); avoid criticism (negative reinforcement); allow for mistakes.
- Assess for ↓ motivation (distraction, changing subject).

Infection Control

Standard Precautions: Tier 1

- Perform hand hygiene before and after care and when soiled; most important way to prevent infection.
- Use personal protective equipment (PPE) if touching, spilling, or splashing of blood or body fluids is likely; use gloves, gown, mask, goggles, face shield, apron, head and foot protection.
- Discard disposable items and soiled tissues in fluid-impermeable bag and contaminated items in biohazard red bag.
- Dispose sharps in a sharps container; do not recap used needles.
- Hold linen away from body; place linen in fluid-impermeable bag in a covered hamper; keep linen hamper in hall, not in client rooms; do not let hampers overflow.
- Place lab specimens in a leak-proof transport bag without contaminating the outside; label with biohazard sticker and client information.
- Assign client to private room if hygiene practices are unacceptable.

Transmission-Based Precautions: Tier 2

Airborne

- Used for microorganisms that spread through air (droplet nuclei <5 mcg) such as TB, measles, chickenpox.
- Private room; negative air pressure room; door closed; high-efficiency disposable mask (replace when moist) or particulate respirator such as for TB; mask on client when transporting.

Droplet

- Used for microorganisms spread by large-particle droplets (droplet nuclei >5 mcg) such as pneumonia (streptococcal, mycoplasmal, meningococcal), rubella, mumps, influenza, adenovirus.
- Private room if available or cohort clients; wear mask when entering room or when within 3 feet of client; may keep door open; mask on client when transporting.

Contact

- Used for microorganisms spread by direct or indirect contact such as methicillin-resistant *S. aureus* (MRSA), vancomycin-resistant enterococcus (VRE), vancomycin intermediate-resistant *S. aureus* (VISA), enteric pathogens (*E. coli, C. difficile*), herpes simplex, pediculosis, hepatitis A and E, varicella zoster, respiratory syncytial virus.
- Private room or cohort clients; gown; gloves; dedicated equipment; maintain precautions when transporting.

Neutropenic Precautions

- For individuals with compromised immune system.
- Use standard precautions, contact precautions to prevent exposure to drug-resistant organisms.
- Caregivers and visitors should be free of communicable illnesses.
- Private room if possible; ensure room is meticulously clean.
- Teach to avoid sources of potential infection such as crowds, confined spaces (airplane, theaters), raw fruits and vegetables, flowers and plants.

Surgical (Sterile) Asepsis

- Check expiration date; ensure packages are dry, intact, stain-free.
- Label solutions with date, time, initials; discard after 24 hr (criteria for medicated and antiseptic solutions may differ); avoid touching bottle rim; inner cap turned up when on table.
- Place sterile equipment inside the outer 1 inch of sterile field.
- Ensure that sterile objects touch only another sterile object.
- Open sterile packages away from sterile field.
- Keep sterile field in line of vision.
- Position solution closest to client; keep field dry and free of moisture.
- Don sterile gloves without contaminating sterile surfaces.
- Keep sterile gloved hands and equipment above level of waist.
- Keep tip of sterile forceps lower than hand holding the forceps.
- Avoid talking, coughing, or sneezing around a sterile field.
- Discard sterile objects that become contaminated or if in doubt.

Basic Nursing Measures

Principles of Body Mechanics

- Follow principles and maintain functional alignment: ↑ balance, movement, physiological function; avoid stress on muscles, tendons, ligaments, bones, joints; avoid twisting body; use supportive devices.
- Keep weight within the center of gravity; avoid reaching.
- Spread feet apart to widen base of support.
- Use large muscles of legs for power.
- Flex knees and hold objects being lifted close to body (lowers center of gravity and keeps weight within base of support).
- Raise bed to working height; transfer client from higher surface to lower surface (uses gravity).
- Use internal girdle to stabilize pelvis when lifting, pulling, stooping.
- Use body weight as a force for pushing and pulling; lean forward and backward or rock on feet.
- Pull, push, roll, or slide rather than lift; face direction of movement.
- Use assistive devices to lessen strain on self (mechanical lift, sit-to-stand lift).

Fall Prevention

- Assess for risk factors: History of falls; ↓ sensory perception; weakness; orthostatic hypotension; ↓ mobility; ↓ LOC; ↓ mental capacity; ↑ anxiety; confusion; meds (diuretics, opioids, antihypertensives).
- Orient to bed and room; teach use of ambulatory aids and call bell; answer call bell immediately.
- Keep bed in lowest position unless receiving care.
- Raise 3 of 4 side rails; raise 4 rails if it is client's preference or if ordered (4 raised rails are considered a restraint).
- Lock wheels on all equipment; ensure that equipment is intact.
- Keep call bell, bedside and overbed table, and personal items in reach.
- Keep floor dry and free of electric cords and obstacles; use night-light.
- Encourage use of grab bars, railings, and rubber-soled shoes.
- Stay with client in bathroom or shower (need order for shower).
- Teach fall-prevention techniques such as rising slowly.
- Use monitoring device that will alert the nurse if a client attempts to ambulate unassisted.

Fire Safety

- Stay calm; keep halls clear; do not use elevator; stay close to the floor (smoke rises); know location, use of alarms/extinguishers.
- Evacuate clients in immediate danger first and then ambulatory, those needing assistance, and finally bedbound clients.
- **Class A fire:** Wood, textiles, paper trash; use water extinguisher.
- **Class B fire:** Oil, grease, paint, chemicals; use dry powder and CO_2 extinguisher (water will spread fire); avoid touching horn of CO_2 extinguisher because it can freeze tissue.
- **Class C fire:** Electrical wires, appliances, motors; use dry powder or CO_2 extinguisher (water will cause electrocution).
- **RACE: R**escue clients in danger; **A**ctivate alarm; **C**ontain fire (close doors and windows); **E**xtinguish fire if small; **E**vacuate horizontally and then vertically.

Pain Management

Pain Rating Scales

FACES Pain Rating Scale

Wong-Baker FACES® Pain Rating Scale
0
No Hurt
2
Hurts Little Bit
4
Hurts Little More
6
Hurts Even More
8
Hurts Whole Lot
10
Hurts Worst

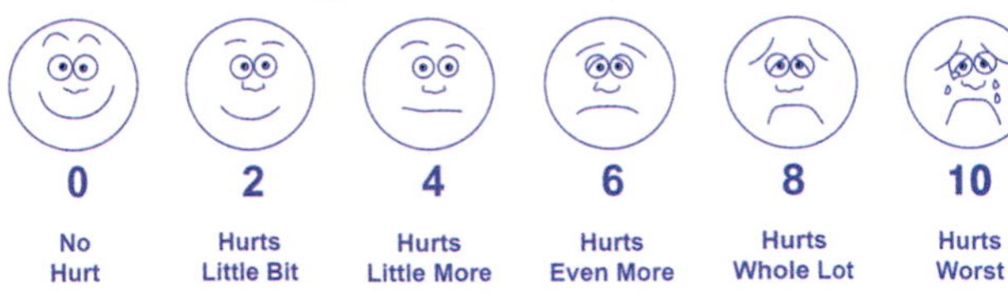

PQRST Pain Rating Scale

P: Provokes/point: What causes the pain? Point to the pain.
Q: Quality: Is it dull, achy, sharp, stabbing, pressuring, deep, etc.?
R: Radiation/relief: Does it radiate? What makes it better or worse?

S: Severity/S&S: Rate pain on 0–10 scale. What S&S are associated with the pain, such as dizziness, diaphoresis, dyspnea, or abnormal VS?

T: Time/onset: When did it start? Is it constant or intermittent? How long does it last? Sudden or gradual onset? Frequency?

Numerical Pain Rating Scale

Request client to rate pain on a scale of 0–10; 0 reflects no pain and 10 excruciating pain.

Nursing Care for Clients in Pain

- **Assess pain**: Presence, severity, characteristics (see pain rating scales, pp. 21–22).
- **Validate client's pain**: Accept that pain exists.
- **Provide comfort**: Positioning, rest.
- **Relieve anxiety**: Answer questions, provide emotional support.
- **Teach client**: Relaxation—rhythmic breathing, guided imagery; ask for meds as pain begins to increase rather than waiting.
- **Provide cutaneous stimulation**: Backrub, heat and cold therapy.
- **Decrease irritating stimuli**: Bright lights, noise, ↑↓ room temperature.
- **Use distraction for mild pain**: Music, TV, reading, imagery.
- **Explore alternative therapies with client and health-care team**: Therapeutic touch, aromatherapy, acupressure, acupuncture, chiropractic, magnetotherapy, Reiki.
- **Give prescribed medications**: Analgesics, opioids, antispasmodics; meds remain in the body longer when older or obese.
- **Evaluate client response**: Document, modify plan, if needed.

Nursing Care for Clients in Seclusion or Restraints

Types

- Physical, environmental, or chemical intervention that ↓ movement.
- Seclusion: Client placed in safe room to limit exposure to environmental stimuli and others.
- Physical restraints: Devices used to ↓ movement, such as vest, mitt, wrist, elbow, belt, mummy.
- Chemical restraints: Meds to calm disruptive or combative behavior that may cause harm to self or others.

Nursing Care

- Document behavior requiring need and failure of deescalation techniques and use of less-invasive measures to protect client.

- In an emergency: Obtain order from primary health-care provider within 1 hr of institution of seclusion or restraint application; serial evaluations as per hospital policy, laws, regulations, and/or accreditation standards.
- Nursing care related to application of restraints.
  - Ensure functional alignment before applying.
  - Follow directions (correct size, snug but does not limit respirations or occlude circulation, apply vest with V opening in front).
  - Pad under wrist when using wrist or mitt restraints.
  - Secure straps with slipknot to bed frame.
  - Assess respiratory and circulatory status routinely.
  - Remove restraint every 1–2 hr, assess skin, massage area, perform ROM.
- Nursing care related to seclusion.
  - Place in safe room; may include removal of possessions and certain attire.
  - Monitor continuously by staff or use of audio and video equipment.

Nursing Care for Clients With Visual Impairments

- Knock on door; greet client by name; identify self; explain purpose.
- Do not touch until client understands your name and purpose.
- Approach in an unhurried manner; use clear, simple sentences.
- Stay within client's field of vision; approach from strong side.
- Orient to room, location, and use of call bell.
- Provide a predictable environment; remove all hazards.
- Limit noise and distraction in environment; explain unusual noises.
- Ensure eyeglasses are clean, accessible, and protected when stored.
- Inform of location of food on meal tray; use numbers on a clock.
- Ambulate client by walking slightly in front while client holds your arm; never try to push or guide from behind; inform of doors, steps.
- Make it clear to client when conversation is over or when leaving area.

Nursing Care for Clients With Hearing Impairments

- Greet client by name; identify yourself and your purpose; ↓ environmental noise when communicating.
- Use touch appropriately to alert client that you are about to talk.
- Face client directly; avoid turning away from client while you are speaking; avoid covering your mouth with your hand to facilitate lipreading.
- Talk in a normal tone at a moderate rate; speak clearly; articulate consonants carefully; do not overly articulate or yell.

- Use gestures and facial expressions to convey message.
- Encourage use of hearing aid; facilitate repair of nonworking aids.
- Remove hearing aid when showering or washing hair.
- Follow manufacturer's directions to insert, remove, clean, or store aid.

Nursing Care of Older Adults (>65 Yr)

Demographic Data

About 70% rate themselves as healthy; majority live in the community; increasingly more live in independent or assisted-living communities; 4.1% in nursing homes.

Physical Changes

Gradual ↓ in physical abilities; close vision impairment **(presbyopia)**; ↓ hearing, especially for high-pitched sounds; ↓ subcutaneous tissue; ↓ muscle strength; ↓ balance and coordination; ↓ immune response; one or more chronic health problems.

Psychosocial Issues

Conflict is ego integrity vs. despair; reminisces about past; personality does not change but may become exaggerated; adjusting to aging, ↓ health, quality of life, retirement, fixed income, death of spouse or friends, change in residence, own mortality; may become focused on bodily needs and comforts; sexual expression (love, touching, sharing, intercourse) important and related to identity.

Cognitive Status

Intelligence does not ↓; mental acuity slows (↑ time to learn and problem solve); long-term memory better than short-term memory.

Reaction to Illness and Hospitalization

Illness and recuperation longer due to ↓ adaptive capacity; ↑ feelings of inadequacy and mortality; may ↑ self-absorption, social isolation, frustration, anger, depression, especially if retirement goals are denied; unfamiliar environment may cause confusion, anxiety; chronic illness, pain, or impending death may cause dependence, hopelessness; may accept and prepare for death.

General Nursing Care

- Understand commonalities of aging, but approach each person as unique.
- Avoid stereotyping because it denies uniqueness; ↓ access to care impacts negatively on individual.
- Ensure access to health care and social services, especially in home; critical illnesses deserve aggressive treatment, if desired.

Common Problems Associated With Aging

Bowel and Bladder Incontinence

Not part of aging process; may be aggravated by ↓ muscle tone of anal and urinary sphincters and prostatic hypertrophy.

- **Nursing care:** Ensure screening for UTI, bladder and prostate cancer; assist with hygiene and skin care; institute bowel or bladder retraining.

Adverse Drug Effects

Multiple health problems require ↑ prescriptions **(polypharmacy)** with ↓ coordination among primary health-care providers; ↓ hepatic and renal function results in drug accumulation; ↑ paradoxical drug effects.

- **Nursing care:** ↑ coordination of health care; identify unnecessary or excessive doses of meds; assess for adverse and toxic effects.

Falls and Accidents

Occur due to sensory impairments (vision, hearing, sensation), postural changes, ↓ muscle strength and endurance, orthostatic hypotension, neurological and cardiovascular decline.

- **Nursing care:** Assist with ambulation; teach safety precautions such as use of grab bars, railings, walker; rise slowly; keep feet apart for a wide base; give up driving when impairment jeopardizes safety.

Infection

Increased risk due to ↓ immune response; ↓ pulmonary elastic recoil, ↓ lung capacity, and ↑ residual lung capacity → retain secretions and ↑ risk of respiratory infection.

- **Nursing care:** Teach preventive measures such as hand hygiene, avoiding crowds, smoking cessation; getting pneumonia and flu vaccines.

Cognitive Impairment

Not part of aging process.
Delirium is an acute, reversible state of agitated confusion.
Dementia is a chronic, progressive, irreversible disorder.
Sundowning syndrome is confusion beginning in late afternoon or evening.

- **Nursing care:** See Nursing Care for Clients With Decreased Cognition in Mental Health Tab, p. 163.

Alcohol Misuse

Associated with depression, loneliness, lack of social support.

- **Nursing care:** Explore effective coping strategies; refer to AA.

Risk of Dehydration
Occurs due to ↓ thirst mechanism; ↓ ability to concentrate urine; med side effects.

- **Nursing care:** Encourage intake of at least 2 L fluid daily; teach to seek care if vomiting or diarrhea occurs >24 hr.

Risk of Suicide
Associated with multiple losses (loved ones, health); lack of social support; depression; feelings of hopelessness; isolation.

- **Nursing care:** Assess for suicide risk; provide reality orientation; validation therapy; reminiscence; support body image; encourage psychological counseling; obtain prescription for antidepressant; refer to social service agency.

Sexual Responsiveness/Erectile Dysfunction
Sexual response takes longer due to ↓ estrogen and testosterone, chronic health problems, and drug side effect; unavailable partner; ↓ cognition.

- **Nursing care:** Provide for privacy and dignity; maintain nonjudgmental attitude; ↑ verbalization of concerns; suggest use of lubricants, penile prostheses, meds to increase erectile function.

Sexually Transmitted Infections (STIs)
Need for sexual expression continues; ↑ society recognition that sex is natural and acceptable even if single by choice or death of spouse.

- **Nursing care:** Maintain nonjudgmental attitude; teach about STI prevention.

Leading Causes of Death
Heart disease, then malignant neoplasms, chronic lower respiratory disease, cerebrovascular disorders, Alzheimer disease, diabetes mellitus, influenza and pneumonia, nephritis, or unintentional injury.

- **Nursing care:** Focus on health promotion, smoking cessation, ↑ exercise, weight control, adequate nutrition, screening programs to identify problems early, health-care supervision to manage chronic conditions.

Common Human Responses and Related Nursing Care

Vital Signs

Temperature
Afebrile

- **Oral:** 97.5°F–99.5°F
- **Rectal:** 0.5°F–1°F more than oral route

Hyperthermia: >99.5°F–100.4°F
Hypothermia: <97.5°F

Pulse

Normal: 60–100 beats per minute
Tachycardia: >100 beats per minute
Bradycardia: <60 beats per minute
Thready: Weak, feeble
Bounding: Forceful, full
Dysrhythmia: Irregular pattern
Pulse deficit: Difference between radial and apical rates

Respirations

Eupnea: Expected rate 12–20 breaths per minute
Tachypnea: >20 breaths per minute
Bradypnea: <12 breaths per minute
Apnea: Absence of breathing
Hyperventilation: ↑ rate and depth
Hypoventilation: ↓ rate and depth
Kussmaul: Deep and rapid; associated with metabolic acidosis
Cheyne-Stokes: Rhythmic waxing and waning from deep to shallow followed by a temporary period of apnea
Orthopnea: Requires upright position to breathe
Dyspnea: Difficulty breathing

Blood Pressure

Normal: SBP <120 mm Hg; DBP <80 mm Hg

- Cuff width should be 40% of upper arm circumference.
- Place arm at heart level; erroneous ↓ BP if arm is above heart; erroneous ↑ BP if arm is below heart.

Prehypertension: SBP 120–139 mm Hg or DBP 80–89 mm Hg
Stage 1 hypertension: SBP 140–159 mm Hg or DBP 90–99 mm Hg
Stage 2 hypertension: SBP ≥160 mm Hg or DBP ≥100 mm Hg
Hypertensive emergency: SBP ≥180 mm Hg or DBP ≥110 mm Hg
Pulse pressure: Difference between systolic and diastolic pressures

Fever

- ↑ temp; low-grade fever is 99°F–101°F; high-grade fever >101°F
- **Etiology**: Bacterial, viral, or fungal infection; DVT; med side effects; tumor
- **S&S**: Fatigue; weakness; flushed, dry skin

Nursing Care

- Assess VS and WBCs; evaluate meds for possible drug-induced fever.
- Obtain specimens such as sputum, blood, or urine for C&S; chest x-ray.

- Perform focused assessments: ↓ breath sounds; crackles; rhonchi; stiff neck; headache; photophobia; irritability; confusion; check IV site, incisions, and wounds for infection; legs for DVT such as redness, warmth, swelling, tenderness; UTI such as burning on urination, cloudy, greenish/reddish color urine; GI S&S such as diarrhea, N&V, abdominal discomfort.
- Institute seizure precautions for infants and toddlers if temperature is >101.8°F.
- Encourage coughing and deep breathing; ↑ fluid intake.
- Give prescribed antipyretics, antibiotics, tepid bath, hypothermia blanket.
- Change IV site if indicated.

Constipation

- ≤2 stools a wk; difficult passage of hardened, dry stool; intractable constipation **(obstipation)**.
- **Etiology**
  - Ignored urge; ↓ fluids or fiber in diet; ↓ mobility; weak abdominal or pelvic floor muscles; med side effects such as opioids, iron, MAO inhibitors; anal lesions; pregnancy; laxative or enema abuse; F&E imbalance; intestinal obstruction.
  - **Infant and child**: Formula feeding; breastfed infants may have ↓ BMs due to digestibility of breast milk; stool-withholding behavior.
- **S&S**: Hard/dry feces; distended abdomen; rectal pressure; back pain; straining at stool; anorexia; blood-streaked stools; ↓ bowel sounds.

Nursing Care

- Assess stools for frequency, amount, color, consistency, shape.
- Assess bowel and dietary habits.
- Teach to ↑ intake of fiber such as whole grain cereal, bran, vegetables, raw fruit, dried prunes; avoid binding foods such as rice, bananas; ↑ fluids; ↑ activity.
- Teach to respond to urge; avoid straining to ↓ risk of dysrhythmias; encourage sitting position and regular time (best in a.m. or after a meal); ↑ relaxation and privacy.
- Teach parents of infants that transient constipation resolves spontaneously and mild constipation resolves with introduction of solid foods; inform them that rectal stimulation with cotton-tipped applicator or thermometer is contraindicated because it can cause pain and anal fissures.
- Give prescribed stool softeners, laxatives, cathartics, or enemas.

Diarrhea

- Passage of fluid or unformed stool >3 a day.
- **Etiology**

  Acute (sudden onset): Viral, bacterial, or parasitic pathogen (usually spread via fecal-oral route or direct person-to-person contact); contaminated food or water; spicy, greasy food; raw seafood; excessive roughage; anxiety; side effects of antibiotics, laxatives, cathartics; environment (attends day care, recent travel); hyperosmolar enteral feedings.

  Chronic (persistent, recurrent): Malabsorption syndrome; food allergies such as lactose, gluten; inflammatory bowel disease such as ulcerative colitis, Crohn disease; AIDS.
- **S&S:** Frequent, loose stool; foul-smelling, bulky stool **(steatorrhea)** indicates malabsorption; perianal excoriation; abdominal pain or cramps; flatus; abdominal distention; ↑ bowel sounds; N&V; anorexia; ↓ weight; fatigue and lethargy; ↑ T; ↑ P; ↑ R; manifestations of dehydration.

Nursing Care

- Assess stools for frequency, amount, color, consistency; VS; S&S of dehydration.
- Provide oral rehydration therapy.
- Assess perianal skin breakdown; provide skin care.
- Ask about dietary intake and recent foreign travel; teach about ordered dietary restrictions such as lactose—milk and dairy products; gluten—wheat, rye, barley.
- Obtain stool specimen for C&S, ova and parasites; obtain specimen before giving prescribed antibiotic.
- Encourage breastfeeding mother to continue breastfeeding.
- Give prescribed antidiarrheals, antibiotics, IV fluids, electrolytes.
- Institute contact precautions as indicated.

Hemorrhage

- Bleeding that compromises tissue and organ perfusion.
- **Etiology**

  External: Surgical and traumatic wounds.

  Internal: Blunt trauma; cancer; ruptured aneurysm; GI perforation; thrombolytic therapy.

- **S&S**: Rapid, thready P; ↑ R; ↓ BP; narrowing pulse pressure; excessive blood loss; capillary refill >3 sec; ↓ peripheral pulses; cool, moist, pale, mottled, or cyanotic skin; thirst.
  Early CNS S&S: ↓ LOC; anxiety; irritability; restlessness.
  Late CNS S&S: Confusion; lethargy; combativeness; coma.

Nursing Care

- Apply direct pressure; reinforce dressing (removal may dislodge clot).
- Assess VS, I&O, lab results such as arterial blood gases, RBC, Hct, Hb, potassium.
- Maintain airway; give O_2.
- Ensure 18-gauge IV access; give prescribed IVF, blood and blood products, colloidal products, vasoconstrictors, cardiac stimulants.

Shock

- Acute circulatory collapse; ↓ O_2 to cells, tissues, and organs.
- **Etiology**
  Hypovolemic: Blood loss; dehydration.
  Neurogenic: Spinal cord injury; anesthesia.
  Anaphylactic: Exposure to antigen causing release of histamine.
  Septic: Infection; endo/exotoxin release.
  Cardiogenic: Heart fails as a pump.
- **S&S of all types**: ↓ BP, urinary output; rapid, thready P; capillary refill >3 sec; cool, pale, mottled, or cyanotic skin; change in mental status.
  Hypovolemic: ↓ peripheral pulses.
  Neurogenic: Tachycardia or bradycardia.
  Anaphylactic: Anxiety; throat tightness; stridor; tachypnea; diaphoresis; flushing; urticaria; coma.
  Septic: Fever; tachycardia; tachypnea.
  Cardiogenic: Distended jugular and peripheral veins; pulmonary edema.

Nursing Care

- **Emergency intervention**: Establish airway; suction if needed; give O_2 via nonrebreather mask 10–15 L/min; use supine position with legs elevated unless airway compromised, then low Fowler; maintain IV access with 18-gauge needle; prepare for code, intubation, central venous access; give prescribed IVF and emergency meds; transfer to ICU.
- **Ongoing assessments**: ECG; hemodynamic monitoring; LOC; orientation; VS; pulse oximetry (may be unreliable due to ↓ peripheral perfusion); I&O; skin for color, temperature, turgor, moistness.

- **Specific to types:**
  Hypovolemic: Control bleeding if present; give prescribed colloids, plasma expanders, and/or blood products.
  Neurogenic: Spinal stabilization; give prescribed vasopressors.
  Anaphylactic: Give prescribed epinephrine, antihistamines, steroids.
  Septic: Give prescribed volume replacement, antibiotics, vasopressors, antipyretics.
  Cardiogenic: Give prescribed vasopressors, cardiotonics, antidysrhythmics.

Infection

- Entry and multiplication of a pathogen in tissue; can be local or systemic or progress from local to systemic such as UTIs that can spread to kidneys and bloodstream; infection is accompanied by the inflammatory response.
- **Etiology:** Invasion by bacterial, viral, or fungal pathogen; ↓↑ age and immunocompromised clients have ↑ risk.
- **S&S**
  Local: Erythema; edema; tenderness; heat; ↓ function; purulent exudate; positive culture; S&S also depend on tissue involved.
  Systemic: ↑ VS; chills; diaphoresis; malaise; ↑ WBCs; positive culture; occasionally headache; muscle/joint pain; changes in mental status.

Nursing Care

- Assess VS, S&S of inflammation and infection.
- Obtain C&S before first dose of antibiotic if infection is suspected.
- Avoid excess bedcovers; change linen if diaphoretic.
- Promote rest and immobilization.
- Give prescribed O_2, IVF, ↑ oral fluids, ↑ protein, vitamin C, wound care.
- Transmission-based precautions as indicated.

Inflammatory Response

- Local vascular response to protect and repair tissue; inflammatory response can occur with or without an infection.
- Progression of response:
  - Offending factor precipitates release of histamine, prostaglandin, bradykinin, and serotonin, which cause blood vessel dilation and ↑ vascular permeability.
  - Fluids, protein, and cells move from the intravascular compartment to interstitial tissue, causing local edema, heat, redness.

  - ↑ interstitial fluid and histamine put pressure on and irritate nerve endings, resulting in pain; pain and edema ↓ function.
  - Formation of inflammatory exudates such as pus and serum occurs.
- **Etiology**: Physical trauma, chemical agents, microorganisms, external radiation.
- **S&S**: Local edema; heat; redness; slight ↑ T; pain; ↓ function; exudate may be clear, plasmalike **(serous)**; pink with RBCs **(serosanguineous)**; yellowish green with WBCs and bacteria **(purulent, pus)**; ↑ T and purulent exudate indicate infection.

Nursing Care

- Assess for S&S of inflammation and infection; wound characteristics.
- Provide ordered wound care; D/C IV if S&S noted at insertion site.
- Elevate area if possible to ↓ edema; immobilize area to ↓ pain.
- Give prescribed antipyretics, anti-inflammatories, antibiotics.
- Perform prescribed thermal applications:

  Cold: At time of injury to ↑ vasoconstriction, which ↓ pain and edema.

  Warm: After 24–48 hr to ↑ circulation, which removes debris and localizes inflammatory agents.

Nausea and Vomiting

- Unpleasant wavelike sensation in throat and epigastrium **(nausea)**; ejection of GI contents through mouth **(vomiting, emesis)**; when ejected with force **(projectile vomiting)**; vomiting ↑ risk for aspiration resulting in atelectasis, pneumonia, asphyxiation; complications include dehydration, electrolyte imbalances, metabolic alkalosis.
- **Etiology**: Gastroenteritis; motion sickness; pain; stress; med side effects; pregnancy; GI obstructions such as pyloric stenosis, tumors, intussusception, volvulus; neurological causes such as ↑ ICP, head trauma, vascular headache; GI diseases such as appendicitis, peptic ulcers.
- **S&S**: N&V; salivation; ↑↓ P; pallor; diaphoresis; hyperactive, high-pitched bowel sounds; abdominal pain; signs of F&E imbalance such as hypokalemia, metabolic alkalosis; visible peristaltic waves with projectile vomiting.
- **Color of vomitus**:

  Red—frank bleeding.

  Coffee grounds—blood acted on by gastric enzymes.

  Green bilious—contains bile.

Nursing Care

- Stay with client; provide physical and emotional support; ↓ environmental stimuli.
- Maintain airway; ↑ HOB or use side-lying position to prevent aspiration.
- Assess emesis amount and characteristics; note if vomiting is projectile.
- Keep NPO; assess hydration status, I&O, VS, electrolytes, daily weight.
- Assess abdomen for distention, tenderness, bowel sounds.
- Assess in relation to food, meds, toxic substances.
- Provide oral and physical hygiene; lubricate lips with water-soluble jelly.
- Notify primary health-care provider; obtain prescription for alternate route for oral meds.
- Give prescribed IVF, antiemetic; reintroduce ordered fluids and foods slowly.

Deficient Fluid Volume (Dehydration)

- ↓ intravascular, interstitial, and/or intracellular fluid.
- **Types:**
  Isotonic: Fluid and electrolyte deficits in balanced proportions.
  Hypotonic: Electrolyte deficit exceeds fluid deficit.
  Hypertonic: Fluid loss exceeds electrolyte loss.
- **Etiology:** ↓ fluid absorption; ↓ fluid intake; GI losses from vomiting; diarrhea; nasogastric tube suction; ↑ urine output due to DM and inappropriate ADH secretion; diaphoresis or excessive evaporative losses from fever, hyperventilation; ↑ environmental temperature; hemorrhage.
  Infant: Use of radiant warmer or phototherapy.
- **S&S:** Vary by degree of dehydration; dry mucous membranes; furrowed tongue; ↑ thirst (not reliable in older adult); rapid weight loss; muscle weakness; lethargy; flat neck veins in supine position; narrow pulse pressure; orthostatic hypotension; urinary output exceeds intake if this is the cause of the deficient fluid volume.

Assessment Factor	Mild Dehydration	Moderate Dehydration	Severe Dehydration
% of fluid loss	Infant: 5%–6% Child: 3%–4% Adult: 2%–3%	Infant: 10% Child: 6%–8% Adult: 5%–6%	Infant: ≥15% Child: ≥10% Adult: >8%
Fluid volume loss	<50 mL/kg	50–100 mL/kg	>100 mL/kg
Blanch test	<2 sec	2–3 sec	>3 sec
Skin turgor has delayed return to normal after pinch **(tenting)**	**Estimate % of total body weight loss** (not accurate in older adults) <2 sec: <5% 2–3 sec: 5%–8% 3–4 sec: 9%–10% >4 sec: >10%		
Skin color	Normal	Pale	Gray, mottled
Fontanels (infants)	Normal or depressed	Depressed	Depressed
Eyeballs	Normal or soft	Soft, sunken	Soft, sunken
Blood pressure	Normal	Normal or decreased	Decreased
Pulse	Normal or ↑ rate, strong strength	↑ rate, weak strength	↑ rate, easily obliterated on palpation (thready)
Respirations	Normal or ↑ rate	↑ rate	↑ rate
Urine output	Slightly ↓	Mild oliguria	Marked oliguria, anuria

Nursing Care

- Assess for S&S; determine degree of dehydration.
  Child or adult: 2.2 lb = 1 L of fluid.
  Infant: 1 g wet diaper weight = 1 mL urine.
- Monitor I&O.
- Assess VS every 15–30 min until stable and then routine.
- Weigh routinely.
  Infant or child: Every 2 hr.
  Adult: Daily.
- Give prescribed oral replacement therapy.
  Infant or child: 50–100 mL/kg for mild to moderate dehydration.
  Adults: Encourage twice usual daily intake (at least 3,000 mL).

- Give prescribed IV fluid replacement for severe dehydration.
  Infant or child: 1–3 boluses of NS or lactated Ringer, 20–30 mL/kg.
  Adult: Normal saline or Ringer solutions.
- Give prescribed sodium bicarbonate to correct metabolic acidosis; potassium replacement once kidney function and adequate circulation are ensured; rapid fluid replacement is contraindicated with hypertonic dehydration because of risk of water intoxication.
- Assess for S&S of water intoxication: ↑ urine output, irritability, somnolence, headache, vomiting, seizures.

Orthostatic Hypotension (Postural Hypotension)

- ↓ BP when rising from lying down to sitting or sitting to standing due to peripheral vasodilation without a compensatory ↑ cardiac output.
- **Etiology:** Older age; immobility; hypovolemia; anemia; dysrhythmias; med side effect (opioids, antihypertensives, diuretics).
- **S&S:** light-headedness; vertigo; weakness; cool, pale, diaphoretic skin.

Nursing Care

- Assess for ↑ P and ↓ BP when changing position.
- Teach to rise slowly, sit for 1 min before standing, resume prior position if dizzy.
- Assist to bed, chair, or floor if falling; if ↓ BP continues, assess for ↓ LOC, neurological status, cardiac status, S&S of dehydration; notify primary health-care provider.

Altered Level of Consciousness (LOC)

Assess Level of Arousal

- Alert: Follows commands.
- Lethargic: Is drowsy, drifts off to sleep.
- Stuporous: Requires vigorous stimulation for a response.
- Comatose: Does not respond to verbal stimulus or pressure on sternum or nail bed.

Use a Stimulus to Precipitate a Response

- Move from least to most intrusive stimulus.
- Verbal—"Open your eyes"; tactile—touch; painful—pressure, pain.

Use the Glasgow Coma Scale

- Assesses eye, motor, and verbal responses to stimuli; numbers applied to various responses; the ↓ number, the ↓ LOC.
- Assesses client with head injury for ↑ ICP.

The General Adaptation Syndrome

- Stress → body wear that can be internal/external, physical/emotional, helpful/harmful, or realistic/exaggerated; generalized, nonspecific response regardless of type of stress.
- Influenced by type of stress, severity of stress, duration of stress, and/or multiplicity of stressors.
- Endocrine and sympathetic nervous systems have primary role in response.
  - Alarm: ↑ BP, P, and R, mental activity, blood glucose level; ↓ urine output; dilated pupils.
  - Resistance or adaptation: BP, P, and R return to normal; achieves homeostasis.
  - Exhaustion: ↑ P, ↑ R, ↓ BP, ↓ ability to adapt.

Grief and Loss

- **Grief**: Subjective state of emotional, physical, and social responses to loss of something valued; may be real, substantiated by others (death of a loved one); may be perceived, not identified by others (loss of masculinity after a prostatectomy).
- **Anticipatory grief**: Work of grieving before loss occurs.
- **Complicated grief**: Distress when bereavement fails to follow normative expectations that results in functional impairments.
- **Delayed or inhibited grief**: Absence of S&S of grief when loss occurs due to denial, ↓ resources to cope with loss, ↑ need to resume role.

Kübler-Ross Stages of Grieving

Stage and Response	Nursing Care
Denial: "Not me"; unable to believe loss; may exhibit cheerfulness.	• Explore own feelings about death and dying; accept but do not strengthen denial. • Encourage communication.
Anger: "Why me?"; questioning; resists loss with hostility/anger.	• Recognize anger is form of coping. • Do not abandon client or become defensive. • Help others to understand client's anger.

Stage and Response	Nursing Care
Bargaining: "Yes me, but"; barters for time and may express guilt for past behavior.	• Assist with expression of feelings such as guilt, fear, sadness. • Help with unfinished business if appropriate.
Depression: "Yes me"; realizes full impact; grieves future losses; may talk, withdraw, cry, or feel extremely lonely.	• Convey caring; use touch; sit quietly. • Acknowledge sad feelings. • Accept and support grieving.
Acceptance: "OK, me"; accepts loss; may have ↓ interest in activities and people; may be quiet or peaceful.	• Support completion of personal affairs. • Support family participation in care. • Do not abandon client and family. • Help family understand and allow client's withdrawal.

Nursing Care for Clients Who Are Grieving

- Assess for stage of grieving; identify expected grieving behaviors; provide adequate time to grieve.
- Encourage expression of feelings such as fears, helplessness, anger, guilt; support interactions between client and family.
- Support honest review of loss; promote review of positive and negative aspects.
- Identify use of unhealthy defenses (substance misuse, social isolation, somatic concerns).
- Support cultural and spiritual rituals.
- Offer opportunity for parents to hold child who dies; provide memorabilia such as lock of hair, blankets, ID bracelet, footprints if desired by parents.
- Help identify personal, social, and community support systems.
- Encourage client to seek grief counseling or attend support group if desired.

Cultural Diversity and Spirituality/Religion

Culture

- **Culture**
  - Values, beliefs, and traditions shared by members of a group; may reflect individual variations.
  - Learned through life experiences; basis for self-identity.
  - Complex, dynamic, and exists on many levels: Language; status within a family; communication styles; spacial orientation; nutritional preferences; orientation to time; rituals for transition to adulthood; health beliefs and practices.
  - Culturally competent nursing care holistically respects values, beliefs, and traditions of individual clients; avoids ethnocentric and stereotypic thinking as well as racism.

Spirituality/Religion

- **Spirituality**
  - Essence that integrates one's biopsychosocial journey through life; issues are faith, hope, and love.
  - Defines personal meaning, fulfillment, and satisfaction, which gives strength and significance to one's life.
- **Religion**
  - Organized system of attitudes, beliefs, and practices; demonstrates faith in and worship of a God or higher power.
  - Has theories related to God, authoritative sacred writings, ceremonies and rituals, concepts of either salvation (Judeo-Christian religions) or enlightenment (Eastern religions), and doctrines about a soul and its relationship to death, judgment, and eternal life (Western concepts).

Common Beliefs of Specific Cultural Groups

African American (Black)

- Families tend to be matriarchal; strong family ties; many people may be at bedside.
- Tend to be present rather than future oriented.
- May believe illness is due to disharmony; believe in prayer, herbs, magic rituals, Voodoo, laying on of hands; may be enthusiastically vocal when grieving.
- May oppose abortion due to religious, moral, cultural beliefs.

Amish

- Families are patriarchal; women have status and respect; 3-generational families.

- Not outwardly demonstrative; quiet, modest manner; stoical toward suffering and grief.
- Prefer birth and death to occur at home; neighbors provide physical and emotional support.
- Accept anesthesia, surgery, blood transfusions, organ transplantation except the heart ("soul of the body").
- Limit end-of-life care to save assets for the living; may be afraid of disability but not death.

Asian American

- Several generations may live together; respect for elders; subordinate to authority.
- Value self-respect and self-control; may stoically cope with disability, pain, grief.
- May avoid eye contact out of respect; if asked "Do you understand?" may inappropriately respond "Yes" to avoid loss of face.
- Females may request female health-care providers.
- Believe illness is disharmony of yin and yang; history of Eastern medicine (e.g., application of heat and cold, herbs, acupuncture, amulets).

European American/Non-Hispanic White

- Value independence, individuality, autonomy; emphasize achievement, youth, and beauty.
- Maintain direct eye contact; readily disclose personal information.
- Future oriented but balance the past with the present.
- Believe health is a balance between physical and emotional well-being.
- Seek health care in a variety of settings; accept new technology.
- Accept alternative therapies: Acupuncture, chiropractic, aromatherapy, herbs.

Hispanic/Latino

- Extended family members tend to live together; emphasis is on the group.
- Celebrate a girl's coming of age on 15th birthday (Quinceanera).
- Believe health is gift from God; illness is an imbalance in the body (hot or cold, wet or dry) or punishment.
- Fatalistic but believe in miracles, wearing of religious medals, prayer, and hot/cold therapies.
- May be enthusiastically vocal when grieving.

Native American

- Original inhabitants of North America; many prefer name specific to their cultural heritage (e.g., Navajo Indians, the largest tribe).
- Most tribes are matrilineal; family unit is nuclear family and female relatives; respect elders.
- Present rather than future oriented; punctuality not important.

- Avoid eye contact; tend not to share thoughts and feelings outside tribe; comfortable with silence.
- Believe health is living in harmony with nature (Mother Earth); illness associated with disharmony or evil spirits.
- Believe in a spiritual power, folk medicine, rituals, chanting, dancing, meditation, herbs, amulets.

Common Beliefs of Specific Religions

Buddist

- Admire Buddha (Enlightened One) as a way of life.
- Believe in avoiding evil, being moral and pure, helping others.
- Believe in multiple cycles of life; goal is to reach eternal life without further reincarnation (nirvana).
- Accept illness is part of life; do not offer prayers for healing; accept modern medicine and technology.
- The Tibetan Book of the Dead is read on 7th day after death to release the person's soul from the nether world (Tibetan Buddhists).

Christian Scientist

- Form of Christianity that teaches dependence on God, not the medical community, for health care.
- Do not smoke tobacco or drink alcohol and may not drink tea or coffee.
- Believe illness is due to lack of knowledge, fear, or sin; prayer and Christian Scientist remedies will alleviate illness.
- Prohibit surgery, drug therapy, but allow setting fractures.
- May require legal intervention for children whose parents refuse life-saving treatment.

Hindu

- Believe in Brahman, the universal life force; may revere several gods.
- Goal is relief from cycle of death and reincarnation, leading to higher status in next life.
- May wear religious thread around wrist or body; vegetarians; eat sweets and yogurt at all meals.
- Eat only with the right hand because left hand is used for toileting; prefer to wash in free-flowing water.
- Believe illness caused by actions in past life and supernatural causes that imbalance bile, phlegm, and wind (body humors); pain is due to anger of a higher power and must be endured.
- Require same-gender caregiver; females wear saris that cover body except for arms and feet.
- Prohibit abortion, circumcision, suicide, euthanasia; permit birth control, organ donation, blood transfusions.
- Cremate body 24 hr after death to release body from connection with earth.

Islam

- Most Arabs and Muslims are united by the Islam faith.
- Believe in 5 pillars of faith: Follow Allah and Muhammad; pray facing Mecca 5 times a day; help the poor; fast during Ramadan; make a pilgrimage to Mecca at least once.
- Husbands are decision makers; women do not make autonomous health-care decisions.
- Females prefer female caregivers, expose only their face, wear a leather bag with religious articles.
- May not practice birth control (strict Muslims) but allow abortion for health reasons.
- Position body or face toward Mecca when dying; family member provides ritual bath after death.

Jehovah's Witness

- Live according to commandments in Old and New Testaments.
- Allow birth control, autopsy, cremation.
- Forbid sterilization, abortion, organ transplantation, food with blood (animals must be bled according to custom), blood transfusions, blood products.
- May require legal intervention for children whose parents refuse life-saving treatment.

Jewish

- Believe in only one God and the Torah and Old Testament to show how to live.
- Consist of Orthodox (most strict), Conservative, and Reformed (least strict); observe Sabbath on Saturday.
- Orthodox and Conservative members may follow strict laws of Kashrut (kosher diet): Prohibit pork, shellfish, meat unless it is bled via custom, and meat and dairy at same meal or prepared with same dishes, pots, and utensils; females may wear wig and clothing covering body and extremities.
- Practice sexual self-denial during menstruation, followed by a ritual bath.
- Male newborns circumcised on 8th day after birth (Bris) and females named in synagogue on first Sabbath after birth; religious rite of passage at puberty (Bar or Bat Mitzvah).
- Prohibit tattoos, suicide, euthanasia, embalming, cremation; permit abortion to save mother's life.
- Buried within 24 hr of death; observe mourning period (sit Shiva) where loved one is memorialized.

Mormon (Church of Jesus Christ of Latter-Day Saints)

- Believe in Jesus, one God, and sacred writing of the Book of Mormon.
- Follow strict health code; forbid alcohol, coffee, cola, tea, overeating; observe monthly fasting.
- Wear a sacred undergarment that is removed only for bathing; may be removed for surgery.
- Permit circumcision, organ transplantation, autopsy, and cremation if required by law.
- Forbid abortion, sterilization, drug misuse, smoking tobacco.

Protestant

- Denominations include Lutheran, Presbyterian, Baptist, Episcopal, Methodist.
- Believe Jesus' death atoned for sins of men and women; makes redemption possible.
- Believe in scriptures in Holy Bible and Books of Doctrine specific to denomination.
- May attend services, celebrate Christmas and Easter, receive Communion.

Roman Catholic

- Believe in Father, Son, and Holy Spirit; redemption comes from Jesus, the son of God.
- Priests administer sacraments of Baptism, Reconciliation, Eucharist, Anointing of the sick, and Matrimony; Bishops administer sacraments of Confirmation and Holy Orders.
- Member of the faith can administer Baptism to a neonate if critically ill.
- Religious service is Holy Sacrifice of the Mass; bread/wine transformed into body/blood of Christ and distributed via wafers (Eucharist, Holy Communion) and sips of wine.
- Do not eat meat on certain Fridays during seasons of penance (Lent).
- Accept rhythm method as only acceptable birth control.
- Prohibit sterilization, abortion, suicide, euthanasia.

Seventh-Day Adventist

- Believe in infallibility of Scripture; salvation comes through faith in Jesus Christ.
- Hold Sabbath on Saturday; spend the day worshiping and resting.
- Believe prayers and anointing with oil promote healing.
- Prohibit alcohol, tobacco, caffeine, drug misuse, tattoos, body piercing, euthanasia.
- Allow birth control, abortion when medically necessary.
- Follow kosher dietary laws; most are vegetarians.
- Consider death to be like sleep; body and soul remain together until Christ comes again.

Culturally and Spiritually Competent Nursing Care

- Be sensitive to individual needs of clients based on their culture and spirituality/religion; do not allow personal beliefs to influence care (nonjudgmental care).
- Involve person in a position of authority to be involved in decisions with consent of client.
- Ensure modesty; allow personal clothing when more covering than a hospital gown is required.
- Arrange for a caregiver of the same gender when desired by client.
- Arrange for a dietician to collaborate with client to meet dietary preferences.
- Explore feelings and promote problem solving when a recommended health-care intervention is prohibited by a client's culture or religion.
- Handle religious articles with respect.
- Arrange for a spiritual advisor to visit and perform rituals or administer sacraments; provide time and privacy for cultural/spiritual interventions; avoid bathing for several hours if anointed with oil.

Prenatal Period: Fertilization to Start of Labor

Signs of Pregnancy

- **Presumptive signs:** Absence of menses **(amenorrhea);** 1st awareness of fetal movement **(quickening)** by 16–20 wk; N&V; urinary frequency; breast tenderness; fatigue.
- **Probable signs:** Softening of cervix **(Goodell sign);** bluish-purple mucous membranes of cervix, vagina, vulva **(Chadwick sign);** softening of lower-uterine segment **(Hegar sign);** floating fetus rebounds against examiner's fingers **(ballottement);** positive pregnancy test.
- **Positive signs:** Fetal heart sounds; fetal movement; ultrasound of fetus.

Prenatal Physiological Progression

- Ovum expelled from graafian follicle **(ovulation);** then sperm unites with ovum **(fertilization)** in fallopian tube within 24 hr.
- Fertilized ovum attaches to uterine endometrium **(implantation).**
- Conceptus called embryo (1st 8 wk), then fetus.
- **Trimesters:** 1st (0–15 wk); 2nd (16–27 wk); 3rd (28–37/40 wk).
- **Nägele Rule:** Expected date of birth (EDB); add 7 days to 1st day of last menstruation, subtract 3 mo, add 1 yr.
- Cells differentiate wk 3–8 **(organogenesis);** negative influences such as meds and illness may cause defects in embryo **(teratogens).**
- Fetal heart audible with Doptone after 12 wk.
- Fetal lungs produce pulmonary surfactants at 24–28 wk.
- Brown fat deposits begin at 28 wk; most weight gain in 3rd trimester.

Signs and Symptoms of Impending Labor

- Fetal presenting part descends into true pelvis **(lightening).**
- Cervix thins and shortens **(effacement);** external os opens **(dilation).**
- Mild, irregular uterine contractions (preparatory contractions, formerly Braxton Hicks).
- Energy spurt **(nesting),** usually 24–48 hr before labor.
- Expulsion of mucous plug, usually 24–48 hr before labor.

Prenatal Maternal Changes

Endocrine

- Placenta secretes human chorionic gonadotropin (hCG); used for pregnancy screening; has role in a.m. nausea.
- Progesterone and estrogen from corpus luteum in 1st trimester; from placenta in 2nd and 3rd trimesters.

- Thyroid, parathyroids, pancreas ↑ secretions; need for ↑ insulin.
- Estro levels ↑; excess in maternal saliva may indicate preterm labor.
- Labor initiated by posterior pituitary oxytocin; ↓ progesterone; ↑ estrogen; ↑ prostaglandins.

Nursing Care

- Obtain specimens for screening tests.

Circulatory

- Cardiac output ↑ 30%–50%; blood volume ↑ 50% and RBCs ↑ 30%; because the plasma volume increase exceeds the RBC increase, hemodilution occurs resulting in a decrease in blood levels of RBCs, Hb, and Hct **(physiological anemia);** ↓ Hct level; WBCs ↑ to 12,000 mm^3.
- Palpitations in 1st trimester are due to SNS stimulation; in 3rd trimester are due to ↑ thoracic pressure.
- Heart rate ↑ 10–15 bpm; ↓ BP in latter half of pregnancy; HR may ↑ 40% with multiple fetuses.
- Supine hypotension syndrome **(vena cava syndrome):** Weight of uterus on vena cava ↓ venous return to heart and ↓ placental blood flow; S&S include ↓ BP, light-headedness, palpitations.
- Fibrinogen and other clotting factors ↑.
- Varicose veins of legs, vulva, perianal area **(hemorrhoids)** due to pressure of uterus on pelvic blood vessels.
- Edema of extremities last 6 wk due to circulatory stasis.

Nursing Care

- Teach to ↑ fluids, change positions slowly, elevate legs, wear antiembolism stockings, avoid prolonged sitting and crossing legs; give prescribed anticoagulant.
- For DVT: Maintain BR, give prescribed anticoagulant.

Respiratory

- O_2 consumption ↑ 15% by 16–40 wk.
- Nasal congestion and epistaxis due to ↑ estrogen levels.
- Dyspnea due to enlarged uterus pressing against diaphragm; subsides when lightening occurs around 38 wk.

Nursing Care

- Teach to balance rest and activity; avoid large meals.
- Suggest to blow nose gently; use saline nasal spray.

Reproductive

- Amenorrhea; leukorrhea.
- ↑ vaginal acidity protects against bacterial invasion.
- Cervical and uterine changes: Goodell, Chadwick, Hegar signs.
- Uterus in pelvic cavity at 12–14 wk; then in abdominal cavity to umbilicus at 22–24 wk and almost xiphoid process at term.

- Breast changes: Fullness; tingling; soreness; darkening of areolae and nipples; nipples more erect; veins more prominent; reddish stretch marks; Montgomery follicles enlarge.

Nursing Care
- Assess fundal height.
- Suggest side-lying, vaginal rear entry for intercourse.
- Teach not to douche; use a supportive brassiere and cotton underpants.

Gastrointestinal
- Nausea without vomiting **(morning sickness)** and ↑ salivation due to hormonal changes.
- Food cravings; eating substances not normally edible **(pica)**.
- Heartburn and gastric reflux due to delayed emptying of stomach and pressure of uterus.
- Flatulence due to ↓ GI motility, air swallowing.
- Constipation due to ↓ peristalsis, pressure of uterus, hemorrhoids.

Nursing Care
- Teach to avoid gastric irritants, gas-forming foods, antacids containing sodium.
- Remain upright 1 hr after meals; small, frequent meals; dry crackers before arising if nauseated; ↑ fiber, fluid, walking to prevent constipation.
- For hemorrhoids: Avoid straining at stool and prolonged sitting; use warm sitz baths or ice packs; anesthetic ointments as prescribed.

Urinary
- Urinary frequency in early and late pregnancy due to enlarging uterus.
- Bladder capacity ↑ to 1,500 mL due to ↓ bladder tone; may lead to stasis and infection.
- ↓ renal threshold may cause glycosuria and mild proteinuria.

Nursing Care
- Teach to void every 2 hr and on urge to prevent stasis.
- Assess for glycosuria due to diabetes and proteinuria due to preeclampsia.

Integumentary
- Blotchy, brownish skin over cheeks, nose, forehead **(melasma)**; pigmented line from symphysis pubis to top of fundus in midline **(linea nigra)**.
- Stretch marks over abdomen, thighs, breasts **(striae gravidarum)** due to adrenocorticosteroids during 2nd half of pregnancy.
- ↑ perspiration; oily skin; hirsutism; acne vulgaris.

Nursing Care
- Teach that integumentary changes are common.
- Explain changes generally subside after birth; striae slowly lighten.

Musculoskeletal

- Softening of ligaments and joints, mainly symphysis pubis and sacroiliac joints; backache due to lordosis and changes in center of gravity; leg cramps due to hypocalcemia and uterus pressing on pelvic nerves.

Nursing Care

- Encourage intake of calcium-rich foods and perinatal vitamin.
- Teach body mechanics, avoid high-heeled shoes and lifting.

Nutritional Needs

- 25–35 lb gain: 2–5 lb/wk in 1st trimester; 3/4 lb/wk in 2nd to 3rd trimesters.
- **Calories:** ↑ 300 calories daily to total of 2,500 calories daily.
- **Protein:** 60 g daily, an ↑ of 14 g daily above prepregnant level.
- **Carbohydrates (CHO):** Adequate to meet requirements; complex CHO preferred.
- **Fats:** 30% of daily caloric intake; 10% should be saturated.
- **RDA vitamins/minerals:** Intake of balanced diet; perinatal vitamin with 400 mcg folic acid; sodium is never completely restricted but avoid excess.

Nursing Care

- Teach to have well-balanced diet, avoid dieting.
- Teach to take multivitamin containing 400 mcg folic acid daily before conception and during pregnancy to prevent fetal neural tube defects.

Prenatal Health Promotion

- **Travel:** Lap belt under abdomen and shoulder belt between breasts; stand and walk briefly every hr; airlines may restrict travel close to EDB.
- **Smoking:** Avoid to prevent spontaneous abortion, ↓ birth weight, apnea in newborn.
- **Employment:** Avoid excessive standing or work that causes severe physical strain or fatigue.
- **Alcohol:** Avoid to prevent preterm birth; ↓ birth weight; fetal alcohol effect (FAE); fetal alcohol syndrome (FAS).
- **Illicit drugs:** Avoid to prevent teratogenic effect; ↓ birth weight; small for gestational age (SGA); fetal addiction or dependency.
- **Caffeine:** ↑ risk of spontaneous abortion and intrauterine growth restriction; Food and Drug Administration recommends ≤2–3 servings (200–300 mg) daily.
- **Artificial sweeteners:** Studies uncertain but moderation is advised; avoid aspartame when mother has phenylketonuria (PKU).

Tests Performed During Pregnancy

Human Chorionic Gonadotropin (hCG)
- Tests for pregnancy; detectable 8 days after conception.
- Produced by cells covering the chorionic villi of placenta.
- Slowly ↑ or ↓ levels: Threatened abortion, ectopic pregnancy.
- ↑ levels: May indicate ectopic pregnancy; hydatidiform mole; Down syndrome.

Maternal Serum Alpha-Fetoprotein (AFP) Screening
- Fetal protein used to screen for neural tube defects.
- Ranges identified for each wk of gestation.
- Peak concentrations at end of 1st trimester.
- 16–18 wk optimum time for testing.
- ↑ levels: Risk of open neural tube defect.
- ↓ levels: Risk of Down syndrome; when ↓ levels persist, ultrasound for structural anomalies and amniocentesis for chromosomal analysis.

Chorionic Villus Sampling
- Reflects fetal chromosomes; DNA; enzymology.
- Placental tissue aspirated at 10–12 wk.
- Earlier testing time than amniocentesis permits earlier decision regarding termination; ↓ risk of 1st trimester spontaneous abortion; costs less than amniocentesis.
- Complications: Infection; preterm labor; Rh sensitization.

Nursing Care
- Obtain consent.
- Encourage full bladder to serve as acoustic window.
- Assess VS; absence of uterine cramping.
- Provide emotional support; ensure genetic counseling if appropriate.
- Teach that spotting of blood for 3 days is expected after transcervical route; report flulike symptoms and vaginal discharge of blood, clots, tissue, or amniotic fluid; avoid sexual activity, lifting, or strenuous activity until spotting resolves.

Biophysical Profile (BPP)
- Indicated when there are S&S of fetal compromise.
- Ultrasonography assesses fetal breathing movements and tone, amniotic fluid volume, and gross body movement.
- Non-stress test assesses FHR reactivity.
- Fetus status reflected numerically like Apgar score.
- Reflects central nervous system integrity; indicator of fetal crisis or demise.

Nursing Care
- Same as fetal ultrasound; provide emotional support.

Percutaneous Umbilical Blood Samplings (PUBS)

- Fetal cord blood assessed at >17 wk; identifies some maternal and fetal problems.
- Complications: Fetal/maternal bleeding, infection, thrombosis, preterm labor.

Nursing Care

- Obtain consent; full bladder may be necessary; assess uterine activity, FHR, and FHR reactivity.
- Teach to take antibiotics, T twice daily; report vaginal bleeding.

Fetal Ultrasound

- Serial exams document progress, gestational age, placenta location, fetal position, presentation.
- Assesses FHR, breathing movements, amniotic fluid index; estimates birth weight; visualizes multiple fetuses, maternal pelvic masses, gross fetal structural parts and abnormalities; pockets of amniotic fluid; fetal demise.

Nursing Care

- Provide education based on findings; emotional support.
- Transabdominal: Drink 1–2 L fluid 1 hr before test to fill bladder.
- Transvaginal: Empty bladder to ↑ view of uterus.
- Place a wedge underneath maternal hip if in 3rd trimester to ↓ compression of the vena cava.

Amniocentesis

- Analysis of amniotic fluid.
- **14–17 wk:** Identifies chromosomal and biochemical disorders such as Down syndrome and neural tube defects, fetal age, gender, ↑ bilirubin such as Rh disease, and intra-amniotic infections.
- **32–39 wk:** Lecithin/sphingomyelin (L/S) ratio of 2:1, phosphatidyl glycerol (PG) present, and lamellar bodies of over 35,000 particles/mcL; all indicate lung maturity.
- Complications: Preterm labor; leaking amniotic fluid and infection rare.

Nursing Care

- Obtain consent.
- **14–17 wk:** Ensure bladder is full to raise uterus toward abdominal cavity.
- **Second half of pregnancy**
  - Tell client to empty bladder to ↓ confusion with uterus; hip roll to ↓ hypotension.
  - Assess maternal VS, fetal cardiac activity.
  - Teach that mild cramping is common; fluid leakage usually is self-limiting.
  - Instruct to avoid intercourse, heavy lifting, strenuous activity for 24 hr after test; report ↑ T, persistent cramping, or vaginal discharge.
  - Ensure genetic counseling if appropriate; provide emotional support.

Amniotic Fluid Tests

- **Nitrazine test:** Test tape turns blue; indicates likely ruptured membranes.
- **Fern test:** Fern pattern of cervical mucus under microscope; indicates likely ruptured membranes.

Nursing Care

- Assist with dorsal lithotomy position; encourage coughing to ↑ fluid expulsion.
- Touch nitrazine tape to vaginal secretions; for fern test, use cotton-tipped applicator to collect secretions and draw over glass slide.

Fetal Fibronectin (fFN)

- Swab of vaginal and cervical secretions done at 22–31 wk; fFN leaks with amniotic sac separation; presence may predict labor onset.

Nursing Care

- Assist with dorsal recumbent or lithotomy position.
- Collect sample like a Pap smear.

Nonstress Test (NST)

- Done after 26–28 wk; Doppler transducer records FHR in relation to fetal movement; indicates reassuring or nonreassuring fetal status.
- Test results
  - **Reactive NST:** Two accelerations (↑ of 15 bpm for 15 sec) in 20 min and normal baseline FHR; predictive of fetal well-being.
  - **Nonreactive NST:** Failure to meet reactive criteria over 40 min; vibroacoustic stimulus for 1 sec may be used to startle fetus, which can be repeated two times; nonreassuring sign of fetal status or fetus may be sleeping.
  - **Inconclusive:** <2 accelerations in 20 min; accelerations do not meet reactive criteria; inadequate quality recording for interpretation.

Nursing Care

- Place in left lateral position to ↓ vena cava compression; attach transducer and tocodynamometer to abdomen; teach to press event button with fetal movement.

Contraction Stress Test (CST)

- Contractions stimulated and fetal response monitored; done after nonreactive NST; identifies if fetus can withstand ↓ O_2 during stress of contraction; can precipitate labor.
- Test results
  - **Negative:** Normal baseline FHR, FHR accelerations with fetal movement, and no late decelerations with three contractions in 10 min indicates healthy fetus; oxytocin discontinued; IV continued until uterine activity returns to prior status; fetus likely to survive labor if it occurs within 1 wk with no maternal or fetal change.

- **Positive:** Late decelerations with 50% of contractions is a nonreassuring fetal sign; assess mother and fetus; prepare for cesarean.
- **Suspicious:** Late decelerations with less than half the contractions.

Nursing Care

- Obtain consent; place in semi-Fowler position with lateral tilt; attach Doppler transducer to abdomen; take baseline and every 30 min maternal VS and FHR.
- Assist with stimulation; assess IV site and mother for S&S of preterm labor.

Fetal Movement Count

- 28 wk fetal movement counted by client at same time daily; more testing indicated for ≤3 fetal movements.

Nursing Care

- Teach to assume a comfortable position; hands on abdomen; count number of fetal movements in 1 hr.

Doppler Studies (Umbilical Vessel Velocimetry)

- Measures blood flow velocity and direction in uterine and fetal structures.
- ↓ umbilical vessel flow seen in intrauterine growth restriction (IUGR), preeclampsia, eclampsia, post-term, anomalies of cord or placenta.

Nursing Care

- Same as fetal ultrasound.

Potential Problems During Pregnancy

Disseminated Intravascular Coagulation (DIC)

- ↑ clotting in microcirculation; ↓ platelets and clotting factors → bleeding and thromboemboli in organs; ↑ risk for DIC with abruptio placentae.
- **S&S**: Bleeding, petechiae, ecchymosis, purpura, occult blood, hematuria, hematemesis, shock, ↑ PT, ↑ PTT, ↓ platelet count, ↓ Hct and ↓ fibrinogen levels; may have catastrophic hemorrhage and S&S of multiorgan dysfunction.

Nursing Care

- Assess for S&S, VS changes, shock.
- Give O_2, prescribed meds and blood products; protect from injury.

Fetal Demise: Fetal Death in Utero

- Birth of dead fetus >20 wk gestation or weight ≤350 g **(stillbirth)**.
- **S&S**: No fetal movement or FHR; ↓ fundal height; ↓ fetal growth; may spontaneously go into labor within 2 wk or may be induced.

Nursing Care

- Assess for S&S of fetal death, infection.
- Assist with procedure for removal of uterine contents: D&C, suction curettage, induction of labor.
- Encourage expression of feelings; support grieving and memories such as seeing, holding, naming, memory box (pictures, blanket, clothing, ID bands, hair lock).
- Provide for privacy; ensure family needs are met; refer to support group.

Hyperemesis Gravidarum

- Intractable N&V beyond 1st trimester causing F&E and nutritional imbalance.
- **S&S**: N&V; ↓ weight; deficient fluid volume; electrolyte and acid–base imbalances; ↑ Hct; ketonuria; headache; fatigue.

Nursing Care

- Assess for S&S.
- Maintain NPO until dehydration resolves and 48 hr after vomiting stops; encourage dry diet if tolerated; advance to small amounts of alternating fluids and solids as prescribed; minimize environmental odors.
- Give prescribed IV fluid and electrolytes, antiemetic, antisecretory agent.

Multiple Gestation

- Multiple fetuses due to multiple ovulation, splitting of fertilized egg(s), or multiple in vitro implantations.
- **S&S**: Excessive fetal activity and uterine size; ↑ weight; multiple FHRs; palpation of 3–4 large fetal parts in uterus.

Nursing Care

- Assess VS, fetal growth, S&S of preterm labor, nonreassuring fetal signs.
- Prepare for cesarean birth; give prescribed oxytocic meds postpartum to prevent hemorrhage because excessive uterine distention → atony.

Rh Incompatibility (Isoimmunization)

- Occurs when Rh-negative (Rh-) mother has Rh-positive (Rh+) fetus; 1st pregnancy no effect on fetus.
- Maternal exposure to Rh+ fetal blood stimulates maternal antibody production; in next pregnancy, antibodies enter fetal circulation and attack fetal erythrocytes causing immature RBCs **(erythroblastosis fetalis)**; severe forms → fetal hypoxia, heart failure, anasarca, respiratory distress, death.
- Early detection and treatment with intrauterine fetal transfusions ↑ positive outcomes.
- *Prevention:* Rh immunoglobulin (RhoGAM) administered to Rh- mother ≤72 hr after birth, miscarriage, abortion, ectopic pregnancy, chorionic villus sampling or amniocentesis with an Rh+ infant; protects fetus in next Rh+ pregnancy.

Nursing Care of Mother

- Give prescribed Rh immunoglobulin with 1st pregnancy at 28th wk and after birth with Rh+ fetus and after events indicated in 4th bullet above.
- Give prescribed Rh immunoglobulin at prescribed intervals especially during 2nd half of subsequent pregnancies.

Nursing Care of Neonate

- *Phototherapy:* Remove clothing; turn frequently; monitor jaundice, Hct, bilirubin levels; protect eyes (close eyes, apply patch, change patch every 8 hr); expect green stools, dark urine due to photodegradation products.
- *Assess for S&S of severe incompatibility:* Severe anemia; heart failure; anasarca; respiratory distress; circulatory collapse.

Ectopic Pregnancy

- Implantation outside uterus; mid-fallopian tube most common site.
- **S&S**: Early signs may be obscure; spotting after 1–2 missed periods; sudden, knifelike right or left lower abdominal pain radiating to shoulder (tube rupture); rigid abdomen; shock with obscured hemorrhage.

Nursing Care

- Assess for S&S, VS for shock, pain pattern, anxiety.
- Give prescribed transfusions, pain meds, RhoGAM to Rh-negative client if appropriate; prepare client for surgical repair or removal of tube.

Infections That Are Teratogenic

Toxoplasmosis

- Mother: Protozoal infection; transmitted via feces of infected cats, raw meat, contaminated food or surfaces; can cause spontaneous abortion in early pregnancy.
- Neonate: Maternal treatment prevents problems; no maternal treatment → intellectual disability, neurological impairment, ↓ birth weight, vision problems, hearing loss.
- **Nursing care**
  - Mother: Teach to avoid cat litter; cook meat well; wash fruits/vegetables; wear gloves gardening; cover child sandboxes.
  - Mother/newborn: Administer prescribed spiramycin (need FDA approval) if fetus tests negative; pyrimethamine and sulfadiazine after 16th wk if fetus tests positive; taken by mother and newborn for 1 yr.

Rubella

- Viral infection rare due to measles, mumps, rubella (MMR) vaccine given during infancy and childhood; if contracted during pregnancy teratogenic in 1st trimester; can cause congenital defects in heart, lungs, ears, eyes, brain.

Cytomegalovirus (CMV)

- Mother: Viral infection acquired via respiratory or sexual route; treated with hyperimmune globulin 100 units/kg with normal ultrasound of fetus and 200 units/kg with fetal signs of CMV on ultrasound.
- Fetus/neonate: Virus acquired via transplacental route; contact with infected blood/genital secretions during birth; breast milk; can cause intellectual disability, hearing loss, heart defects, death of neonate.
- **Nursing care**
  - Mother: Teach to avoid others with flulike infections; give prescribed meds.
  - Neonate: Ganciclovir or valganciclovir for severe congenital CMV infection.

Genital Herpes

- Mother: Virus causes painful, draining vesicles on external genitalia, vagina, cervix; antiviral given to prevent outbreak at birth; cesarean if having outbreak at birth.
- Fetus: Fetal–neonatal risk greater when 1st maternal outbreak occurs during pregnancy; fatal or permanent CNS damage if infected during vaginal birth.
- **Nursing care**
  - Mother: Use contact precautions and prepare for cesarean birth during active infection; teach meticulous hand hygiene, not to kiss infant if a cold sore is present; continue antiviral med after birth.
  - Fetus: Separate from mother with active lesions; give antiviral med after birth.

Human Immunodeficiency Virus (HIV)

- Mother: Viral infection; ↑ transmission risk with high viral load and prolonged ruptured membranes; antiviral therapy in 2nd to 3rd trimesters.
- **Nursing care**
  - Mother: Encourage prenatal care, taking of all meds to ↓ viral load, health promotion to ↓ opportunistic infections; instruct to avoid breast-feeding; encourage continuation of med regimen; refer for HIV counseling especially if acquired via risky behavior.
  - Neonate: Give prescribed zidovudine for 6 wk after birth ↓ HIV by 66%; switch to prescribed multiple HIV meds if HIV infection present 4 mo after birth.

Vena Cava Syndrome (Supine Hypotensive Syndrome)

- Partial occlusion of vena cava from pressure of uterus.
- **S&S**: ↑ P; ↓ BP; N&V; diaphoresis; respiratory distress; fainting; nonreassuring fetal signs.

Nursing Care

- Position on left side to shift weight of fetus off inferior vena cava.
- Assess VS, FHR, S&S of shock; give O_2.

Hypertensive Disorders in Pregnancy

- Maternal BP ≥140/90 mm Hg.
- Risk factors: Primipara <17 yr, >35 yr, multipara, DM, chronic HTN, multiple fetuses, trophoblastic or kidney disease, inadequate nutrition, Rh incompatibility.
- May cause maternal and fetal morbidity and are main cause of maternal death.

Chronic Hypertension

- BP ↑ 140/90 mm Hg before pregnancy or before 20 wk and persists for 12 wk postpartum; no excess protein in urine.

Gestational Hypertension

- BP ≥140/90 mm Hg 1st time after 20 wk; BP ↓ to normal ≤12 wk postpartum; no excess protein in urine.

Preeclampsia Toxemia (PET)

- *PET with proteinuria 20 wk or later:* BP ≥140/90 mm Hg 2 times 4 hr apart.
- *PET without proteinuria 20 wk or later:* Same BP as PET with proteinuria plus any of the following—thrombocytopenia, ↓ renal or liver function, pulmonary edema, or cerebral or visual S&S.
- *Severe PET:* SBP ≥160 mm Hg, DBP ≥110 mm Hg; 3–4+ proteinuria, massive generalized edema, oliguria, sudden large ↑ weight, CNS irritability.

PET Superimposed on Chronic Hypertension

- HTN before pregnancy; worsening ↑ BP; proteinuria ≥20 wk; OR ↑ platelets with HTN and proteinuria before 20 wk.

Eclampsia

- Seizures not attributed to other causes in woman with PET.
- **HELLP syndrome:** Hemolysis of red blood cells, Elevated Liver enzymes, Low Platelets; variant of severe preeclampsia; multiorgan failure.

Nursing Care for Clients With a Hypertensive Disorder

- Assess VS and BP every 15 min when critical, then every 1–4 hr; assess edema (I&O, daily weight); CNS irritability such as vision problems and hyperreflexia; proteinuria; fetal status; hematological studies; signs of bleeding or labor.
- Institute seizure precautions; provide quiet environment; limit visitors.
- Encourage ↑ protein and moderate sodium intake; give O_2, prescribed antihypertensive (hydralazine, labetalol, nifedipine) and in severe preeclampsia magnesium sulfate.
- Assess for magnesium sulfate toxicity: Depressed or absent deep tendon reflexes; R <12 bpm; drug blood level >8 mg/dL (therapeutic

range 48 mg/dL); keep calcium gluconate available as antidote for magnesium sulfate.

- Maintain bedrest in side-lying position during labor and birth; be prepared for cesarean birth; assess for 48 hr postpartum.
- Provide emotional support.

Incompetent Cervix

- Premature dilation-effacement of cervix; cervix may be sutured closed **(cerclage)** usually at 10–14 wk gestation; sutures are removed at 37 wk.
- **S&S**: Painless contractions; vaginal bleeding 18–28 wk; fetal membranes observed through cervix.

Nursing Care

- Assess for S&S, nonreassuring fetal signs; maintain bedrest; prepare for suturing of cervix.
- Postop cerclage: Maintain BR for 24 hr; assess for ruptured membranes, contractions, vaginal bleeding; teach to avoid intercourse, lifting, prolonged standing as ordered.

Termination (Abortion and Assisted Abortion)

- Spontaneous or planned expulsion of products of conception.
- Treatment: Mifepristone 1st 9 wk; vacuum aspiration 1st 12 wk; D&C 12–14 wk; dilation and evacuation 14–21 wk; late-term abortion after potential fetal viability requires labor induction; some states prohibit late-term abortion unless mother's life is in danger.

Nursing Care

- Assess VS, S&S of bleeding and infection, expelled products, pain, F&E balance.
- Teach to report heavy bleeding, severe back or abdominal pain, T ≥100.4°F, foul-smelling vaginal discharge.
- Give prescribed RhoGAM to Rh-negative mother; support grieving.

Labor and Birth

Stages of Labor

Nursing Care Common to All Stages

- Establish trust; answer questions; support mother and coach; inform parents and primary health-care provider of progress.
- Use standard precautions.
- Assess contractions; dilation; engagement; position and presentation; fetal and maternal VS (assess between contractions, normal FHR 120–160 bpm); S&S of dehydration, edema.

- Provide prescribed fluids; encourage voiding every 1–2 hr.
- For ↓ BP: Turn on side and retake.
- For pulse oximetry <90% provide O_2.
- For ruptured membranes: Assess for prolapsed cord; meconium-stained amniotic fluid (a nonreassuring fetal sign); S&S of infection; fetal monitoring: See Fetal Heart Rate Monitoring, p. 59.

Stage 1: Begins With Regular Contractions and Ends With Fully Dilated and Effaced Cervix

Phase and Description	Nursing Care
Early phase: Mild to moderate contractions; every 15–30 min, 15–30 sec long; dilation 0–3 cm. **Mother:** Alert; excited; verbalizes concerns; may rest or sleep; uses relaxation techniques.	• Encourage ambulation and upright position if no ruptured membranes. • Review breathing and focusing techniques. • Offer prescribed fluids and food. • Assess fetal presentation and position **(Leopold maneuvers)**.
Active phase: Moderate to strong contractions; every 3–5 min, up to 60 sec long; dilation 4–7 cm; membranes may rupture. Scant to moderate mucoid, bloody show; toward end of active phase, contractions increase in intensity and frequency (some refer to this as transition); contractions every 1–2 min, 45–60 sec long; dilation 8–10 cm. **Mother:** Alert; more demanding; anxious; restless; may seek pain relief; uses breathing and focusing techniques. Toward end of active phase restless; agitated; may have sudden N&V; rectal pressure; difficulty focusing and following directions.	• Assist with position changes, hygiene, oral care; provide prescribed fluids. • Provide counterpressure to sacrococcygeal area, pillow support, and backrubs. • Offer and explain prescribed pain meds. • Talk through contractions. • Initiate hydrotherapy if desired. • Encourage breathing and focusing techniques. • Stay with client; accept irritability. • Use relaxation techniques such as effleurage between contractions. • Teach to pant to avoid premature pushing. • Provide supportive care for N&V and pain relief as indicated. • Prepare for birth.

Stage 2: Begins When Cervix Is Fully Dilated and Effaced and Ends With Birth of Fetus

Description	Nursing Care
Progress determined by descent through birth canal **(fetal station)**; strong contractions every 2–3 min, 60–90 sec long; ↑ bloody show; fetal head visible **(crowning)**. **Mother**: Relaxes between but pushes with contractions; may report severe pain or burning sensation as perineum distends.	• Perform assessments every 5 min; assess FHR before, during, and after contractions. • Note duration, intensity, frequency of contractions with continuous monitoring device. • Assist to position that aids pushing. • Assess for crowning; encourage panting during contraction because it avoids precipitous birth; bearing down with contractions promotes birth. • Prepare for birth; offer mirror to see birth.

Stage 3: Begins at Birth of Neonate and Ends With Delivery of Placenta

Description	Nursing Care
Contractions every 3–4 min. Firming and upward movement of fundus; rush of blood from vagina; lengthening umbilical cord; ↓ bleeding as uterus shrinks. May have perineal laceration or prophylactic incision **(episiotomy)**.	• Assess neonate (see Apgar, p. 71 and Assessment of the Newborn, p. 72). • Assess mother: VS, fundal tone, contractions until placental delivery. • Assist to bear down to deliver placenta. • Give prescribed oxytocic and analgesic. • Keep mother and neonate warm. • Promote bonding before eye prophylaxis. • Put to breast or skin to skin if desired. • Assess parental reaction.

Recovery Stage: First 4 Hours After Placental Delivery

Description	Nursing Care
↓ BP and slight tachycardia expected. Fundus midline, halfway between umbilicus and symphysis pubis; fundus should remain firm and contracted. Red lochia **(lochia rubra)** scant to moderate amount. Expected blood loss 250–500 mL.	• Assess VS every 15 min for 1 hr. • Fundus: Should be 2 fingerbreadths below umbilicus. • Bleeding: <2 pads/hr, no free-flow or clots with fundal massage. • Perineum: No bulging, slight bruising, sutures intact if present. • Bladder: Spontaneous voiding >100 mL; nondistended; uterus above umbilicus and to the right of midline indicates a full bladder; encourage voiding or catheterize if prescribed. • Discomfort: Tolerable, <3 on 0–10 pain scale; generally no severe pain. • Provide hygiene.

Fetal Heart Rate (FHR)

FHR Monitoring

- **FHR monitoring:** Number of fetal heartbeats per min; reflects fetal status and, indirectly, a supportive or nonsupportive uterine environment.
- **Auscultation:** Obtained by Doppler at 10–12 wk; obtained by fetoscope at 16–20 wk.
- **Intrapartum electronic monitoring:** Patterns reflect expected and abnormal fetal responses during labor; frequency and duration of contractions; FHR variability.
- **External monitor:** Ultrasound transducer on abdomen over fetal heart; tocotransducer over uterine fundus.
- **Internal monitor:** Electrode attached to fetal scalp after rupture of membranes.

FHR Patterns

- **Baseline FHR:** FHR between contractions.
- **Normal FHR:** 120–160 bpm after 12 wk; can be ↑ for short periods <10 min.
- **Tachycardia:** Sustained FHR >160 bpm for >10 min; etiologies: early fetal hypoxia, immaturity, amnionitis, maternal fever, terbutaline, diphenhydramine.
- **Bradycardia:** Sustained FHR <120 bpm for >10 min; etiologies: late or profound fetal hypoxia, maternal hypotension, prolonged cord compression, meds, anesthetics.

- **Accelerations:** ↑ FHR 15 bpm and duration of 15 sec; begins with contraction onset and returns to baseline at end of contraction; this is expected.
- **Decelerations:** ↓ FHR in response to onset, peak, or relaxation of contractions or fetal activity.
  - **Early onset:** Fetal head compression; generally benign. **During 2nd stage:** If close together, stop client from pushing until FHR returns to normal; rule out cephalopelvic disproportion if head is above ischial spines.
  - **Variable:** Rapid onset and rapid return with variable relationship to contraction; OK if FHR baseline is acceptable; if it lasts >30 sec or recovery to baseline is slow, notify primary health-care provider because it may indicate cord compromise (cord prolapse, around fetal neck or shoulder, knotted). **If due to cord compression:** Stop oxytocin; place in lateral position; provide O_2 and IV fluids; prepare for cesarean birth if not corrected.
  - **Late onset:** Starts at height of contraction and returns to baseline after contraction ends; reflects uteroplacental insufficiency.

Interventions Associated With Labor

Labor Induction

- Vaginal insertion of med to ripen cervix: misoprostol; dinoprostone.
- ↑ contractions once uterus is inducible: Amniotomy; oxytocin.
- Indications: Post-term, preeclampsia, eclampsia, intrauterine growth restriction, DM, fetal demise.
- Contraindications: Placenta previa, prolapsed cord, transverse fetal lie, active genital herpes, vertical cesarean scar, nonreassuring fetal signs, cephalopelvic disproportion.
- Complications: Contractions <2 min apart or lasting >90 sec **(uterine tetany)**; nausea; ↓ urine output.

Nursing Care

- Assess fetal and maternal response; discontinue oxytocin with uterine tetany.
- Place in left side-lying position; give O_2; prepare for cesarean birth if prescribed.

Augmentation of Labor

- Accelerate labor once it has begun; give prescribed oxytocin.
- Indications: Prolonged or dysfunctional labor, failure to dilate.
- Contraindications, complications, and nursing care same as labor induction.

Artificial Rupture of Membranes (AROM, Amniotomy)

- Indications: Hasten labor; permit internal fetal monitoring.
- Complication: Risk for infection the longer it takes to give birth.

Nursing Care

- Assess for cord prolapse and FHR.
- Maintain horizontal position; provide perineal care.

Forceps and Vacuum-Assisted Birth

- Forceps: Instruments used to encircle fetal head; gentle pulling on handles helps extract neonate from birth canal.
- Vacuum: Soft cup applied over posterior fontanel; gentle traction applied during a contraction; discontinued after 3 pulls, 20 min, 3 cup detachments or observed scalp trauma; helps extract neonate from birth canal.
- Maternal indications: Prolonged 2nd stage, fatigue, maternal illness.
- Fetal indications: Nonreassuring FHR.
- Complications: Vaginal and rectal lacerations, fetal injury.

Nursing Care

- Assess for S&S of complications.
- Provide emotional support.
- Forceps: Assess FHR to ensure cord is not compressed.
- Vacuum: Teach that the temporary swelling of infant's head **(chignon)** will resolve in 1–7 days.

Cesarean Birth

- Birth via abdominal incision; low transverse incision most common; vertical incision ↑ risk of uterine rupture in future pregnancies.
- Indications: Stalled labor progress **(dystocia)**, repeat cesarean birth, breech presentation, fetal compromise, active genital herpes, placenta previa, abruptio placentae, cord prolapse, preeclampsia, eclampsia.
- Complications: Wound infection, dehiscence, hemorrhage, bladder or bowel injury, thrombophlebitis, pulmonary embolus, fetal injury or aspiration.

Nursing Care

- Place emphasis on healthy neonate and mother; assess for S&S of complications.
- Teach about surgery, anesthesia, recovery.

Labor and Birth: Analgesia and Anesthesia

Epidural Block/Infusion

Injection of anesthetic into epidural space to ↓ pain of labor and birth; most common intervention for pain relief during labor.
Advantages: Titratable level; client is awake; nausea and sedation are minimal; urge to push may be preserved; no headache.
Disadvantages: Maternal ↓ BP; labor progress and fetal descent may be slowed; less effective pushing in 2nd stage; may cause N&V, pruritus, urinary retention.

Nursing Care

- Have client void before; assess for bladder distention routinely.
- Minimize hypotension by giving 500–1,000 mL IV fluids 15–30 min before placement as prescribed; maintain side-lying position; alternate sides.
- Assist to side-lying or sitting position and support during insertion (client must remain still); time insertion between contractions.
- Use an infusion pump; ensure catheter placement remains intact.
- Assess VS before, every 1–2 min for 1st 10 min, and then every 5–15 min (may cause ↓ BP and respiratory depression); follow standing prescriptions if ↓ BP occurs: terminate infusion; give O_2 by mask; maintain Trendelenburg position; give bolus of crystalloid fluid; notify primary health-care provider.
- Maintain continuous electronic fetal monitoring.
- Assess pain control; notify primary health-care provider if breakthrough pain occurs because dose is ↓ than therapeutic.
- Assess level of sensation and ability to move feet and legs (recovery takes several hr).
- Ensure 2 people assist with 1st ambulation after the birth.

Regional Anesthesia (Pudendal Block)

Anesthetic agent injected into vaginal wall; ↓ pain of birth.

Advantages: Does not alter maternal VS or FHR; minimal complications; client is awake; effective up to 1 hr.

Disadvantages: May affect only 1 side of the perineum.

Nursing Care

- Assess effectiveness.
- Ensure thermal injury does not occur if cold application is used to ↓ inflammation.

Spinal Block

Agent injected into spinal fluid; anesthesia for cesarean birth and occasionally for vaginal birth with midforceps delivery or vacuum extraction.

Advantages: Ease of administration, immediate onset, client is awake, smaller med volume, less shivering, little placental transfer.

Disadvantages: Finite duration, possible severe maternal hypotension and total spinal anesthetic response, may ↓ ability to push.

Nursing Care

- Hypotension: Give 500–1,000 mL IV fluids 15–30 min before block.
- Assist to side-lying or sitting position during insertion (client must remain still); time insertion between contractions.
- Insert urinary retention catheter before cesarean birth.
- Assess VS before insertion and routinely thereafter.
- Move client with caution because of temporary leg paralysis.
- Vaginal birth: Assist to sitting position for 1–2 min after block so that solution migrates toward sacral area before side-lying; maintain continuous electronic fetal monitoring; encourage bearing down during contractions.

- Cesarean birth: Assist to supine position, with a left lateral tilt, so that cephalad spread of anesthesia occurs.
- Interventions after birth: Maintain BR for 6–12 hr; ensure 2 people assist with 1st ambulation; assess for urinary retention because sensation and control may not return for 8–12 hr; catheterize as prescribed.

General Anesthesia

Induced unconsciousness; requires intubation with cuffed endotracheal tube, ventilation, oxygenation.

Advantages: Total pain relief; optimum operating conditions.

Disadvantages: Client is not awake; may cause ↓ maternal respirations, vomiting, aspiration, uterine atony; may cause fetal depression.

Nursing Care

- Maintain supine position with left-lateral tilt; insert IV line; give prescribed prophylactic antacid.
- Preoxygenate 3–5 min with 100% O_2; maintain cricoid ring pressure to occlude esophagus until cuff of endotracheal tube is inflated.
- When extubated, maintain airway; give O_2; assess VS, ECG, pulse oximetry; keep suction and resuscitative equipment available.

Problems During Labor and Birth

Abruptio Placentae

Partial, marginal, complete separation of placenta from uterine wall >20th wk and before birth; rare.

S&S: Painful vaginal bleeding (concealed bleeding if margins are intact), rigid abdomen, shock, rapid uterine contractions, nonreassuring fetal signs.

Nursing Care

- Assess for S&S, VS, FHR, bleeding, pain, uterine activity, I&O; serum studies for DIC, PT, PTT.
- Maintain bedrest; give prescribed O_2 and IV blood products; prepare for cesarean birth.

Amniotic Fluid Embolism

Escape of amniotic fluid into maternal circulation → pulmonary embolus; 80% fatal; ↑ risk of abruptio placentae and hypertonic labor; rare.

S&S: Chest pain, respiratory distress, cyanosis, rapid shock, ↑ anxiety, feelings of doom, cardiovascular collapse, coagulopathy.

Nursing Care

- Assess for S&S during 3rd and 4th stages of labor; provide aggressive resuscitation if necessary.
- Give prescribed IV fluids, blood products to control coagulopathy, cardiac meds to improve heart function, O_2.

Breech Presentation

Fetal presenting part is buttocks, legs, feet, or combination thereof; risk for cord prolapse, fetal hypoxia and injury, maternal injury.
S&S: Identified via Leopold maneuvers; fetal heart tone above umbilicus; meconium without nonreassuring fetal signs; vaginal exam.

Nursing Care

- Assess for S&S; VS; nonreassuring fetal signs; progress of labor.
- Assess birth canal for cord prolapse when membranes rupture.
- Provide pain relief for "back labor" such as massage, prescribed IV meds or anesthesia.
- Set up for both vaginal and cesarean birth; give emotional support.
- Give prescribed nitroglycerin for rapid uterine relaxation if head becomes trapped.

Premature Rupture of Membranes (PROM)

Ruptured membranes before start of labor.
S&S: Leaking amniotic fluid from vagina; confirmed with fern or nitrazine test.

Nursing Care

- Establish time of rupture; avoid unnecessary vaginal exams.
- Assess for cord compression, FHR, maternal VS, S&S of infection.
- At term and no labor within 12–24 hr: Assist with induction. <37 wk: Maintain BR in hospital in attempt to delay labor until 24 or more wk; give prescribed steroids for fetal lung development, prophylactic antibiotics to prevent infection.

Placenta Previa

Low lying: Placenta in close proximity but not covering os; placenta moves away from os as uterus stretches during 3rd trimester **(migrating placenta)**.
Marginal: Edge of placenta extends to os and may extend onto os during dilation.
Partial: Os is incompletely covered by placenta.
Total: Placenta completely covers os.
S&S: 3rd trimester painless bright red bleeding, soft uterus, anemia, ultrasound confirmation.

Nursing Care

- Maintain BR; avoid vaginal exams; assess VS, FHR, blood loss.
- Give prescribed IVs and transfusions for excessive blood loss.
- Give prescribed betamethasone to ↑ fetal lung maturity; prepare for preterm or cesarean birth.

Precipitous Labor and Birth

Birth with <3–5 hr labor.
S&S: History of rapid labor; rapid dilation and fetal descent; rapid contractions with ↓ relaxation between each; risk for fetal intracranial hemorrhage and anoxia; risk for maternal laceration and hemorrhage.

Nursing Care

- Remain with client; encourage panting with contractions.
- Use palm of hand to support fetal head during birth; do not stop birth of fetus.

Prolapsed Cord

Umbilical cord below presenting fetal part.

S&S: Prolonged variable decelerations; baseline bradycardia; observation of cord protruding through cervix.

Nursing Care

- Lift presenting part away from cord gently, which relieves pressure.
- Provide O_2; elevate client's hips while on side to ↑ placental perfusion.
- Assess FHR.
- Notify primary health-care provider immediately; prepare for possible cesarean birth.

Ruptured Uterus

Complete or partial separation of uterine tissue from stress of labor or trauma such as scar of previous cesarean.

S&S: Silent or dramatic; sudden extreme pain; hypotonic or absent contractions; indications of shock such as ↓ BP, ↑ P, pallor, cool clammy skin; may or may not have nonreassuring fetal signs.

Nursing Care

- Prevention: Explore cesarean versus vaginal birth after previous cesarean birth; prevent or limit uterine hyperstimulation.
- After rupture: Give O_2; prepare for laparotomy for uterine repair or hysterectomy; give prescribed blood or blood products; provide emotional support.

Cephalopelvic Disproportion (CPD)

Fetus larger than pelvic diameters; pelvic inlet and/or pelvic outlet diameter narrowed due to small, abnormally shaped or deformed maternal pelvis.

S&S: Prolonged or arrested 1st or 2nd stage of labor; impaired fetal descent; measurements indicating small pelvic size.

Nursing Care

- Assist with ultrasound to identify pelvic size.
- Assess for nonreassuring fetal signs; prepare for cesarean birth.

Dystocia

Painful or prolonged labor (≥24 hr) due to conditions such as large fetus, cephalopelvic disproportion, malpresentation, abnormal contractions, multiple fetuses.

Maternal S&S: Exhaustion; extreme pain; ↑ P; contractions with ↑ frequency and ↓ intensity; weak, inefficient, or stopped contractions; cervical trauma.

Fetal S&S: ↑ FHR; nonreassuring signs; fetal demise.

Nursing Care

- Assess for S&S; progress of labor; S&S of infection.
- Evaluate response to prescribed uterine stimulant; ensure client does not have a contraindication—cephalopelvic disproportion, malpresentation, hypertonic or hyperactive uterus, placenta previa, prolapsed cord, genital herpes.
- Provide pain relief measures.
- Assist with ultrasonography to identify pelvic size.
- Have O_2 and resuscitation equipment available.
- Assess neonate for extent of head molding, caput succedaneum, cephalhematoma.

Preterm Labor

Start of labor before EDB due to conditions such as multiple gestation or abortions, maternal illness with ↑T, opioid use, bacteriuria, pyelonephritis, bacterial vaginitis, smoking, HTN, DM, pregnancy complications.

S&S: Contractions between 20–37 wk with 2 cm dilation and 80% effacement; contractions every 10 min lasting 30 sec or longer.

Nursing Care

- Maintain lateral recumbent position and quiet environment; provide prescribed tocolytic agents such as ritodrine, terbutaline, magnesium sulfate, indomethacin, nifedipine to suppress labor.
- Give prescribed betamethasone to ↓ severity of fetal respiratory distress syndrome 24–48 hr before probable birth.
- Assess FHR, maternal VS, progress of labor.
- Assess for respiratory depression with magnesium sulfate and tachycardia with terbutaline and ritodrine.

Postpartum: First 6 Weeks After Birth

Maternal Changes During Postpartum

Vital Signs

T ≤100.4°F during 1st 24 hr due to exertion and dehydration; BP returns to baseline; P 50–70 bpm for 6–10 days due to ↓ blood volume and ↓ cardiac effort.

Nursing Care

- Assess VS every 4–8 hr.
- Complete focused assessment if ↑ T (infection), ↑ P, and ↓ BP (hemorrhage).

Fundus

Intermittent contractions return uterus to prepregnant state **(involution)**; 12 hr after birth, uterus is up to or 1 fingerbreadth (FB) above umbilicus; descends 1 FB daily; remains firm and in midline; not felt by 7–9 days.

Nursing Care

- Assess fundal height; massage uterus if boggy but avoid overstimulation.
- Give prescribed oxytocic agent.
- Have client void if uterus is elevated and deviated to the right of midline.
- Teach multipara and breastfeeding mothers that afterpains may accompany involution.

Vaginal Discharge

Red 2–3 days **(lochia rubra)**; pinkish brown 3–10 days **(lochia serosa)**; whitish yellow 10–21 days **(lochia alba)**.

Nursing Care

- Assess for excessive Peri-Pad saturation (1 pad in 15 min is excessive); check linen under buttocks for blood; assess for S&S of shock.
- Check lochia for color, amount, clots, odor; should progress from rubra to serosa and finally to alba; teach to notify the primary health-care provider if lochia returns to an earlier stage, is excessive, or has an offensive odor.
- Flush perineum routinely and after toileting; change Peri-Pad after toileting and prn.
- Teach menstruation returns in about 6 wk when not breastfeeding and 24 wk when breastfeeding.

Perineum

May be bruised, edematous.

Nursing Care

- Assess for hematoma; hemorrhoids; perineum for **R**edness, **E**cchymosis, **E**dema, **D**ischarge, **A**pproximation **(REEDA)**.
- Apply prescribed cold treatment 1st 24 hr for 15 min on, 45 min off, then warm sitz baths 2 to 4 times daily; use anesthetic spray or witch hazel pads.

Breasts

Soft 1st 2 days; engorgement 3rd to 5th day due to vasodilation and ↑ milk volume.

Nursing Care

- Encourage wearing supportive bra; use cool applications such as fresh cabbage leaves inside bra.
- Teach to avoid breast stimulation such as warm shower and stroking.
- For breastfeeding mother, see Breastfeeding and Nursing Care Related to Breastfeeding, pp. 80 and 81.
- For nonbreastfeeding mother, see Formula Feeding and Nursing Care Related to Formula Feeding, p. 83.

Circulatory

↑ WBC, ↓ RBC, and ↓ Hb by 4th day; ↑ fibrinogen and ↑ platelets by 1st wk; blood volume returns to baseline by 3rd wk.

Nursing Care

- Monitor WBC, RBC, Hb; assess for S&S of thrombophlebitis.
- Encourage early ambulation and ↑ fluid intake; promote rest.

Urinary

Diuresis in 1st 24 hr ≥1 L urine; ↓ bladder tone, perineal edema, or regional anesthesia may cause retention; urinary retention displaces uterus up and to right of the midline, which may cause impaired involution of the uterus.

Nursing Care

- Assess I&O, VS.
- Encourage to void; call primary health-care provider if client has not voided within 6–8 hr; catheterize if prescribed.

Gastrointestinal

↑ hunger and thirst; ↑ need for protein and calories to support involution and recovery; usually no BMs for several days due to ↓ food during labor, fear of pain (hemorrhoids), ↓ peristalsis during pregnancy.

Nursing Care

- Provide nutritious diet; assess BMs.
- Encourage fluids, fiber, and activity to prevent constipation; give prescribed stool softener, suppository, or enema.

Integumentary

↑ diaphoresis in 1st 24 hr; pigmentation changes such as striae, linea nigra, and darkened areolae begin to fade; separation of rectus abdominis muscles **(diastasis recti)** may be evident.

Nursing Care

- Promote hygiene.

Parental Emotional Changes

Phases of Maternal Adjustment

- **Dependent (taking-in)**: 1st 24–48 hr; fatigued but exhilarated; reviews birth process; focuses on self; dependent.
- **Dependent-independent (taking-hold)**: Starts on 2nd–3rd day; lasts 10–14 days; begins care of self and infant; eager to learn; still needs nurturing; may have beginning S&S of postpartum depression.
- **Interdependent (letting-go)**: 3rd–4th wk; focuses on family as a unit; reasserts relationship with partner; resumes sexual intimacy.

Stages of Transition to Fatherhood

- **Stage 1 (Expectations)**: Preconception of future; initial excitement.
- **Stage 2 (Reality)**: Realization that expectations not based on fact; feelings of sadness, ambivalence, jealousy, frustration; desire to be more involved.

- **Stage 3 (Transition to mastery):** Conscious decision to take control and become involved with infant.

Nursing Care of Parents

- Encourage attachment and bonding such as eye contact, touching, skin-to-skin contact, rooming-in, infant care.
- Support adjustment to change in role, self-concept.
- Assess interactions with infant; observe for S&S of maternal depression or psychosis (see Major Depressive Disorder, p. 148 and Nursing Care for Clients Who Are Withdrawn in Mental Health Tab, p. 166).
- Notify primary health-care provider if postpartum depression or psychosis is suspected.

Problems During Postpartum Period

Cystitis

Bladder infection.

S&S: Pain or burning on urination, fever, frequency, hematuria.

Nursing Care

- Assess for S&S, distention, fundal height; obtain urine C&S.
- ↑ fluids to 3,000 mL daily; encourage frequent and complete emptying of bladder.
- Give prescribed antibiotics.

Perineal Hematoma

Collection of blood in connective tissue due to episiotomy, prolonged labor, or use of forceps.

S&S: Perineal or rectal pain or pressure; bulging mass in perineum with discoloration; ↓ urinary output; shock.

Nursing Care

- Assess for S&S; apply ice and give analgesics or blood products as ordered.
- Catheterize client; prepare for surgical ligation or evacuation.

Postpartum Hemorrhage

Bleeding due to uterine atony, laceration, or inversion of uterus during 1st 24 hr; may be caused by retained placental fragments after 1st 24 hr.

S&S: ≥500 mL vaginal bleeding.

Nursing Care

- Stay with client; massage fundus; assess for bleeding such as changing Peri-Pads more often than every 1–2 hr initially then every 3–4 hr; monitor changes in VS, ↓ Hb and Hct levels indicating hemorrhage.

- Monitor I&O; provide ordered IV fluids; prepare to give prescribed uterine stimulant (oxytocin, methylergonovine, ergonovine, carboprost) and blood transfusions.

Puerperal Infection

Reproductive organ infection usually after 24 hr and within 10 days after birth.
S&S: ↑ T, chills, pelvic or abdominal pain, vaginal discharge, ↑ WBC.

Nursing Care

- Assess for S&S, VS, I&O.
- Enhance comfort, keep warm, encourage 3 L fluid daily; ↑ calorie and protein intake; give prescribed antibiotics and antipyretics.

Pulmonary Embolism (PE)

Blood clot in lungs from uterine and/or pelvic vein thrombosis that dislodges.
S&S: Dyspnea, ↑ P and R, crackles, cough, chest pain, hemoptysis, anxiety.

Nursing Care

- Assess for S&S of hypoxia; give O_2; ↑ HOB.
- Give prescribed IV fluids, anticoagulants, streptokinase to dissolve clot(s).
- Notify primary health-care provider immediately.

Subinvolution

Delay of uterus to return to prepregnancy size or condition.
S&S: Prolonged or ↑ lochial discharge, excessive bleeding, uterine pain on palpation, large boggy uterus.

Nursing Care

- Assess for S&S, VS, bleeding; perform firm fundal massage.
- Give prescribed uterine stimulant (ergonovine, methylergonovine), antibiotics.
- Prepare for D&C to remove placental fragments.

Thrombophlebitis

Inflammation and clot formation inside a vessel caused by venous stasis and hypercoagulation; confirmed by Doppler ultrasound.
S&S: Pain or tenderness in lower extremity with heat, redness, swelling.

Nursing Care

- Assess for S&S; PT; PTT; maintain BR; elevate leg.
- Give prescribed analgesics and anticoagulants; generally IV heparin 5–7 days followed by warfarin for 3 mo.
- Apply warm, moist heat; do not dorsiflex client's foot or rub area (may cause thrombus to become an embolus); apply antiembolism stockings before getting OOB when prescribed.
- Teach safety related to anticoagulants such as use of soft toothbrush and electric razor.

The Newborn

Apgar Score

Sign	Possible Scores			Assessments	
	0	**1**	**2**	**1 min**	**5 min**
Respiratory effort	Absent	Slow, irregular, weak cry	Strong, loud cry		
Heart rate/ pulse	Absent	<100 bpm	>100 bpm		
Muscle tone/ activity	Flaccid	Limited movement, some flexion of extremities	Active movement		
Reflex irritability	None	Grimace, limited cry	Cry		
Color/ appearance	Pale, blue	Pink torso, blue extremities	Pink torso & extremities		
TOTAL SCORE					

Rating Total Scores

Normal 7–10 **Moderate Depression 4–6** **Aggressive Resuscitation 0–3**

Periods of Reactivity

First Period of Reactivity: 1st 6–8 hr after birth.

- 1st Stage: First 30–60 min after birth most awake, active, strong sucking reflex; HR may be 160–180 bpm and irregular; R may be >80 breaths per min; transient nasal flaring and grunting; bowel sounds are active.
- 2nd Stage: Follows 1st stage; lasts 2–4 hr; HR and R gradually ↓ to baseline; sleeps 30 min to 4 hr; difficult to awaken; no interest in sucking.

Nursing Care

- 1st Stage: Encourage parent-newborn interaction such as eye-to-eye contact, touching, rocking, singing; encourage breastfeeding if desired; provide privacy.

- 2nd Stage: Avoid undressing and bathing neonate; encourage skin-to-skin contact (kangaroo care); allow neonate and parents to rest.

Second Period of Reactivity: Awakens from 2nd stage; lasts 2-6 hr.

- Alert; ↑ response to stimuli; may have ↑ R and HR, apneic episodes, mild cyanosis, mottling; may gag, choke, and regurgitate; may pass meconium stool and 1st void; sucking, rooting, swallowing indicates readiness for feeding.

Nursing Care

- Maintain airway; stimulate during apneic episodes.
- Encourage breastfeeding if desired; document 1st void and meconium stool.

Assessment of the Newborn

Normal and Abnormal Characteristics of the Neonate

Weight, Length, Gestational Age	
Expected Characteristics	**Variations/Abnormalities**
Term: Birth 37–42 wk gestation. **Appropriate for gestational age (AGA)**: 10th to 90th percentile for gestational age. **Birth weight**: 2,500–4,000 g; loss of 10% in 1st few wk; regained in 10–14 days. **Crown-to-rump length**: 31–35 cm; approximately equal to chest circumference. **Head-to-heel length**: 48–53 cm. **Head circumference**: 33–35 cm. **Chest circumference**: 30.5–33 cm.	**Intrauterine growth restriction (IUGR)**: Fetal weight <10th percentile of expected weight for gestational age. **Preterm**: Birth at <37 wk gestation. **Post-term**: Birth >42 wk gestation. **Small for gestational age (SGA)**: Birth weight <10th percentile for gestational age. **Large for gestational age (LGA)**: Birth weight >90th percentile for gestational age. **Low birth weight (LBW)**: Birth weight ≤2,500 g. **Very low birth weight (VLBW)**: Birth weight ≤1,500 g.
Vital Signs	
Expected Characteristics	**Variations/Abnormalities**
Axillary temp: 97.7°F–98.9°F.	**T**: Hyperthermia, hypothermia.
Apical pulse: 100–180 bpm after birth, 120–140 bpm when stabilized; murmurs may reflect incomplete closure of fetal shunts.	**Apical pulse**: *Tachycardia*: >160–180 bpm. *Bradycardia*: <80–100 bpm, irregular rhythm. *Sinus arrhythmia*: HR ↑ on inspiration and ↓ on expiration.

Vital Signs (con't)	
Expected Characteristics	**Variations/Abnormalities**
Respirations: 30–60 bpm; shallow, irregular and abdominal; bilateral bronchial breath sounds. **Blood pressure:** Oscillometric—65/41 mm Hg in arm and calf at 1–3 days of age. **Activity/crying:** May ↑ T, P, R, and BP. **Preterm:** ↓ respiratory effort may require O_2 and ventilation; ↓ brown fat and subcutaneous tissue → T instability.	**Respirations:** *Tachypnea*: >60 bpm. *Apnea*: No breathing >20 sec; nasal flaring, retractions, diminished breath sounds, expiratory grunting, inspiratory stridor, wheezing, crackles. **Blood pressure:** Oscillometric systolic pressure in calf 6–9 mm Hg less than the pressure in an arm may be sign of coarctation of aorta.

Skin	
Expected Characteristics	**Variations/Abnormalities**
Bright red, puffy, smooth skin becomes pink, flaky, and dry by 3rd day. Grayish white, cheesy deposit covering skin **(vernix caseosa).** Fine, downy hair on shoulders, back, and face **(lanugo);** amount ↓ as gestational age ↑. Cyanosis of hands and feet **(acrocyanosis).** Transient mottling **(cutis marmorata)** due to stress, overstimulation, cool environment. Neonatal jaundice after 1st 24 hr **(physiological jaundice, icterus neonatorum).** **Preterm:** Wrinkled and translucent; abundant lanugo; eyebrows absent; extensive vernix.	Ecchymoses and petechiae. Generalized cyanosis, pallor, mottling, grayness. When lying on side, lower half of body becomes pink and upper half is pale **(harlequin color change).** Progressive jaundice, especially during 1st 24 hr usually due to Rh or ABO incompatibility. Tenting of skin may indicate dehydration. Light brown spots **(café-au-lait spots).** Port-wine stain ***(nevus flammeus).*** Strawberry mark ***(nevus vasculosus).*** Tiny white papules on cheeks, chin, nose **(milia).** Flat, deep pink localized areas usually on back of neck ***(telangiectatic nevus,* stork bite).**

Continued

Skin (con't)

Expected Characteristics	Variations/Abnormalities
Post-term: Dry, cracking, parchmentlike skin without vernix or lanugo; greenish-tinged skin due to meconium staining.	Irregular areas of deep blue pigmentation usually in sacral or gluteal areas **(Mongolian spots).**

Posture

Expected Characteristics	Variations/Abnormalities
Slight flexion of extremities. Holds head erect momentarily; turns head from side to side when prone; may have brief tremors. **Preterm:** Limp extended limbs; legs abducted.	Limp extended extremities; marked head lag **(hypotonia).** Tremors; twitches; startles easily; arms and hands flexed; legs extended **(hypertonia).** Asymmetric or opisthotonic posturing.

Head Shape and Circumference

Expected Characteristics	Variations/Abnormalities
Circumference: 33–35 cm. Fontanels are flat, soft, and firm; bulge when crying. **Anterior fontanel:** Diamond-shaped 1–1.75 in; closes in 9–18 mo. **Posterior fontanel:** Triangle-shaped 0.2–0.4 in; closes in 2–3 mo. **Face:** Symmetry of face as neonate cries. **Head lag:** Head lags behind trunk when moved from supine to a sitting position; disappears at 3–4 mo as neck muscles strengthen. **Preterm:** Head large compared to chest; small fontanels; hair like matted wool. **Post-term:** Hair may be profuse.	Molding may occur with vaginal birth. Head circumference <10th percentile may indicate microcephaly or >90th percentile may indicate hydrocephalus. Bulging or depressed fontanels when quiet. Widened sutures or fontanels; fused sutures. Asymmetry of face as neonate cries. Diffuse edema of soft scalp tissue that crosses suture line **(caput succedaneum).** Hematoma between periosteum and skull bone **(cephalhematoma);** unilateral and does not cross suture line. **Intracranial hemorrhage:** Muscle twitching; seizures; cyanosis; breathing abnormal; shrill cry. **Head lag:** Persists after 4 mo; may indicate autism spectrum disorder, neurological problem.

Eyes	
Expected Characteristics	**Variations/Abnormalities**
Lids edematous. Absence of tears. Blink, corneal, and pupillary reflexes present. Funduscopic exam reveals red reflex. Undeveloped fixation on objects. Epicanthal folds in neonates of Asian descent.	Absence of reflexes. Purulent discharge. Epicanthal folds in non-Asians may indicate Down syndrome. Unable to follow bright light. Unable to close one eye with drawing of mouth to one side and inability to wrinkle forehead **(facial palsy)** due to trauma to 7th cranial nerve with vaginal birth or use of forceps.

Ears	
Expected Characteristics	**Variations/Abnormalities**
Startle reflex with loud noises. Ear cartilages formed, pinna flexible; top of pinna on horizontal line with outer canthus of eye. **Preterm:** Ear cartilages undeveloped, ear may fold easily.	Absence of startle reflex in response to noise. Low placement.

Nose	
Expected Characteristics	**Variations/Abnormalities**
Compressed and bruised. Nostrils patent with thin white discharge; sneezing.	Nonpatent nostrils. Purulent or copious nasal discharge. Flaring of nares.

Mouth	
Expected Characteristics	**Variations/Abnormalities**
Intact, arched palate with uvula in midline. Frenulum of tongue and upper lip. Extrusion, gag, rooting, and sucking reflexes present.	Incomplete closure of lip **(cleft lip)**; incomplete closure of palate or roof of mouth **(cleft palate)**. Enlarged, protruding tongue; profuse salivation may indicate Down syndrome.

Continued

Mouth (con't)	
Expected Characteristics	**Variations/Abnormalities**
Minimal salivation. Vigorous cry.	Cry: Absent, weak, high-pitched. White patches on oral membranes and tongue **(candidiasis, thrush)**.

Neck	
Expected Characteristics	**Variations/Abnormalities**
Short, thick with multiple skin folds. Tonic neck reflex present.	Excessive skin folds. Absence of tonic neck reflex.

Chest	
Expected Characteristics	**Variations/Abnormalities**
Anteroposterior and lateral diameters equal. Xiphoid process evident. Bilateral areola and breast bud tissue 0.5–1 cm; breast tissue ↑ as gestational age ↑. Mild sternal retractions on inspiration. **Preterm**: Absent or ↓ breast tissue.	Depressed sternum, funnel chest **(pectus excavatum)**; pigeon chest **(pectus carinatum)**. Wide-spaced nipples, extra nipples **(supernumerary nipples)**. Milky discharge from breast **(witch's milk)**. Marked sternal retractions during inspiration. Asymmetric chest expansion.

Abdomen	
Expected Characteristics	**Variations/Abnormalities**
Umbilical cord: Bluish white; two arteries and one vein. Presence of bowel sounds. **Liver**: Palpable 2–3 cm below right costal margin. **Spleen:** Tip palpable left costal margin by 1 wk. **Kidneys:** Palpable 1–2 cm above umbilicus. **Preterm**: ↓ bowel sounds.	Presence of one artery in cord. Umbilical hernia obvious when crying. Cord bleeding or hematoma. Gap between recti muscles **(diastasis recti)**. Abdominal distention; absent bowel sounds. Visible peristaltic waves. Enlarged liver or spleen.

Back and Rectum	
Expected Characteristics	**Variations/Abnormalities**
Spine intact. Trunk incurvation **(Galant)** reflex present. Patent anal opening. Passage of meconium within 24 hr. Anal constriction when touched **(anal wink).**	External saclike protrusion along spinal column **(spina bifida).** Dimple with tuft of hair along spine **(pilonidal cyst);** may indicate underlying spina bifida occulta. No trunk incurvation reflex. No anal opening **(imperforate anus).** No meconium passed within 24–48 hr; may indicate Hirschsprung disease.

Extremities	
Expected Characteristics	**Variations/Abnormalities**
Symmetrical with full ROM; 10 fingers and toes; feet flat; creases on anterior 2/3 of sole. **Preterm:** Fine wrinkles; flexing of hand toward forearm creates angle that ↓ with ↑ in gestational age **(square window sign).** Elbow in relation to midline when arm is drawn across chest: The farther the elbow passes the midline, the ↓ gestational age **(scarf sign).** **Post-term:** Long fingernails.	Extra digits; fused/webbed digits. Palmar simian crease may indicate Down syndrome. ↓ ROM; fractures of clavicle, humerus, or femur; signs of paralysis. Audible click on flexion and abduction of hips **(Ortolani sign)** and unequal gluteal or leg folds may indicate developmental dysplasia of the hip. Fixed plantar flexion with medial deviation **(clubfoot, talipes equinovarus).** Flaccid arm with elbow extended and hand internally rotated **(Duchenne-Erb paralysis)** due to birth trauma. Tremors, hypertonicity, restlessness, and high-pitched shrill cry may indicate opioid withdrawal.

Male Genitalia	
Expected Characteristics	**Variations/Abnormalities**
Urethral opening at tip of penis. Scrotum developed; pendulous, multiple rugae, and contains testes. May be unable to retract foreskin.	Urethra opens on ventral surface **(hypospadias)** or dorsal surface **(epispadias).** Ventral curvature of penis **(chordee).** Fluid in scrotum **(hydrocele).**

Continued

Male Genitalia (con't)	
Expected Characteristics	**Variations/Abnormalities**
Urination within 24 hr. **Preterm**: Scrotum undeveloped.	Testes not palpable. Ambiguous genitalia. No urination within 24 hr.
Female Genitalia	
Expected Characteristics	**Variations/Abnormalities**
Urethral opening between clitoris and vagina. Labia majora developed; nonprominent clitoris. Urination within 24 hr. **Preterm:** Labia majora incompletely developed; clitoris prominent.	Enlarged clitoris with urethral opening at tip. Fused labia; no vaginal opening. Blood-tinged or mucoid vaginal discharge **(pseudomenstruation).** Ambiguous genitalia. No urination within 24 hr.

Reflexes in the Neonate

Reflex Name	Physical Response
Babinski	When stimulating outer sole of foot from heel upward and across ball of foot toward large toe, the large toe dorsiflexes and toes flare; persists 1 yr.
Blink	When startled or quick movement is made toward eye, eyelids close; persists for life.
Corneal	When cornea is directly stimulated, eyelids close; persists for life.
Crawl	When placed on abdomen, arms and legs make crawling motions; persists 6 wk.
Extrusion	When tongue is touched, tongue moves forward out through the lips; persists 4 mo.
Gag	When stimulating posterior pharynx, choking occurs; persists for life.
Grasp	When palm **(palmar reflex)** or sole of foot **(plantar reflex)** is stimulated at base of digits, fingers and toes flex in griplike motion; persists 3 mo and 8 mo, respectively.

Reflex Name	Physical Response
Moro (startle)	When stimulated by noise or jarring, arms extend and abduct with fingers forming a C while knees and hips flex slightly, arms return to chest in an embracing motion; persists 3–4 mo.
Step (dance)	When supported under both arms with feet against firm surface, feet will make stepping movements; persists 3–4 wk.
Pupillary	When retina stimulated by light, pupil constricts; persists for life.
Rooting	When touching cheek or lips, head turns toward touch and mouth opens in attempt to suck; lasts 3–4 mo, may persist 1 yr.
Sucking	When object touches lips or is placed in mouth, sucking is attempted; persists through infancy.
Tonic neck (fencing)	When supine with head turned to one side, extremities on same side straighten and extremities on opposite side flex; persists 3–4 mo.
Trunk incurvation (Galant)	When stroking infant's back alongside spine, hips move toward stimulated side; persists 4 wk.

Nursing Care of the Newborn

- **Patent airway**: Suction mouth and then nasal passages; insert bulb syringe or DeLee catheter alongside of mouth to avoid gag reflex; use side-lying position with roll behind back.
- **Identification**: Apply matching ID bracelets to newborn and mother with name, sex, date, and time of birth, ID number (significant others may also wear bracelets); obtain newborn footprint on form with mother's fingerprints, name, date, time of birth; identify before mother and newborn are separated.
- **Body temperature**: Dry baby thoroughly; put on a cap; place on mother's abdomen; cover with warm blanket in an Isolette or unclothed under radiant warmer; assess T (use axillary or ThermoProbe) every hr until stable; rectal route contraindicated. Newborn is unable to shiver and breaks down brown fat to produce energy for warmth; stress ↑ need for O_2 and upsets acid–base balance.

- **Eye prophylaxis:** Insert ophthalmic antibiotic such as 0.5% erythromycin into lower conjunctiva of each eye; prevents gonorrheal or chlamydial infection of eyes **(ophthalmia neonatorum)** contracted during vaginal birth; insert after parent–newborn attachment is facilitated.
- **Vitamin K:** Give IM dose of vitamin K to promote normal clotting; vitamin K is produced in GI tract when bacterial formation occurs after ingesting breast milk or formula, usually by 8th day.
- **Umbilical cord:** Clamp for 24 hr until cord is dry; assess for bleeding or infection; clean cord with soap and water after each diaper change; place diaper below umbilical cord stump; continue care until cord falls off naturally in about 10–14 days. Teach parents related principles.
- **Bathing:** Bathe with warm water and mild soap to remove amniotic fluid, blood, vaginal secretions, skin residue; keep environment warm and draft-free to ↓ chilling; dry and swaddle infant; sponge bathe daily—tub bath after cord falls off and circumcision is healed usually within 2 wk. Teach parents related principles.
- **Circumcision:** Assess for edema, redness, bleeding every 30 min for 2 hr, then every 2 hr for 24 hr, then with each diaper change; assess urination (<6 diapers a day may indicate urethral occlusion); change dressing as ordered such as 3 times on 1st day and then daily for 3 days; apply petroleum jelly with or without gauze; avoid disrupting yellowish exudate that appears on 2nd day, because this is part of the healing process; apply diaper loosely to ↓ pressure and friction; give prescribed analgesic. Teach parents related principles. Support desire of parents who are Jewish to have circumcision conducted by a mohel during a ceremony on the 8th day of life (Bris, Brit Milah Ceremony).

Infant Feeding

Breastfeeding

Maternal Benefits

↑ attachment; releases oxytocin, promotes uterine contraction and involution (lochia flow may ↑); extends suspension of ovulation **(anovulation)** beyond 4–6 wk; contraception should be discussed with primary health-care provider if desired; convenient and economical; ↓ risk of breast and ovarian cancer.

Newborn Benefits

↑ attachment; optimum nutritional value for 1st 6 mo of age; provides immunological components such as passive immunity via IgE, IgM, and IgA immunoglobulins, macrophages, leukocytes, lymphocytes, and neutrophils; ↓ incidence of morbidity and mortality.

Contraindications

Mother: HIV positive (except in developing countries where HIV is prevalent because the benefits outweigh the risk); active TB; opioid addiction; breast abnormalities from trauma, burns, radiation; chronic disease that interferes with lactation or maternal status; taking meds excreted in breast milk that are harmful to infant; inadequate maternal fluid and/or nutrition intake.

Newborn: Anomalies that prevent ingestion such as cleft palate or inborn errors of metabolism that cause negative response to breast milk; preterm infant may not have energy to suck; breast milk may be given by bottle or gastric tube.

Nursing Care Related to Breastfeeding

Initial Assessment

- Determine mother's desire to breastfeed, level of anxiety, condition of nipples, maternal and infant physical status, family support.

Teach Self-Breast Care

- Cleanse with water daily; avoid soap and alcohol because of drying effect.
- Wear a supportive brassiere day and night.
- Wear nursing pads to absorb leaking milk; allow nipples to air-dry several times a day.

Teach Breastfeeding Techniques

- Begin breastfeeding as soon as possible, preferably in birthing room.
- Offer breast every 2–3 hr or on demand; infant feeding cues include sucking movements and hand-to-mouth motions.
- Assume comfortable position such as semi-reclining or sitting; place infant with entire body facing breast using cradle, side-lying, or football hold.
- Alternate starting breast and use both breasts at each feeding to ↑ milk production.
- Stimulate rooting reflex and direct nipple and entire areola into open mouth above tongue **(latching-on)**. Nipple stimulation or emotional response to infant precipitates tingling sensation in breast as milk enters ducts and is secreted from breasts **(let-down reflex)**.
- Burp infant during and after feeding; rub or pat back while infant sits on mother's lap, flexed forward to allow for assessment of airway.
- Place in infant seat or supine with head of mattress slightly elevated after feeding to ↓ regurgitation and reflux.
- Pump milk and store for future use if desired; refrigerate for 72 hr or freeze for ≤6 mo; date each bottle; use oldest 1st; do not warm in microwave.
- Evaluate maternal and neonate response to breastfeeding.
- Document knowledge and demonstration of effective breast care, breast pumping, and breastfeeding.

Problems Encountered With Breastfeeding

Breast Engorgement

Breasts are swollen, hard, hot, tender and may be dry and red due to vascular congestion before secreting milk; usually occurs 3–5 days postpartum.

Nursing Care

- Encourage breastfeeding every 2 hr and to empty breasts entirely by pumping if necessary; otherwise back pressure on full milk glands ↓ milk production.
- Apply ice between feedings 15 min on and 45 min off; avoid heat because it will ↑ vascular congestion.

Inverted Nipples

Nipples are below surface of surrounding skin.

Nursing Care

- Wear breast shield to draw nipple out.
- Use electric breast pump before attempting latching-on.
- Apply ice, tug and roll nipple with hands before feeding.

Sore or Cracked Nipples

Nipple irritation resulting in discomfort or pain.

Nursing Care

- Alternate infant position; use less-sore nipple 1st; use breast shield.
- Ensure infant has the areola and not just the nipple in the mouth.
- Apply ice before feeding to ↑ nipple erectness and ↓ soreness OR breast massage and warm compress before feeding to ↑ let-down reflex.
- Analgesic 1 hr before feeding to ↓ soreness.
- Apply breast milk to nipples and air-dry at end of feeding.

Mastitis

Infection of breast; often occurs 2–3 wk after birth when breastfeeding; flulike clinical manifestations; ↑T; local heat and swelling; discomfort or pain.

Nursing Care

- Assess for S&S.
- Apply heat or cold as prescribed; give prescribed analgesics and antibiotics.
- Encourage continued lactation or use of breast pump every 4 hr; suggest use of supportive bra; teach hand and breast hygiene.

Formula Feeding (Bottle-Feeding)

Benefits
More freedom for mother; permits feeding by significant others; allows for accurate assessment of intake; special formulas can be given for infants with allergies or inborn errors of metabolism; appropriate for infants with congenital anomalies such as cleft palate.

Contraindications
Cost of formula and equipment; lack of time or ability to prepare, store, and refrigerate bottles of formula; potential for contaminated water supply.

Nursing Care Related to Formula Feeding

Teach Regarding Formulas
- Formula should yield 110–130 calories and 130–200 mL of fluid/kg of body weight.
- From birth to 2 mo, 6–8 feedings of 2–4 oz of formula may be ingested in 24 hr.
- Formula may be ready-to-feed, concentrated, or powdered; sterilization may be necessary if water source is questionable; prepare 1 day supply at a time and discard if not used within 48 hr.
- Regular cow's milk not appropriate <12 mo of age because of ↑ protein and ↑ calcium and less vitamin C, iron, and carbohydrates than breast milk.

Teach Formula-Feeding Techniques
- Warm bottle by placing it in warm water; never use microwave.
- Sprinkle a few drops on wrist to test T.
- Offer bottle every 2½–4 hr or on demand; start with 3 oz in each bottle.
- Always hold infant because propping bottle may cause aspiration.
- Support entire length of body with head elevated and attempt eye-to-eye contact.
- Enlarge nipple hole size for infant with ↓ sucking reflex or ↓ energy if advised by primary health-care provider.
- Keep nipple filled with formula to ↓ air ingestion; burp during and after feeding.
- Place in infant seat or supine with head of mattress slightly elevated after feeding to ↓ regurgitation and reflux.
- Discard unused formula with each feeding.
- Evaluate maternal and neonate response to formula feeding.
- Document knowledge and demonstration of effective formula preparation and feeding techniques.
- Teach to seek medical attention if infant has bottle-feeding problems (irritability, diarrhea, reflux, gas); may need to change formula.

Problems Encountered With Formula Feeding

- Overdilution of formula → inadequate gain in weight.
- Underdilution of formula → excess gain in weight.
- Infant may not tolerate fats or carbohydrates found in formula.
- Bacterial contamination during preparation and storage may occur.

Contraception

- Prevention of conception via various methods, techniques, or devices.
- Client generally chooses method consistent with religious beliefs, cultural traditions, preference of partner, medical indications.
- *Hormonal:* Oral monophasic, biphasic, triphasic formulation (combined estrogen and progestin in different doses and cycles); medroxyprogesterone (Depo-Provera); etonogestrel implant (Implanon). Contraindicated with ≥ 35-yr-old smoker; history of thromboembolism.
- *Devices:* Copper IUD (ParaGard) and hormonal IUD (Mirena).
- *Natural:* Rhythm (abstinence just before and during ovulation), basal body temp (safest time for intercourse after T drops 3–4 days after ovulation up to menstruation), cervical mucus (becomes abundant, clear, wet 3–4 days before, during and a few days after ovulation which is most unsafe time for intercourse).
- *Emergency contraception-hormonal:* Levonorgestrel; prevents implantation; begin within 72 hr after intercourse; 75% effective.

Nursing Care

- Emphasize consistent and correct use to ↑ effectiveness.
- Discuss types and teach information related to each.
- Teach ↑ risk of pregnancy with hormonal methods and concurrent use of antibiotics, phenobarbital, phenytoin, rifampin.
- Teach certain methods must be used consistently and correctly to ↑ effectiveness; condom is only method that provides some protection from STIs.
- *Hormonal:* Report breakthrough bleeding, S&S of thromboembolism; teach to stop smoking.
- *Etonogestrel implant:* Assess implant site at mid upper arm for inflammation.

Age-Appropriate Vital Sign Ranges

	Heart Rate	Respirations	Blood Pressure (Systolic/Diastolic)
Newborn	80–180	30–60	60–80/30–60
Toddler	80–110	24–32	90–100/50–65
School-Age	60–110	18–26	95–110/55–70
Adolescent	50–90	16–20	110–120/60–80
Adult	60–100	12–20	110–140/60–90

Immunization Schedule—United States, 2016

Recommended Immunization Schedule for Persons Age 0–18 Years

Recommended Immunization Schedule for Persons Aged 0–6 Years UNITED STATES • 2016

These recommendations must be read with the footnotes that contain number of doses, interval between doses, and other important information. See original source for footnotes and recommendations associated with these immunizations and the schedule for those whose immunizations fall behind or start late: http://www.cdc.gov/vaccines/schedules/downloads/child/0-18yrs-schedule.pdf

Vaccine / Age	Birth	1 month	2 months	4 months	6 months	9 months	12 months	15 months	18 months	19–23 months	2–3 years	4–6 years
Hepatitis B[1] (Hep B)	Hep B	Hep B			Hep B							
Rotavirus[2]			RV	RV	RV*							
Diphtheria, Tetanus, & Acellular Pertussis[3]			DTaP	DTaP	DTaP			DTaP				DTaP
Haemophilus influenzae type b[4]			Hib	Hib	Hib*		Hib					Hib
Pneumococcal conjugate[5]			PCV	PCV	PCV		PCV					PCV
Inactivated Poliovirus[6]			IPV	IPV	IPV							IPV
Influenza[7]					Influenza (Yearly)							
Measles, Mumps, Rubella[8]					MMR		MMR					MMR
Varicella[9]							Varicella					Varicella
Hepatitis A[10]							HepA (2 doses)				HepA Series	
Meningococcal[11]			MCV4								MCV4	
Pneumococcal polysaccharide[5]											PPSV23	

*certain vaccine products only

Recommended ages for all children

Certain high-risk groups

Additional dose needed for certain versions of vaccine

Recommended Immunization Schedule for Persons Aged 7–18 Years UNITED STATES • 2016

These recommendations must be read with the footnotes that contain number of doses, interval between doses, and other important information. See original source for footnotes and recommendations associated with these immunizations and the schedule for those whose immunizations fall behind or start late: http://www.cdc.gov/vaccines/schedules/downloads/child/0-18yrs-schedule.pdf

Vaccine / Age	7–10 years	11–12 years	13–15 years	16–18 years
Haemophilus influenzae type b[4]	HiB	HiB	HiB	HiB
Pneumococcal conjugate[5]	PCV	PCV	PCV	PCV
Influenza[7]	Influenza (Yearly)	Influenza (Yearly)	Influenza (Yearly)	Influenza (Yearly)
Hepatitis A[10]	Hep A	Hep A	Hep A	Hep A
Meningococcal[11]	MCV4	MCV4	MCV4	MCV4
Tetanus, Diphtheria, Acellular Pertussis[3]		Tdap		
Human Papillomavirus[13]		HPV (3 dose series)		
Pneumococcal polysaccharide[5]	PPSV23	PPSV23	PPSV23	PPSV23

Legend: Recommended ages for all children (orange); Certain high-risk groups (purple); Additional dose needed for certain versions of vaccine (green)

MCV4 at 11–12 and 16–18 years, Influenza (Yearly), Tdap and HPV (3 dose series) are shown as recommended ages for all children; all other entries are for certain high-risk groups.

Nursing Care Related to Administration of Immunizations

- Assess for contraindications: High fever; acquired passive immunity (maternal antibodies, blood transfusions, immunoglobulin); immunosuppression; previous allergic response; pregnancy—measles, mumps, and rubella vaccinations.
- Follow schedule approved by the Advisory Committee on Immunizations Practices of the Centers for Disease Control and Prevention (CDC). See vaccine schedule in menu of CDC official site http://www.cdc.gov.
- Use appropriate-length needle to reach muscle to ↓ local reactions.
- Use age-appropriate muscle—vastus lateralis or ventrogluteal for infants; deltoid may be used ≥18 mo.
- Apply topical anesthetic spray at injection site; inject slowly.
- Teach side effects: Systemic—low-grade T; Local—tenderness, erythema, swelling; Behavioral—drowsiness, irritability, anorexia.

Growth and Development

Infant: 1–12 Months

Physical

- Weight triples; chest approaches head circumference; 6–8 teeth.
- Turns from abdomen to back by 5 mo and back to abdomen by 6 mo.
- Sits by 7 mo.
- Crawls, pulls self up, and uses pincer grasp by 9 mo.
- Walks holding on by 11 mo.

Psychosocial

- Task: Development of trust that → faith and optimism; support task by meeting needs immediately.
- Oral stage: Provide pacifier for comfort and to meet oral needs.
- Egocentric; smiles and focuses on bright objects by 2 mo; laughs by 4 mo; separation anxiety begins by 4–8 mo; fears strangers by 6–8 mo—provide consistent caregiver.
- May have security object—keep object available.

Cognitive

- Sensorimotor phase; reflexes replaced by voluntary activity.
- Beginning understanding of cause and effect by 1–4 mo.
- Knows objects moved out of sight still exist **(object permanence)** by 9–10 mo.

Language

- Crying signals displeasure 1st 6 mo.
- Babbles by 3 mo; imitates sounds by 6 mo; reacts to simple commands by 9 mo; says one word by 10 mo; says 3–5 words and understands 100 by 12 mo.

Play

- Plays alone **(solitary play)**; involves own body; becomes more interactive and shows toy preferences by 3–6 mo; involves sensorimotor skills by 6–12 mo—ensure play is interactive, recreational, and educational.
- Toys: Large enough to prevent aspiration; simple because of short attention span; black and white or bright mobiles, stuffed animals, rattles, teething rings, push-pull toys, blocks, and books with textures.

Injury Prevention

- *Suffocation/aspiration:* Avoid prone position, pillows, excessive bedding, tucked-in blankets, baby powder, propping bottles, latex balloons, buttons, plastic bags; use cribs with stationary side rails, corner posts no higher than 1/16 inch above end panel, and vertical slats ≤2⅜ inch apart.
- *Motor vehicle:* Use rear-facing car seat until child is 2 yr old or exceeds height and weight indicated by manufacturer (usually 22–35 lb); do not leave in car unattended.
- *Falls:* Supervise when on raised surface; place gates at top and bottom of stairs; use restraints with infant seat, high chair, walker, or swing.
- *Poisoning:* Store agents in high, locked cabinet; avoid secondhand smoke; keep poison control center number by telephone.
- *Burns:* Set water heater at ≤120°F; test water before bath; use bathtub not sink for baths; avoid exposure to sun; do not use microwave to warm bottle; put inserts in electric outlets, and install smoke and heat detectors throughout house.
- *Drowning:* Supervise when in or near water such as bathtub, toilet, bucket, pool, lake; keep toilet lid down with safety lock; know CPR.

Reaction to Illness, Hospitalization, Pain

- Before 6 mo, recognizes pain; not troubled by intrusive procedures.
- S&S of pain: High-pitched cry, irritability, tearing, stiff posture, fisting, brows lowered and drawn together, eyes tightly closed, mouth open, difficulty sleeping and eating.
- Nursing care
  - Meet needs immediately to ↑ trust.
  - Provide nipple dipped in sucrose solution during painful procedure; administer prescribed pain med.

Toddler: 12–36 Months

Physical

- ↓ growth rate; birth weight quadruples by 2.5 yr.
- Anterior fontanel closed by 18 mo; chest circumference greater than head circumference.
- ↓ appetite **(physiological anorexia)**; 20 teeth.
- ↓ naps; day bowel and bladder control at 2 yr; night control by 3–4 yr.
- ↑ taste preferences; walks by 14 mo; runs by 18 mo.
- Mastery of gross and fine motor movements.

Psychosocial

- Task: Autonomy → self-control—encourage independence.
- Anal stage of development.
- Differentiates self from others; notes sex role differences; explores own body.
- Withstands short periods of delayed gratification and parental separation.
- Negativistic—give choices, avoid frustration, provide for safety while ignoring tantrum.
- Needs routines and may suck thumb for comfort—support routines.
- May fear sleep, engines, and animals; may have a security object.
- Sibling rivalry with newborn—supervise interaction, give individual attention, include in newborn care, provide doll for imitative play.

Cognitive

- Continuation of sensorimotor phase.
- Preconceptual thought by 2–4 yr; beginning of memory.
- ↑ sense of time; asking why and how by 2 yr; magical thinking.
- ↑ concept of ownership ("mine"); beginning conscience.

Language

- Comprehension; 4–6 words by 15 mo; ≥10 at 18 mo; >300 at 2 yr.
- Talks incessantly; sentences by 2 yr.

Play

- Plays alongside, not with, other children **(parallel play)**; imitative.
- Types of play: Interactive, recreational, and educational.
- Interactions: Alone, peers, adults.
- Environments: Home, park, preschool.
- Activities: Quiet, active, structured, unstructured—provide varieties of play.

- Toys
  - Physical: Push-pull objects; pounding board, pedal-propelled toys, balls.
  - Social/creative: Telephone, dolls, safe kitchen utensils, dress-up, trucks.
  - Fine-motor skills: Crayons, nesting blocks, tactile such as finger paints and clay.
  - Cognitive: Simple puzzles, picture books, appropriate TV programs and videos.

Injury Prevention

- ↑ risk due to desire for independence, lack of judgment, immature physical abilities.
- *Motor vehicle:* Use forward-facing seat for all children who are 2 yr old or have exceeded height and weight recommended for rear-facing seat even if under 2 yr of age; use forward-facing seat until child exceeds recommended height and weight (usually 20–40 lb) and then use belt-positioning booster seat; do not leave in car unattended.
- *Drowning:* Supervise when in or near water; fence or cover pool and hot tub; toilet seat down with safety lock; know CPR.
- *Burns:* Turn pot handles to back of stove; front guards on radiators, space heaters, fireplaces; keep appliance cords, candles, and iron out of reach.
- *Poisoning:* Store agents in high, locked cabinet; avoid secondhand smoke; keep poison control center number by telephone.
- *Suffocation/aspiration:* Avoid foods that may occlude airway such as nuts, grapes, hot dogs, hard candy; keep garage door openers inaccessible; avoid toy boxes with heavy hinged lids, clothing with drawstrings, appliances that cannot be opened from inside.
- *Bodily damage:* Avoid running with objects in mouth and jumping near doors or furniture with glass; hold pointed objects downward; keep tools and firearms in locked cabinet; keep away from lawnmowers; teach to never go with a stranger or allow inappropriate touching.

Reaction to Illness, Hospitalization, Pain

- Fears punishment, the unknown, separation, immobilization, isolation.
- Altered rituals ↑ stress; regresses when anxious.
- Stages of separation anxiety
  - Protest: Inconsolable crying and rejects others.
  - Despair: Flat affect, unresponsive to stimuli, altered sleep, ↓ appetite.
  - Detachment/denial: Lack of preference for parents; friendly to all.
- S&S of pain: Expresses pain in a word ("ow"), regresses, clings to parent, cries.
- Nursing care
  - Provide consistent routines and caregiver.
  - Encourage parent to stay with child when possible.
  - Ignore regression while praising appropriate behavior.

- Use distraction, massage.
- Administer thermotherapy and meds as prescribed.

Preschooler: 3–5 Years

Physical

- Average ↑ weight 5 lb per yr; ↑ height 2.5–3 inches per yr.
- ↑ immune responses.
- ↑ strength; refinement of gross and fine-motor skills.
- Dresses and washes self; skips, hops, jumps rope, skates, holds pencil and utensils with fingers; uses rounded-tip scissors by 5 yr.
- Potential for amblyopia by 4–6 yr—assess for nonbinocular vision **(strabismus)**.

Psychosocial

- Task: Development of initiative promotes direction and purpose which encourage endeavors.
- Oedipal stage of psychosexual development; attaches to parent of opposite sex while identifying with same-sex parent—encourage imitative and imaginative play; begin informal sex education.
- May have imaginary friend; selfish; impatient; exaggerates.
- Beginning morality (difference between right and wrong); personality developed by 5 yr.

Cognitive

- ↑ preconceptual thought; intuitive thought by 4–5 yr.
- ↑ readiness for learning; curious about immediate world.
- Considers another's views; understands past, present, and future by 5 yr.

Language

- ↑ complexity; uses all parts of speech; asks meaning of new words.
- Knows 900 words by 3 yr; 1,500 by 4 yr; 2,100 by 5 yr.
- Stuttering and stammering common during 2–4 yr.

Play

- Group play without rigid rules **(associative play)**.
- Physical, manipulative, imitative, imaginary play; ↑ sharing by 5 yr.
- Toys
  - *Physical:* Playground, uses sports equipment, bicycles.
  - *Social/creative:* Dress-up, puppets, villages.
  - *Fine motor skills:* Construction sets, simple musical instruments, craft projects.
  - *Cognitive:* Computer games with numbers and letters, simple board games, activity books.

Injury Prevention

- Similar to toddler but not as significant due to ↑ fine and gross motor skills, coordination, balance; ↑ awareness of danger and parental rules.
- *Teach safety habits:* Look both ways crossing street, wear helmets, play in yard or playground; parents should set example of acceptable behavior.
- *Motor vehicle injuries:* Use forward-facing seat until child exceeds recommended height and weight (usually 20–40 lb) and then use belt-positioning booster seat; do not leave in car unattended.
- Teach difference between acceptable and unacceptable touching and to tell parent or a person they trust if they are being touched inappropriately.

Reaction to Illness, Hospitalization, Pain

- Fears intrusive procedures, pain, punishment, rejection, bodily harm, castration, darkness more than separation; may lie about pain to avoid needle.
- S&S of pain: Crying, biting, hitting, kicking.
- Death viewed as temporary.
- **Nursing care**
  - Assess pain using FACES pain rating scale.
  - Explain and demonstrate what may be experienced to ↓ anxiety.
  - Visit hospital before elective procedure or surgery.
  - Support therapeutic play with dolls, medical equipment; use distraction, massage; administer thermotherapy and meds as prescribed.

School-Age Child: 6–12 Years

Physical

- Bone precedes muscular development; fractures at epiphyseal plate may cause unequal limb length if untreated.
- Average ↑ height 2 inches per yr; ↑ weight 4.5–6.5 lb per yr; girls pass boys in height and weight by 12 yr.
- Permanent teeth begin with front teeth.
- Puberty begins earlier in females (about 10 yr) than males (about 12 yr).

Psychosocial

- Task: Achievement of industry → personal and interpersonal competence—recognize accomplishments, avoid comparisons.
- Latent stage of psychosexual development; ↓ egocentricity.
- Identifies with peers of same sex by 6–10 yr; beginning interest in opposite sex by 10–12 yr.
- Develops intrinsic motivation (mastery, self-satisfaction).
- Behaves according to set norms; develops self-image, body image.

Cognitive

- Concrete operations, inductive reasoning, beginning logic by 7–11 yr.
- Grasps concepts of conservation.
- Classifies, serializes, tells time, and reads.

Language

- Vocabulary and comprehension expand.
- Adult speech well established by 9–12 yr.

Play

- ↑ ego mastery, conformity in play, fanatic about rules.
- ↑ peer relationships such as team sports and clubs.
- Collections are more selective; ↑ complexity of board games.
- Engages in hero worship—promote positive role model.

Injury Prevention

- ↑ risk-taking behaviors due to ↑ physical abilities, ↓ parental supervision, inadequate judgment; more injuries in boys than girls.
- *Motor vehicle:* Teach pedestrian skills; play in park, not street; use belt-positioning booster seat when child exceeds recommended weight and height for forward-facing seat; use booster seat until vehicle seat belt fits properly (usually 4 feet 9 inches in height and between 8 and 12 yr of age); then use vehicle-provided lap and shoulder seat belts; all children under the age of 13 should sit in the rear seat using an appropriate restraint.
- *Bodily damage:* Wear eye, mouth, and ear protection with sports; supervise activities such as climbing and gymnastics.
- Teach to go to school nurse if experiencing bullying, sexual harassment, or abuse; never go with a stranger.
- *Toxic substances:* Role-play saying "no" to tobacco, drugs, alcohol.

Reaction to Illness, Hospitalization, Pain

- Fears the unknown, loss of control, dependency, disfigurement, death.
- Typifies death as bogeyman; has realistic concept of death by 9–10 yr.
- S&S of pain: Attempts to cooperate or stays rigid for painful procedures; may cry, yell, resist; clenched fists, gritted teeth, closed eyes.
- Nursing care
  - Assess pain using FACES pain rating scale or numerical scale.
  - Place with age-appropriate roommate; support visits from peers, doing schoolwork.
  - Provide privacy for activities of daily living and procedures.
  - Permit wearing underpants; allow touching of equipment; provide choices; praise attempts at cooperation; encourage expression of feelings; never belittle regression, resistance, crying.
  - Use distraction, guided imagery, soothing music, massage; administer prescribed meds for pain.

Adolescent: 12–21 Years

- Early adolescence (11–14 yr): Changes of puberty and reaction to changes.
- Middle adolescence (15–17 yr): Transition to peer group identification.
- Late adolescence (18–21 yr): Transition into adulthood.

Physical

- Uncoordinated as linear exceeds muscular growth; ↑ strength, especially males.
- Male puberty 12–16 yr: Enlargement of scrotum, testes, and penis; pubic, axillary, facial, body hair; nocturnal emissions, mature spermatozoa; voice deepens; 95% of height by 15 yr.
- Female puberty 10–14 yr: Development of breasts, pubic and axillary hair; 1st menstruation **(menarche)**; ovulation about 12 mo after menarche; 95% of height by menarche.

Psychosocial

- Task: Developing sense of identity → positive self-concept and body image.
- Feels omnipotent; behavior motivated by peer group.
- Resists enforcement of discipline.
- Desires independence but may avoid responsibilities.
- ↑ interest in appearance; ↑ interest in sex (experimentation); forms intimate relationships (opposite sex if heterosexual; same sex if homosexual).

Cognitive

- Formal operational thought; capable of abstract, conceptual, hypothetical thinking; comprehends satire and double meanings.
- ↑ learning through inference vs. repetition and imitation.
- Difficulty accepting another viewpoint; idealistic.
- Develops personal value systems **(value autonomy)**.

Language

- ↑ vocabulary and reading comprehension.
- Experiments with language, uses jargon.

Play

- Individual and team sports provide exercise; ↑ social and personal development and experience of competition, teamwork, and conflict resolution.
- Follows rules of complex games such as Monopoly and chess.

Injury Prevention

- Risk-taking due to feelings of omnipotence, independence, or to impress peers; may experiment with alcohol and/or illegal substances.
- *Motor vehicle:* Assess level of responsibility and ability to resist peer pressure; set limits on driving; encourage wearing lap and shoulder seat belt.

- *Sports:* Encourage warming up and cooling down, playing within abilities, wearing protective gear.
- *Suicide and homicide:* Males more than females; related to economic deprivation, family dysfunction, availability of firearms; assess risk due to frustration, deprivation, aggression, depression, social isolation; lock up firearms.
- Teach to go to school nurse if experiencing bullying, sexual harassment or abuse.
- *Sexually transmitted infections (STIs):* May not seek medical care due to lack of S&S, misinformation, guilt, shame, fear; teach sex education and STI prevention such as abstinence or ↓ number of partners, use of condoms; role-play resisting peer pressure.

Reaction to Illness, Hospitalization, Pain

- Similar to school-age child; ↑ need for independence, privacy, body integrity.
- Fear of disfigurement or ↓ function.
- ↓ need for parental visits, but separation from peers may be traumatic.
- S&S of pain: Physical pain tolerated; stoicism important among males; clenched fist, gritting teeth, self-splinting; ↓ interest and concentration; has realistic concept of death but emotionally may be unable to accept it.
- Nursing care
  - Assess pain using numerical scale.
  - Use distraction, music, massage.
  - Encourage peer relationships.

Genitourinary Malformations

Exstrophy of the Bladder

- Absence of portion of abdominal and bladder walls causing eversion of bladder through opening.

Signs and Symptoms

- Presence of defect; leaking of urine; urine smell due to leaking.
- Associated defects: Pubic bone malformation, inguinal hernia, epispadias, undescended testes or short penis in males; cleft clitoris or absent vagina in females.

Treatment

- Surgical bone repair and closure at birth; 6–12 mo epispadias and continence repair.

Nursing Care

Infant

- Cover bladder with clear plastic wrap or thin film dressing without adhesive.
- Apply prescribed protective barrier to protect skin from urine.
- Assess I&O and drainage from bladder or ureteral drainage tubes.
- Assess bowel function if surgery included resection of intestine.
- Care after surgery for penile lengthening; chordee release; urethral reconstruction similar to hypospadias repair (see Displaced Urethral Openings, p. 98).

Child/Adolescent

- Encourage expression of feelings regarding appearance of genitalia, rejection by peers, ability to function sexually and procreate; care for permanent urinary diversion if present.

Parents

- Support parents coping with child with a defect, multistage surgeries, possible need for permanent urinary diversion, and impact on child's future sexual functioning.
- Teach care of child: S&S of infection; clean intermittent catheterization to empty urinary reservoir.

Cryptorchidism (Cryptorchism)

- One or both testes do not descend into scrotum; risk for cancer of testes.

Signs and Symptoms

- Nonpalpable testes; affected hemiscrotum appears smaller.
- May experience infertility due to exposure of testes to body heat.

Treatment

- Orchiopexy at 6–24 mo to prevent torsion; analgesics; antibiotics.

Nursing Care

- Assess urinary functioning, I&O.
- Prevent contamination of operative site by urine and feces.
- Apply prescribed cool compresses to operative site.
- Give prescribed analgesics, antibiotics.
- Teach parents to assess testes and scrotum monthly and to teach procedure to child when older.

Displaced Urethral Openings

- Abnormal location of urethral opening.
- May reflect ambiguous genitalia.

Signs and Symptoms

- **Hypospadias:** Female has opening in vagina; male has opening on lower surface of penis; penis may have downward curvature **(chordee)** due to fibrous band of tissue; penis appears hooded and crooked; small penis may appear as elongated clitoris.
- **Epispadias:** Occurs only in males; opening on dorsal surface of penis; related to exstrophy of bladder, undescended testes, short penis.

Treatment

- Circumcision delayed to preserve tissue; surgical repair generally at 3 mo.

Nursing Care

Child

Postoperative hypospadias: Assess for S&S of infection; care for indwelling catheter or stent, irrigate if prescribed; avoid tub baths until stent is removed; apply prescribed antibacterial ointment to penis daily; give prescribed sedatives, analgesics, antibiotics.

Postoperative epispadias: See Exstrophy of the Bladder, Nursing Care, p. 97.

Parents

- Support coping with child with a defect, multiple surgeries, and impact on child's future sexual functioning.
- Teach S&S of infection; care of indwelling catheter (avoid kinks in tubing, never clamp).
- Teach to encourage ↑ fluid intake.
- Teach avoidance of straddle toys, sandboxes, swimming, contact sports until permitted.

Urinary Tract Problems

Glomerulonephritis and Nephrotic Syndrome

Glomerulonephritis	Nephrotic Syndrome
• Immune-complex reaction resulting in exudative process that narrows capillaries of glomeruli. • Complication of having an infection in prior 10–14 days; organism is usually group A β-hemolytic streptococcus.	• Metabolic, biochemical, or physiochemical disturbance that occurs in glomerular capillary basement membranes causing ↑ in permeability to protein (albumin).
S&S	**S&S**
• Periorbital edema in a.m., peripheral edema in p.m.; ↓ urine output; dark-colored urine; dysuria; anorexia; pallor; irritability; lethargy; headache; ↑ BP; mild to moderate proteinuria; heart failure. • Peak incidence 6–7 yr of age.	• Periorbital edema in a.m., generalized edema in p.m. → anasarca; ↓ urine output; dark, frothy urine; pallor; fatigue; irritability; anorexia; progressive ↑ weight; normal or ↓ BP; massive proteinuria. • Peak incidence 2–7 yr of age.
Treatment	**Treatment**
• Symptomatic; recovery usually uneventful; fluid intake equal to volume of urine excreted plus insensible loss with oliguria; regular diet; ↓ K and ↓ Na with oliguria; ↓ protein with azotemia; antibiotic for persistent infection; antihypertensive for ↑ BP.	• Regular diet; ↓ Na diet with anasarca; corticosteroids; immunosuppressive if unresponsive to steroids or for relapses; occasionally diuretics, anticoagulants, antihypertensives; plasma expanders with anasarca.

Nursing Care

- Assess VS, particularly ↑ BP with glomerulonephritis and signs of infection with nephrotic syndrome; I&O (weigh diapers); daily weight; extent of edema; abdominal girth; urine for amount, frequency, color, clarity, odor; extent of proteinuria.
- Position in semi- to high-Fowler position with ↑ R or SOB.
- Divide restricted fluid during waking hours; encourage intake of permitted foods; teach fluid and/or dietary restrictions.
- Protect edematous skin: Reposition every 2 hr; elevate scrotum and legs; clean and dry skin and separate skin folds with cotton clothing.
- Encourage rest until proteinuria resolves; provide appropriate age- and activity-level diversions.
- Promote a positive body image regarding physical changes related to edema and steroids.
- Teach parents about meds and their side effects; that irritability and mood swings result from disease and steroids.

Upper Gastrointestinal Tract Problems

Cleft Lip (CL) and Cleft Palate (CP)

- Congenital malformation caused by genetic aberration or teratogens such as meds, viruses, or other toxins.
- **Cleft lip:** Unilateral or bilateral fissure in lip; more common in boys.
- **Cleft palate:** Unilateral or bilateral; complete or incomplete opening in soft and/or hard palate; may include lip; more common in girls.

Signs and Symptoms

- Difficulty feeding: ↓ ability to form vacuum with mouth; may be able to breastfeed.
- Mouth breathing with ↑ swallowed air → distended abdomen and dry mucous membranes.
- Recurrent otitis media and ↓ hearing due to inefficient eustachian tubes.
- Impaired speech due to inefficient muscles of soft palate, nasopharynx; ↓ hearing; misaligned teeth.

Treatment

- Surgical repair of cleft lip within 2–3 mo; palate 9–18 mo.
- Follow up with speech therapist, orthodontist, plastic surgeon.

Nursing Care

Preoperative

- Prevent aspiration: Feed with ↑ HOB; use CL/CP feeding device such as Haberman feeder, Pigeon bottle, Ross Gravity Flow.
- Burp frequently; place in partial side-lying position with ↑ HOB; gently suction oropharynx prn.

Postoperative

- Prevent aspiration (see Preoperative above).
- Prevent trauma to suture line by limiting crying, if possible, and maintaining position of lip-protective device; use elbow restraints if necessary; place on back or position in infant seat.
- Cleanse suture line after each feeding.
- Assess for ↑ swallowing that may indicate bleeding.
- Give prescribed analgesic, sedative, antibiotic.

Parents

- Encourage expression of feelings; show pictures of successful repairs; teach pre- and postoperative care; encourage cuddling to ↑ attachment.

Nasopharyngeal and Tracheoesophageal Anomalies

- Congenital malformation caused by genetic aberration or teratogens such as meds, viruses, or other toxins.
- **Choanal atresia:** Lack of opening between one or both nasal passages and nasopharynx.
- **Chalasia:** Incompetent cardiac sphincter at entrance to stomach.
- **Esophageal atresia:** Failed esophageal development.
- **Tracheoesophageal fistula:** Opening between trachea and esophagus.

Signs and Symptoms

- Respiratory distress, three Cs: Coughing, Choking, Cyanosis.
- Excessive salivation and drooling; abdominal distention.
- During feeding: Choking, coughing, sneezing, regurgitation into mouth/nose.
- Inability to pass a NGT.

Treatment

- Surgical repair.

Nursing Care

Preoperative

- Maintain NPO status; supine with ↑ HOB; assess I&O and pulse oximetry.

- Provide prescribed IVF and antibiotics.
- Suction esophageal pouch as prescribed and oropharynx prn.

Postoperative

- Maintain airway; care for chest tubes if present; change position to prevent pneumonia; give prescribed analgesics and antibiotics.
- Give prescribed gastrostomy feedings until able to tolerate oral feedings; provide mouth care; assess I&O and daily weight.
- Hold, cuddle, provide pacifier for nonnutritive sucking.

Parents

- Encourage expression of feelings; support attachment; encourage cuddling; discuss repair, including stay in ICU.
- Teach postop care such as suctioning, gastrostomy feedings, and skin care.

Hypertrophic Pyloric Stenosis

- Thickened muscle of pyloric sphincter narrows or obstructs opening between stomach and duodenum; presents 1–10 wk after birth.

Signs and Symptoms

- Palpable olive-shaped mass just to right of umbilicus.
- Visible peristaltic waves across abdomen, colicky pain.
- Progressive projectile vomiting, constipation, distention of epigastrium.
- Dehydration, ↓ weight, failure to thrive.
- Metabolic alkalosis: ↑ pH, ↑ bicarbonate, ↓ Na, ↓ chloride, ↓ potassium.

Treatment

- Surgical repair.

Nursing Care

Preoperative

- Keep NPO; provide prescribed IVF to rehydrate and electrolytes to correct imbalances.
- Maintain NGT to decompress stomach.

Postoperative

- Provide prescribed small frequent feedings of glucose, water, or electrolyte solution every 4–6 hr; then formula 24 hr later; ↑ amount and intervals between feedings gradually.

Parents

- Teach care of child; assess and support child-care skills.

Lower Gastrointestinal Problems

Colic

- Paroxysmal abdominal cramping; usually occurs >3 hr a day for >3 days a wk during 1st 3 mo.
- Multicausation theories: Immature nervous system, cow's milk allergy, ↑ fermentation and excessive swallowing of air that ↑ flatus, dietary intake of breastfeeding mother, secondhand smoke.

Signs and Symptoms

- Inconsolable, loud crying; pulls legs up to abdomen.
- Distended tense abdomen, ↑ flatus.

Treatment

- Rule out other causes for infant distress; treat symptomatically, simethicone for flatus.
- No evidence-based role for meds that promote a cure.

Nursing Care

- Obtain history
  - Frequency, duration, characteristics of crying; relationship of crying to time of day and feedings.
  - Infant's diet, breastfeeding mother's diet, stooling and voiding patterns.
  - Sleeping pattern, environmental stimuli.
  - Caregiver behaviors such as methods to ↓ crying, response to crying, smoking.
- Change modifiable causes that may contribute to abdominal pain.
- **Implement 5 Ss**
  - Swaddle tightly in receiving blanket.
  - Sucking: Encourage pacifier, mother's nipple.
  - Side or Stomach lying while monitored.
  - Shushing sounds: Use white noise machine or CD tape.
  - Swinging: Provide rhythmic movements with bed vibrator, swing, or hammock.
- Teach feeding techniques: Proper placement of breast or nipple; give small, frequent feedings slowly; burp often; use bottles that ↓ air swallowing; provide calm environment.
- Apply pressure to abdomen with hand; massage abdomen.
- Eliminate secondhand smoke.
- Encourage parents to seek respite from child care.

Obstructions: Volvulus and Intussusception

- **Intussusception:** Proximal segment of bowel telescopes into a distal segment; often at ileocecal valve; presents at 3–12 mo; requires nonsurgical hydrostatic reduction or surgical repair.
- **Volvulus:** Intestine twists around itself; presents during 1st 6 mo; linked to malrotation of intestine; requires surgical repair.

Signs and Symptoms

- Intussusception triad
  - Acute onset of severe paroxysmal abdominal pain.
  - Palpable sausage-shaped mass.
  - Currant-jelly stools.
- Inconsolable crying, kicking, drawing legs up to abdomen, grunting respirations due to abdominal distention, vomiting, lethargy.
- Untreated: Necrosis, perforation, peritonitis, and sepsis.

Treatment

- Surgical repair of both conditions; hydrostatic reduction for intussusception.

Nursing Care

Preprocedure/Surgery

- Maintain NPO and gastric decompression; give prescribed IVF and electrolytes.
- Give prescribed analgesics, antibiotics.

Postprocedure/Surgery

- Give prescribed IVF and electrolytes.
- Assess VS; amount and characteristics of stool.
- Assess passage of contrast material if hydrostatic reduction used for intussusception.
- Give prescribed oral feedings; encourage breastfeeding to ↓ infant constipation.
- Encourage parental visits to ↓ separation anxiety in older infant.

Intestinal Malformations

Imperforate Anus	Megacolon (Hirschsprung)
Stricture or absence of anus with simple to complex genitourinary and pelvic organ involvement.	Lack of parasympathetic ganglion cells in portion of bowel leads to bowel enlargement proximal to defect.
S&S	**S&S**
• Failure to pass meconium stool, abdominal distention, vomiting. • Meconium on perineum; meconium in vagina or in urine due to a fistula.	• Neonate: Abdominal distention, vomiting, failure to pass meconium within 48 hr of birth, enterocolitis. • Infant/child: Occurs gradually; pellet- or ribbon-like, foul-smelling stool; refusal of food; abdominal distention; chronic constipation; failure to gain weight; S&S of intestinal obstruction.
Treatment	**Treatment**
• Surgical repair depends on extent of anomaly; repair with possible temporary colostomy.	• Resection with temporary colostomy, stool softeners, dietary modifications.

Nursing Care

Preoperative

- Maintain NPO; administer prescribed IVF, electrolytes; assess I&O.
- Implement and maintain prescribed gastric decompression.
- Give prescribed analgesics, antibiotics.
- Assist with diagnostic tests to identify related anomalies.

Postoperative

- Assess VS; amount and characteristics of stool; give prescribed IVF, electrolytes.
- Extent of surgery dictates care: Provide prescribed anal dilations; care for temporary colostomy; implement bowel management program; give prescribed oral feedings; encourage breastfeeding because it ↓ infant constipation.

Parents

- Promote attachment with neonate.
- Encourage visits to ↓ separation anxiety in older infant.

Diabetes Mellitus (DM) in Children

- Disorder of carbohydrate, protein, and fat metabolism causing hyperglycemia that ultimately precipitates multiorgan complications; for more detail, including information about hyperglycemia, hypoglycemia, DKA, HHNS, Somogyi effect, and dawn phenomenon, see Alterations in Blood Glucose Associated With DM in Med Surg Tab, p. 186.
- **Type 1:** Hereditary and environment; 60% of genetic susceptibility related to human leukocyte antigen (HLA); HLA ↑ susceptibility to a trigger such as viruses, cow's milk, or chemical irritants that initiate an autoimmune process that destroys beta cells.
- **Type 2:** ↓ release of insulin and/or insulin secretion is inhibited or inactivated; increasing incidence in school-age children and adolescents; more common with obesity, inactivity, ↑ fat and ↑ calorie diets, and in Native Americans.

Signs and Symptoms

- **Type 1:** Onset is rapid and obvious, three Ps (**P**olyuria, **P**olyphagia, **P**olydipsia), enuresis, fatigue.
- **Type 2:** Onset is gradual, fatigue, obesity, recurrent UTIs and vaginal infections.

Treatment

- Dietary and lifestyle changes; insulin to maintain normal glucose levels.
- A battery-operated pump for continuous insulin delivery via a narrow tube inserted just under the skin is optional.

Nursing Care

- Design strategies appropriate for developmental and cognitive level; use pictures and play; be interactive.
- **Preschoolers:** Teach about DM and food choices on child's cognitive level.
- **School-age children:** Teach self-monitoring of blood glucose, urine testing, and insulin injection such as syringe-loaded injector (Inject-Ease) or self-contained device (NovoPen); S&S of complications.
- **Adolescents:** Explore desire for conformity with peers and nonadherence with medical regimen; ↑ self-care; ↑ motivation with day off or occasional dietary treat.
- **Self-injection of insulin:** Inject same area for 6–8 injections or up to 1 mo; abdomen and thigh best; use shortest, largest-gauge needle possible and pinch technique; insert needle at 90°; track injection sites.

- **Nutrition:** Teach glycemic index of foods, appropriate snacks, sugar substitutes with moderation; support personal and cultural preferences.
- **Exercise:** Encourage daily exercise; additional food intake ½ hr before activity and then every 45 min to 1 hr throughout.
- **Continued supervision:** Promote multidisciplinary approach; refer to American Diabetes Association.

Congenital Heart Defects

Defects With Increased Pulmonary Blood Flow

Ventricular Septal Defect

- Abnormal opening between ventricles; ↑ right ventricular pressure causing pulmonary hypertension and right ventricular hypertrophy.
- S&S: Low harsh murmur throughout systole.

Atrial Septal Defect

- Abnormal opening between atria; right atrial and ventricular enlargement stretches conduction fibers, causing dysrhythmias.
- S&S: Murmur heard high in chest with fixed splitting of 2nd heart sound.

Patent Ductus Arteriosus

- Patency of fetal connection between aorta and pulmonary artery; ↑ left atrial and ventricular workload causing ↑ pulmonary vascular congestion.
- S&S: May be asymptomatic; machinery-type murmur heard in left 2nd or 3rd intercostal space; bounding pulse; widened pulse pressure.

Defects With Decreased Pulmonary Blood Flow

Tetralogy of Fallot

- 4 defects: Pulmonary valve stenosis, ventricular septal defect, overriding aorta, right ventricular hypertrophy.
- S&S: Depends on extent of defects; mild to acute cyanosis; murmur; acute episodes of cyanosis and hypoxia **(blue spells, tet spells)** when energy demands exceed O_2 supply such as when crying or feeding.

Tricuspid Atresia

- Absence of tricuspid valve; no communication from right atrium to right ventricle.
- S&S: Cyanosis, tachycardia, dyspnea.

Defects With Mixed Blood Flow

Transposition of the Great Vessels

- Aorta exits from right ventricle and pulmonary artery exits from left ventricle; no communication between pulmonary and systemic circulation.
- S&S: Mild to severe cyanosis; heart sounds and other S&S depend on associated defects.

Truncus Arteriosus

- Blood from both ventricles enters single great vessel that arises from base of heart directing blood to both pulmonary and systemic circulation; more blood flows to pulmonary arteries because of ↓ resistance than systemic circulation, causing hypoxia.
- S&S: Systolic murmur, single semilunar valve produces loud 2nd heart sound that is not split, variable cyanosis, delayed growth, activity intolerance.

Obstructive Defects

Coarctation of the Aorta

- Narrowing of aorta near insertion of ductus arteriosus causing ↑ pressure proximal to defect and ↓ pressure distal to defect; ↓ blood flow out of ventricles.
- S&S: ↑ BP; bounding radial and carotid pulses; lower extremities have ↓ BP, weak or absent femoral pulses, cool to touch.

Pulmonic Stenosis

- Narrowing of pulmonary valve; resistance to blood flow causing ↓ pulmonary blood flow and right ventricular hypertrophy.
- S&S: Murmur, mild cyanosis, cardiomegaly, or may be asymptomatic.

Aortic Stenosis

- Narrowing of aortic valve; resistance to blood flow, causing ↓ cardiac output; left ventricular hypertrophy; ↑ pulmonary vascular congestion.
- S&S: Murmur, faint pulses, ↓ BP, tachycardia, difficulty feeding, exercise intolerance.

Complications of Congenital Heart Defects

Heart Failure (HF)

- Heart unable to pump blood to meet body's metabolic demands due to ↓ myocardial contractility and ↑ volume of blood returning to heart **(preload)**; ↑ resistance against blood being ejected from left ventricle **(afterload)**.
- S&S: ↑ P; weak peripheral pulses; ↓ BP; gallop rhythm; diaphoresis; ↓ urinary output; pale, cool extremities; fatigue; restlessness; weakness; anorexia.

Pulmonary Congestion

- Excessive amount of blood in pulmonary vascular bed; fluid moves into interstitial spaces when pulmonary capillary pressure exceeds plasma osmotic pressure **(pulmonary edema)**; associated with left-sided HF.
- S&S: ↑ P, dyspnea, retractions in infants, flaring nares, wheezing, grunting, cyanosis, cough, hoarseness, orthopnea, activity intolerance.

Systemic Venous Congestion

- ↑ pressure and pooling of blood in venous circulation.
- Called **cor pulmonale** when due to primary lung disease such as cystic fibrosis.
- S&S: ↑ weight, peripheral and periorbital edema, hepatomegaly, ascites, distended neck veins.

Nursing Care of Children With Congenital Heart Defects

Child

- Assess for S&S specific to defect, hypoxia, squatting, difficulty sucking, pulmonary congestion, systemic venous congestion, HF.
- Assess child
  - VS, heart and breath sounds, pulse oximetry, ECG.
  - I&O, daily weight, maintain prescribed fluid restriction.
  - Electrolyte imbalances, especially hypokalemia (↓ BP, ↑ ↓ P, irritability, drowsiness) → ↑ risk of digoxin toxicity.
- Facilitate breathing: ↑ HOB 30°–45°; avoid constipation and constrictive clothing; provide O_2.
- Provide postoperative nursing care specific to surgical intervention: Palliative shunt or surgical repair.
- Manage hypercyanotic spells **(tet spell)**: Interrupt activity; soothe if crying; hold in knee–chest position with ↑ head to ↓ venous return to heart, which will ↓ preload.
- Provide prescribed small feedings or gavage (usually every 2–3 hr); use soft nipple with large hole to ↓ work of sucking; burp frequently.
- Provide age-appropriate teaching to prepare older child for surgery.

Parents

- Support grieving; discuss specifics of disorder and appropriate care.
- Teach to treat child and siblings equally to ↓ overdependency; set age-appropriate goals within child's activity tolerance; provide consistent discipline to ↓ secondary gains.
- Encourage delegation to prevent parental exhaustion.

Respiratory Problems

Respiratory Tract Infections (RTIs)

- **Nasopharyngitis (common cold)**: Inflammation of nasopharynx.
- **Streptococcal pharyngitis**: Group A β-hemolytic streptococcus (GABHS) infects upper airway; can lead to acute rheumatic fever or acute glomerulonephritis.
- **Tonsillitis**: Inflammation of lymphatic tissue of pharynx particularly palatine tonsils.
- **Influenza**: Influenza virus type A or B → inflammation of respiratory tract.
- **Otitis media**: Acute infection of middle ear usually due to *Streptococcus pneumoniae* or *Haemophilus influenzae.*
- **Bronchiolitis**: Bronchiolar inflammation usually due to respiratory syncytial virus (RSV).
- **Pneumonia**: Inflammation of pulmonary parenchyma.
- **Epiglottitis**: Inflammation of epiglottis.
- **Laryngitis**: Inflammation of larynx.
- **Laryngotracheobronchitis**: Inflammation of larynx, trachea, bronchi; cause identified via C&S; rapid immunofluorescent antibody or enzyme-linked immunosorbent assay techniques for RSV detection.

Factors Influencing Occurrence of RTIs

- **Age of child**: <3 mo protected by maternal antibodies; infant and toddler have ↑ incidence of viral infections; school-age have ↑ incidence of pneumonia and β-hemolytic streptococcus infections.
- **Size of child**: Infants and toddlers have small diameter airways and short, open eustachian tubes, increasing risk of otitis media.
- **Season**: Viral infections particularly respiratory syncytial virus in winter and spring; asthmatic bronchitis in winter.
- **Living conditions**: Secondhand smoke, day-care centers, multiple siblings, crowded conditions.
- **Preexisting medical condition**: Immune deficiencies; malnutrition; allergies; problems such as cystic fibrosis, Down syndrome, asthma.

Common Signs and Symptoms

- Irritability, restlessness, anorexia, malaise, chills, muscular aches, headache.
- Irritation of pharynx and nasal passages, nasal discharge, mouth or breath odor.
- ↑ VS, cough, dyspnea, cervical lymphadenopathy.
- Seizures may occur with T >102°F.

Specific Signs and Symptoms

- *Laryngitis:* Hoarseness.
- *Tonsillitis:* Tonsils covered with exudates.
- *Epiglottitis:* Large cherry-red edematous epiglottis; slow, quiet breathing; agitation; drooling; sore throat; no spontaneous cough.
- *Otitis media:* Pulling at ears or rolling head side to side; earache; sucking or chewing ↑ pain; bulging red eardrum; may exhibit hearing loss, vomiting, diarrhea.
- *Laryngotracheobronchitis (croup):*
  - *Stage I:* Fear, hoarseness, barking cough, inspiratory stridor.
  - *Stage II:* Dyspnea, retractions, use of accessory muscles.
  - *Stage III:* Restlessness, pallor, diaphoresis, ↑ R, S&S of hypoxia, CO_2 retention.
  - *Stage IV:* Cyanosis, cessation of breathing.

Commonalities of Treatment

- Promote respirations: Saline nasal spray; bronchodilators; ↑ HOB; O_2; oropharyngeal suctioning except with croup syndromes.
- ↓ T: Give antipyretics but avoid aspirin to prevent Reye syndrome; cool liquids, chest PT to ↑ expectoration of secretions.
- ↑ hydration: Oral rehydration such as Pedialyte or Infalyte; sports drinks such as Gatorade and Exceed; high-calorie liquids; provide prescribed IVF if unable to drink.
- ↑ rest: BR or quiet activity.
- ↑ comfort: Analgesics, heat, cold, gargles, or troches for sore throat, cough suppressants for dry cough.

Treatment for Specific RTIs

- *Bacterial infections:* Judicious use of antibiotics such as amoxicillin, 2nd-generation cephalosporins or erythromycin; rifampin may be added for GABHS.
- *Tonsillitis:* Surgical removal of tonsils and adenoids (T&A) that obstruct breathing or for recurrent infections.
- *Otitis media:* Antibiotic eardrops, local heat, myringotomy for persistent effusion or hearing loss.
- *Epiglottitis:* Corticosteroids, endotracheal intubation or tracheostomy for severe respiratory distress.
- *Croup:* Corticosteroids, nebulized epinephrine.

Nursing Care

- **Acute care**
  - Institute and maintain droplet precautions.
  - Assess risk for respiratory obstruction.
  - Collect sputum specimen for C&S before beginning antibiotics (best in a.m.).
  - Support parents and child with frightening SOB or airway obstruction.
  - Keep upright (sit on lap), supine, or side-lying position with neck slightly extended **(sniff position)**.
  - Provide prescribed humidified O_2; assess pulse oximetry.
  - ↑ fluids to replace loss from fever, perspiration, ↑ respirations, and to liquefy secretions.
  - Manage secretions (nasal aspirator, oropharyngeal suctioning except with croup syndromes); chest PT.
  - Give prescribed antibiotics, decongestants, analgesics.
  - Maintain BR, calm environment; engage in age-appropriate quiet diversionary activities.
- **Teach preventive measures:** Frequent hand hygiene; containment of soiled tissues; cough or sneeze into tissue or elbow; avoid sharing eating utensils, glasses, or towels; formula-feeding of infants in upright position to ↓ fluid entering eustachian tubes.
- **Postoperative T&A:** Maintain side-lying position with HOB ↑ 30°; discourage coughing, throat clearing, nose blowing; apply ice collar; offer ice chips, ice pops, diluted juice; avoid dairy products or red-colored fluids; give prescribed analgesics; frequent swallowing may indicate bleeding.
- **Postoperative myringotomy:** Place on affected side to ↑ ear drainage; apply prescribed heat or cold; clean and apply moisture barrier to pinna to protect skin from drainage; recognize S&S of ↓ hearing; teach parents to prevent bath and shampoo water from entering ear; feed in upright position; eliminate allergens; encourage follow-up care.

Asthma

- Stimulus causes inflammation that ↑ mucus, mucosal edema, bronchospasm; this traps air in lungs → chronic tissue irritation, scarring, hyperinflation.
- Peak expiratory flow rate: ↓ maximum flow of air forcefully exhaled in 1 min.
- Occurs due to allergens such as mold, pollen, dust mites, and cockroach allergen or nonimmunological stimuli such as infections, exercise, cold air, odors, smoke, stress, and dairy products.
- Characterized by remissions and exacerbations; may be mild and intermittent to severe, persistent, intractable **(status asthmaticus)**.

Signs and Symptoms

- Dyspnea, dry cough, prolonged expirations with wheezing, sternal retractions, flaring nares, barrel chest.
- Prodromal exacerbation: Rhinorrhea; low-grade fever; itching on neck, chest, and upper back; anorexia; headache; irritability; restlessness; fatigue; chest tightness; anxiety.
- Progression of exacerbation: Frothy, clear, gelatinous sputum; productive cough; ↑ R; SOB; pale face with red ears; lips dark red progressing to cyanosis; tripod or orthopneic position; hyperresonance on chest percussion; breath sounds coarse with sonorous crackles.
- Imminent ventilatory failure: SOB with absence of breath sounds.

Treatment

- Removal of stimulus.
- Long-term control meds **(preventer meds)**: Oral or inhaled corticosteroids; NSAIDs to ↓ inflammation and allergic response; bronchodilators; anti-immunoglobulin E antibodies (omalizumab) to prevent an attack. Quick-relief meds **(rescue meds)**: ↓ exacerbations; β-adrenergics, anticholinergics, corticosteroids ↓ bronchospasm.
- Emergency protocol: 3 treatments with short-acting β-adrenergic spaced at 20–30 min; systemic prednisone; and an anticholinergic; hydration with caution to prevent pulmonary edema; O_2 with caution to prevent CO_2 narcosis.
- Allergy-induced asthma: Omalizumab to ↓ immune system reaction; antihistamines, decongestants, corticosteroids, nasal sprays, immunotherapy (allergy shots).

Nursing Care

- Support child and parent in coping with chronic illness and fear due to SOB.
- Prevent exacerbations: Avoid triggers such as dairy products and animals; allergy-proof home such as eliminate carpets, drapes, down bedding; wet-mop floors; assess status via peak expiratory flowmeter (PEFM).
- Care during exacerbation: Provide calm presence; assess cardiopulmonary status; place in high-Fowler position; encourage pursed-lip breathing; give prescribed meds.
- Teach how to use a PEFM:
  - Measures respiratory volume of one forced expiration; begin with indicator at bottom of scale, stand straight, take a deep breath, place mouthpiece in mouth, blow out as hard and fast as possible; note result on scale.
  - Repeat 3 times and record highest value.
    Green: Under control.
    Yellow: Exacerbation; may indicate need to ↑ maintenance dose of meds.
    Red: Severe airway narrowing; give rescue med.

Cystic Fibrosis (CF)

- Causes ↑ viscosity of mucus from exocrine glands and abnormal glandular secretion of ions. It is an autosomal recessive disease.

Effects on Organ Systems

Respiratory System

- Mucus obstructs respiratory passages → ↓ expectoration and ↓ gas exchange.
- Mucus stagnation causes hypercapnia; hypoxia; acidosis; infection.
- ↑ lung dysfunction → atelectasis, emphysema, cor pulmonale, respiratory failure, and death.

Pancreas

- ↓ secretion of chloride and bicarbonate.
- Mucus blocks enzymes from reaching duodenum, causing ↓ digestion of fats, proteins, and CHO; fibrosis may result in DM.

Liver

- Local biliary obstruction; fibrosis causes biliary cirrhosis.

Reproductive System

- Delayed puberty; females may be infertile; males usually sterile due to mucus blocking sperm.

Integumentary System

- ↑ secretion of sodium and chloride in saliva and sweat; hyperthermic conditions cause hyponatremic alkalosis, hypochloremia, and dehydration.

Signs and Symptoms

- Variable; may be asymptomatic for mo or yr.
- Suspected with meconium ileus, failure to regain weight loss at birth, and failure to thrive.
- Frequent RTIs, nonproductive cough, wheezing.
- Chest x-ray shows atelectasis and emphysema; pulmonary function tests reveal small airway dysfunction.
- Foul-smelling, pale, bulky, watery stools **(steatorrhea)**; stools contain ↑ fat and pancreatic enzymes.
- Positive sweat chloride test: Chlorine concentration >60 mEq/L.
- Chronic S&S: ↓ salivation, paroxysmal cough, dyspnea, cyanosis, barrel chest, distended abdomen, thin extremities, clubbing of fingers and toes, rectal prolapse, F&E imbalances, bruising due to ↓ vitamin K.

Treatment

- Oral fluids and mucolytic enzymes to ↓ mucus viscosity; chest PT.
- Bronchodilators, anti-inflammatories, antibiotics, steroids, mucolytics.

- ↑ protein and ↑ calorie diet; salt supplements prn; pancreatic enzymes with meals and snacks to ↓ steatorrhea and ↑ growth; vitamins A, D, E, and K.
- Daily aerobic exercise.
- O_2 therapy, feeding tube, bowel surgery, lung transplant.

Nursing Care

Child

- **Respiratory Functioning**
  - Assess lung sounds; S&S of respiratory distress.
  - Balance rest and activity; ↑ fluids to ↓ mucus viscosity.
  - Teach how to ↑ expectoration such as huffing on expectoration and use of flutter mucus clearance device.
- **GI Functioning**
  - Assess weight, abdominal distention, and stools for characteristics and frequency.
  - Assess for S&S of intestinal obstruction.
  - Teach to ↑ protein and ↑ calories; give pancreatic enzymes with food.
  - Ensure adequate salt intake, particularly in hot weather.
  - Use perianal skin barrier to protect skin from GI enzymes.
- **Psychosocial Support**
  - Provide age-appropriate support to ↑ coping with chronic illness, respiratory equipment, invasive procedures, and infertility.
  - Promote a positive self-image.

Parents

- Assist parents with shock and guilt (each contributed a gene), chronicity of illness, and potential for death.
- Teach chest PT such as postural drainage, percussion, and vibration; perform daily in a.m. and p.m. and between meals to prevent vomiting.
- Teach about ThAIRapy vest to provide chest wall oscillation.
- Teach diaphragmatic breathing and coughing.
- Encourage child's independence; limit overindulgence to ↓ secondary gains.
- Ensure routine immunizations; flu vaccine at 6 mo and then yearly, teach about meds.
- Refer for genetic counseling and to Cystic Fibrosis Foundation.

Blood Disorders

Hemophilia

- X-linked recessive genetic disorder; possible gene mutation.
- Males usually are affected and females are carriers.
- **Hemophilia A (classic hemophilia):** Associated with deficiency of factor VIII.

- **Hemophilia B (Christmas disease)**: Associated with deficiency of factor IX.
- Lack of a blood-clotting factor affects coagulation cascade, prolonging clot formation and bleeding.
- Prenatal testing identifies affected fetus.
- Tests distinguish specific factor deficiencies: PT; PTT; thromboplastin generation test (TGT); whole blood clotting time; prothrombin consumption test; fibrinogen level.

Signs and Symptoms

- Bleeding
  - Into joints **(hemarthrosis)**: Joint stiffness, tingling, ache; followed by warmth, redness, swelling, pain, loss of movement, joint deformities, and impaired growth.
  - Into brain: Headache, slurred speech, ↓ LOC.
  - Into subcutaneous and intramuscular tissue: Ecchymosis, red spots **(petechiae)**.
  - Into GI tract: Black tarry stools, abdominal pain.
  - From nose **(epistaxis)**.

Treatment

- Replacement of missing clotting factor.
- Analgesics to ↓ pain; **RICE** protocol: **R**est, **I**ce, **C**ompression, **E**levation.
- Corticosteroids and nonsteroidal anti-inflammatories for hemarthrosis and inflammation of synovial membranes **(synovitis)**.
- PT; weight control to ↓ stress on joints.

Nursing Care

Child

- Identify bleeding event; provide factor replacement as prescribed.
- Rest joints; ROM after acute episode subsides.
- Prevent bleeding: Teach to use soft toothbrush, water pick, and electric razor; avoid contact sports.
- Encourage to wear medical alert identification.
- Teach to disclose condition before invasive procedures.
- Support child and adolescent in learning self-care.
- Explore coping with chronic disease, vocational, financial, and childbearing issues.

Parents

- Encourage expression of feelings about child with chronic illness, particularly the mother because it is X-linked; refer for genetic counseling.
- Safety-proof house and toys; supervise activity.
- Teach to use acetaminophen for pain and avoid ibuprofen and aspirin which exacerbate bleeding.
- Discuss need for multidisciplinary follow-up.

Anemia

Iron Deficiency	Sickle Cell (SCA)	β-Thalassemia
• Inadequate amount of iron to make hemoglobin (Hb), a component of RBCs, which causes anemia. • Caused by ↓ dietary iron; infant has iron reserve for only 5–6 mo. • Children receiving only milk have no source of dietary iron **(milk babies)**.	• Autosomal recessive disorder: Homozygous client will develop sickle cell anemia; heterozygous client will be a carrier. • More common in African Americans. • HbS forms long, slender crystals causing sickle-shaped RBCs, ↓ RBCs, Hb $<$9 g/dL; precipitated by dehydration; acidosis; ↑ T; hypoxia. • Cloudy mixture with sickle-turbidity test (Sickledex) for newborn screening. • Hb electrophoresis to determine if client is heterozygous or homozygous. • Complications: Problems with bones and joints, CNS, spleen, eyes, liver, reproductive system, kidneys, and lungs (chest syndrome: Pulmonary infiltrate → chest pain, ↑ T, ↑ R, cough, wheezing, hypoxia).	• Autosomal recessive disorder more common in people of Mediterranean descent. • ↓ synthesis of β-chain polypeptides → ↓ globin molecules. • Inability to maintain erythropoiesis commensurate with hemolysis; RBC changes, ↓ Hct, ↓ Hb, ↑ HbF, ↑ $HbgA_2$. • **Thalassemia major (Cooley anemia)** homozygous form that results in death without transfusions.

Continued

Iron Deficiency	Sickle Cell (SCA)	β-Thalassemia
S&S	**S&S**	**S&S**
• Slow onset. • ↑ P, pallor, ↓ motor development, weakness, dizziness. • ↓ RBC, ↓ Hb, ↓ Hct, ↑ total iron-binding capacity, ↓ serum-iron concentration.	• Longer than 6 mo; failure to thrive; ↑ risk of infection. **Vaso-occlusive Crisis** • Pain episode: Sickled cells obstruct blood vessels, causing occlusion, ischemia, and necrosis; pain and swelling of hands and feet; abdominal pain; arthralgia; ↑ T; prolonged penile erection **(priapism)**. **Sequestration Crisis** • Pooling of blood → splenomegaly; hepatomegaly; ↓ BP; lethargy; hypovolemia; shock. **Aplastic Crisis** • Profound anemia due to ↓ RBC production and ↑ RBC destruction; lethargy; SOB; altered mental status; and S&S of HF. **Hyperhemolytic Crisis** • ↑ RBC destruction → jaundice, reticulocytosis; suggests coexisting disorders.	• Fatigue, anorexia, ↑ T. • Bronze, freckled skin. • Splenomegaly, hepatomegaly. • Thickened cranial bones, malocclusion of jaw, chipmunklike facies, ↓ bone growth, bone pain. • Delayed sexual maturation.

Iron Deficiency	Sickle Cell (SCA)	β-Thalassemia
Treatment	**Treatment**	**Treatment**
• Breast milk or 1 L/day of iron-fortified formula for 1st 12 mo. • Ferrous sulfate supplement may cause gastric irritation and greenish/black stools.	**Treatment to Prevent Sickling** • O_2, ↑ fluids, maintenance of electrolyte and acid–base balance, hydroxyurea, erythropoietin. **Treatment During Crisis** • BR to ↓ O_2 demands, rest joints, analgesics, ↑ fluids, correct electrolytes, treat acidosis. • Blood transfusions or exchange transfusions to replace sickle cells; antibiotics; O_2 if SOB; O_2 will not reverse sickling. • Chelation therapy to ↓ iron overload.	• Blood transfusions (may be every 3 wk); vitamin C ↑ iron excretion; chelation therapy. • Splenectomy if splenomegaly interferes with breathing or if RBC destruction is extreme. • Bone marrow transplant.
Specific Nursing Care	**Specific Nursing Care**	**Specific Nursing Care**
• Assess for S&S; give iron-fortified milk and cereals or breast milk. • Give iron via a straw to ↓ staining teeth and with orange juice between meals to ↑ absorption. • Balance activity and rest.	• Assess for S&S; implement interventions to prevent dehydration, acidosis, and ↑ temp, which cause hypoxia precipitating sickling. **During Crises** • Give prescribed meds such as analgesics, antipyretics, and electrolytes; give prescribed IVF and blood transfusions; maintain BR with ↑ HOB; support joints on pillows and when moving.	• Support coping with transfusions and chelation therapy. • Arrange therapy around lifestyle. • Support adolescents with potential infertility. • Teach that screening fetus for β-thalassemia is available.

General Nursing Care for Child With SCA or β-Thalassemia

- Support parents and child coping with a genetic, chronic illness and potential for death during crises.
- Refer for genetic counseling and continued medical care.
- Prevent infection: Give prescribed flu and pneumococcal vaccines; avoid sources of infection.
- Balance activity and rest.
- Teach to avoid contact sports to prevent splenic rupture.
- Support child and adolescent coping with multiple transfusions, delayed sexual maturation, and body-image issues.
- Teach child about disorder and refer to supportive organizations such as Cooley's Anemia Foundation.

Cancer

Leukemia

- Unrestricted proliferation of immature white blood cells (WBCs) in blood-forming tissues.
- Leukocyte count is low and immature cells **(blasts)** are high.
- Blast cells compete for and deprive normal cells of nutrients essential for metabolism, causing anemia from ↓ RBCs, infection from ↓ neutrophils, bleeding from ↓ platelets.
- Leukemic cells may infiltrate other organs such as spleen, liver, lymph nodes, and CNS.

Classification

- Acute lymphoid leukemia (ALL) and acute myelogenous leukemia (AML).
- Each have subtypes that have therapeutic and prognostic implications.

Signs and Symptoms

- Pallor, fatigue, irritability, ↑ T, anorexia, ↓ weight, fever, chills, night sweats.
- Bleeding tendencies: Bruising, bleeding from mucous membranes, petechiae, hemorrhage.
- Bone and joint pain; enlarged liver, spleen, lymph nodes; CNS involvement.
- Usually occurs 2–6-yr-old child; onset is insidious to acute; positive bone marrow test.

Treatment

- Based on staging.
- IV and intrathecal chemotherapy given via 4-phase protocol to achieve remission, ↓ tumor burden, ↓ CNS involvement, and preserve remission.

- Biological and targeted therapy; targeted radiation therapy.
- Bone marrow transplant.

Nursing Care

- Interventions depend on side effects of med regimen, extent of myelosuppression, degree of leukemic infiltration.
- Handle gently to ↓ pain, bleeding, fractures.
- Emotional support for child and parents coping with diagnosis of cancer; invasive tests; chronic course; potential for relapse, death.
- Assess VS especially T and BP; balance rest and quiet play.
- Teach infection prevention such as hand hygiene, avoid crowds and people with an infection.
- Support child coping with side effects of antineoplastic therapies (see Nursing Care for Clients With Cancer or Experiencing Nontherapeutic Effects of Antineoplastic Therapies in Med Surg Tab, p. 172).
- Give prescribed chemotherapeutic and analgesic meds.

Wilms Tumor (Nephroblastoma)

- Malignant tumor of kidney; possibly genetic; usually occurs < age 5 yr.
- Associated with congenital disorders such as genitourinary problems.
- Tumor compresses body tissues, causing secondary metabolic problems.
- May be encapsulated; metastasizes to lung, liver, bone, and brain.

Classification

- Stages I to V, depending on confinement to kidney, extent of metastasis, if tumor is bilateral.

Signs and Symptoms

- Presents as nontender, firm mass deep within unilateral flank.
- Fatigue; ↓ weight; abdominal pain; ↑ T; hematuria; ↑ BP.
- Clinical indicators of lung metastasis: Dyspnea, cough, SOB, chest pain.

Treatment

- Radiation and/or chemotherapy before and/or after surgery.
- Excision of adrenal gland, affected regional lymph nodes, adjacent organs.
- 1 kidney excised if unilateral; 1 kidney excised and partial nephrectomy of less affected kidney if bilateral.

Nursing Care

- Depends on side effects of med regimen and extent of myelosuppression.
- Ensure that all primary health-care providers know not to palpate abdomen to prevent dissemination of cancer cells or rupture of tumor capsule.
- Assess VS, particularly T and BP.
- Teach infection prevention such as hand hygiene, and avoid crowds and people with an infection; provide balance between rest and quiet play.

- Give prescribed chemotherapeutic, analgesic meds.
- Teach turning, coughing, deep breathing to prevent respiratory problems because operative site is close to diaphragm.
- Provide emotional support for child and parents coping with diagnosis of cancer, invasive tests, chronic course, potential for relapse and death.
- Support child who is coping with side effects of antineoplastic therapies (see Nursing Care for Clients With Cancer or Experiencing Nontherapeutic Effects of Antineoplastic Therapies in Med Surg Tab, p. 172).

Neurological Problems

Neural Tube Defects

Maternal Risk Factors

- Folate deficiency; some antiseizure meds; uncontrolled DM; obesity; family history.
- ↑ T, fever, or saunas/hot tub in early weeks of pregnancy.

Spina Bifida Occulta

- Defect of vertebrae with intact spinal cord and meninges.

Signs and Symptoms

- May not be visible or may have superficial signs in lumbosacral area such as tufts of hair, angiomatous nevi, dimple, subcutaneous lipomas.
- Progressive disturbance of gait; ↓ bowel and bladder control.

Spina Bifida Cystica

- Saclike protrusion on back.
- **Meningocele:** Exposed sac contains meninges and spinal fluid.
- **Myelomeningocele (meningomyelocele):** Sac contains spinal cord, nerve roots, spinal fluid, meninges. Myelomeningocele is associated with other malformations such as intestinal, cardiac, renal, urinary, and orthopedic.

Signs and Symptoms

- Vary, depending on anatomical level and extent of defect; sensory disturbances parallel motor impairments.
- Joint deformities due to denervation to ↓ extremities and flexion and extension contractures; talipes valgus or varus contractures; kyphosis; lumbosacral scoliosis; hip dislocation.
- **Defect below 2nd lumbar vertebra:** Flaccid, partial paralysis of legs; varying degrees of ↓ sensation; continuous dribbling of urine and overflow incontinence; no bowel control and possible rectal prolapse.
- **Defect below 3rd sacral vertebra:** No motor impairment; ↓ bowel and bladder control.

Treatment

- Cesarean birth; surgery within 24–72 hr to ↓ stretching of nerve roots and ↓ risk for trauma to sac, hydrocephalus, infection.
- Eventually artificial sphincters and reservoirs may be created surgically.
- *Prevention:* 400 mcg of folic acid daily for all women of childbearing age.

Nursing Care

Infant Preoperative

- Keep naked in radiant warmer to prevent trauma to sac.
- Keep prone even when feeding.

Infant Postoperative

- Place in prone or partial side-lying position.
- Use sterile, moist, nonadherent dressing to site to ↓ drying; change every 2–4 hr.
- Assess for S&S of infection (fever, irritability, lethargy, nuchal rigidity).
- Assess for leaks, tears, abrasions, hydrocephalus, ↑ ICP.
- Keep area free of urine and feces.
- Use Credé maneuver to empty bladder or prescribed straight catheterization.
- Keep hips in slight abduction; perform prescribed PROM to knees, ankles, and feet; for older child, use prescribed braces, walking devices, and wheelchair.

Child

- Teach clean intermittent catheterization; provide emotional support because incontinence is stressful for child's social development.

Parents

- Support coping with decision to abort; lifelong care of infant with multiple neurological, genitourinary, and musculoskeletal problems.
- Involve in care; refer to Spina Bifida Association of America.

Hydrocephalus

- Abnormal ↑ cerebrospinal fluid (CSF) in ventricular system.

Communicating Hydrocephalus

- ↓ absorption of CSF within subarachnoid space.
- Often due to infection, trauma, thick arachnoid membrane or meninges.

Noncommunicating Hydrocephalus

- Obstruction of flow of CSF through ventricular system.
- Usually due to neoplasm, hematoma, or congenital herniation of medulla through foramen magnum.

Signs and Symptoms

- ↑ head size in infant is due to open sutures and bulging fontanels.
- Sclera visible above iris **(sunset eyes)**; retinal papilledema.
- Prominent scalp veins and shiny, taut skin; head lag after 4–6 mo.
- May exhibit attention deficit, hyperactivity, intellectual disability.
- **Clinical indicators of ↑ intracranial pressure**
  - Infant: Projectile vomiting unassociated with feeding; altered feeding behaviors; irritability; high shrill cry; seizures.
  - Older child: Headache usually in a.m., confusion, apathy, ↓ LOC.

Treatment

- Surgical removal of obstruction.
- ↓ excessive CSF by shunting fluid out of the ventricles and to the peritoneum (ventricular peritoneal shunt); shunt revision as the child grows.

Nursing Care

Preoperative

- Maintain Fowler position to permit gravity drainage of CSF.

Pre- and Postoperative

- Assess VS; take serial measures of head circumference (mark site with pen).
- Assess fontanels for bulging daily.
- Assess for clinical indicators of ↑ ICP.
- Support head and neck when holding or moving infant; protect from skin breakdown.
- Keep eyes moist and free from irritation.
- Provide small frequent feedings and schedule care around feedings to ↓ vomiting.

Postoperative

- Place on unoperative side to ↓ pressure on shunt; keep flat to prevent rapid decrease in intracranial fluid that may → subdural hematoma.
- Assess for S&S of infection such as shunt malfunction, fever, wound or shunt tract inflammation, difficulty feeding, vomiting, abdominal pain; most common complication 1–2 mo after surgery.

Anencephaly and Microcephaly

Anencephaly

- Severe defect when neural tube does not close during 3rd–4th wk of pregnancy; absent or reduced cerebrum, cerebellum, skull.
- Small, malformed head and face with thick neck.
- Frequently stillborn; may live several hr to a few days; death usually due to respiratory failure.

Microcephaly

- Neural tube defect where head is significantly smaller than expected.
- Receding forehead; abnormal brain growth.
- Prognosis depends on anomalies.

Risk Factors

- Gene or chromosome mutation; family history.
- Some antiseizure meds, uncontrolled DM, obesity, ↑ T (fever or saunas/hot tub), folic acid deficiency, exposure to Zika virus in utero.

Nursing Care

- Provide infant with palliative care.
- Support parents as they consider decision to abort if condition is identified in utero; in coping with realization that their infant has a fatal/chronic condition; and when considering organ donation.

Cerebral Palsy (CP)

- Impaired movement, posture, muscle tone, coordination.
- May have intellectual, perceptual, language, emotional deficits.
- Multifactorial causes: Cerebral anoxia most significant (traumatic birth), teratogens, brain malformations, intrauterine infections, prematurity, childhood meningitis, toxin exposure.
- Usually diagnosed at end of 1st yr; nonprogressive; most children have average intelligence.

Signs and Symptoms

- Inadequate head control and failure to smile by 3 mo; unable to sit by 8 mo.
- Stiff arms and legs; crossed legs **(scissoring)**; floppiness; arched back positioning.
- Irritability and crying, persistent primitive reflexes (asymmetrical tonic neck, Moro), tongue thrusting and choking after 6 mo, walking on toes, ADHD; seizures.
- **Spastic:** Hypertonicity; ↓ balance, posture, coordination; ↓ fine and gross motor skills.
- **Ataxic:** Wide-based gait; deficient performance of rapid repetitive movements or use of upper extremities.
- **Dyskinetic-athetoid:** Abnormal involuntary movements **(dyskinesia)**; slow, writhing movements **(athetosis)**.
- Drooling and imperfect articulation **(dysarthria)**.
- Mixed type/dystonic: Spasticity and athetosis.

Treatment

- PT (braces, splints), OT (adaptive equipment), speech therapy.
- Surgery: Tendon lengthening, selective dorsal rhizotomy.
- Meds: Skeletal muscle relaxants, antiseizure, botulinum toxin type A.

- Education: Early intervention; individualized education program (IEP).
- ↑ calories for energy expenditure; ↑ protein for muscle activity; ↑ vitamin B_6 for amino acid metabolism.

Nursing Care

- Teach careful eating to ↓ risk of aspiration; safe environment; helmet use.
- Avoid overstimulation; engage in play appropriate for developmental level and ability; be patient with attempts at speech.
- Assist with bowel and bladder training.
- Perform ROM to stretch heel cords and prevent contractures.
- Teach health maintenance and encourage rehab (PT, OT, speech therapy).
- Teach use and care of orthotics, walking aids, adaptive devices.
- Teach side effects of meds.
- Assist parents and child coping with lifelong disability.

Chromosome Disorders

Turner Syndrome

- Abnormal or missing X chromosome; occurs in females.
- **S&S**
  - *Infants:* Lymphedema of hands and feet; low posterior hairline.
  - *Children:* Webbed neck, short stature, shield-shaped chest.
  - *Adolescents/adults:* Undeveloped secondary sex characteristics, amenorrhea, generally infertile, immature, difficulty with social cues, socially isolated behavior, learning disabilities, usually normal intelligence.

Klinefelter Syndrome

- Extra X chromosome; occurs in males.
- **S&S**
  - *Infants/children:* No distinct clinical indicators.
  - *Adolescents/adults:* Tall, thin, with long legs and arms; deficient secondary sex characteristics; infertile; gynecomastia; variable mental impairment; learning disabilities; behavioral problems such as ↓ impulse control and hyperactivity.
- Treatment: Testosterone replacement, breast tissue removal, speech and physical therapy.

Trisomy 21 (Down Syndrome)

- Extra chromosome 21; occurs in males and females.
- **S&S**
  - *Infants/children:* Small head with flat occiput; small nose with flat bridge **(saddle nose)**; inner epicanthic folds; small, low-set ears; short, thick neck; protruding tongue; broad, short hands and feet; transverse palmar crease; hypotonic musculature; hyperflexible; variable mental impairment; congenital anomalies, especially heart; ↓ immune response; difficulty managing oral secretions; ↑ sociability.
  - *Adolescents/adults:* Delayed and/or incomplete sexual development; males usually infertile; females may be fertile; sensory problems such as cataracts and ↓ hearing; short stature; overweight.
- Treatment: Early intervention to maximize potential; pediatric specialists as needed (cardiologist, gastroenterologist, endocrinologist, neurologist, ophthalmologist, audiologist, PT, ST, OT).

Nursing Care for Clients With Chromosome Disorders

Child

- Interact based on developmental level, not chronological age; provide emotional support, encourage independence.
- *When indicated:* Prepare for lack of pubertal changes; teach about prescribed hormone replacement.
- Down syndrome: Maintain airway; protect from infection.

Parents

- Provide emotional support; encourage genetic counseling.
- Help set realistic goals for child; support decision regarding placement; help adolescent/adult manage emerging sexuality and fertility in females with Down syndrome.

Skeletal Malformations

Clubfoot (Talipes Equinovarus) and Developmental Dysplasia of Hip (DDH)

Clubfoot (Talipes Equinovarus)

- Foot in plantar flexion (downward) and deviated medially (inward); rigid or flexible.
- Familial tendency, intrauterine crowding, arrested development.

Signs and Symptoms

- Affected foot/feet smaller, shorter with empty heel pad and transverse plantar crease.
- Unilateral affected extremity may be shorter with calf atrophy; ↑ risk of hip dysplasia.

Treatment

- Serial casts or surgical correction.

Developmental Dysplasia of Hip

- Abnormal development of one or more hip with shallow acetabulum, subluxation, and/or dislocation.
- Physiological, mechanical, genetic causes.

Signs and Symptoms

- **Ortolani sign**: ↓ abduction of affected leg; audible click when abducting and externally rotating affected hip.
- **Galeazzi sign**: Asymmetry of gluteal, popliteal, and thigh folds; apparent shortening of femur.
- **Trendelenburg sign**: Pelvis tilts downward on unaffected side when standing on affected extremity.
- Waddling gait and lordosis when walking.

Treatment

- Brace, serial casts, surgical correction.

Nursing Care for Infant With Clubfoot or DDH

- Ensure casts are reapplied as child grows.
  - Clubfoot: Daily for 2 wk, then every 1–2 wk for total of 8–12 wk.
  - DDH: Hip spica cast changed when needed every 3–6 mo.
- Ensure that splint such as Pavlik harness is applied correctly; splint permits some mobility but prevents hip extension and adduction; straps should be checked every 1–2 wk; worn continuously for 3–5 mo.
- Perform neurovascular check: Blanching, warm toes, mobility of toes, pedal pulse.
- **Cast care**: Place diaper below edge of cast; apply transparent film dressing to form bridge between cast and skin; apply clothing over cast to prevent stuffing of objects down cast; assess for odor that indicates infection.
- **Splint care**: Sponge-bathe; keep straps dry; place diaper below straps; dress in knee socks and undershirt to prevent skin irritation from straps; inspect skin under straps 3 times daily and massage area under straps; feed with head elevated; use football hold when breastfeeding; hold and cuddle infant; provide appropriate toys; involve child in age-appropriate activities.

Scoliosis

- Complex spinal deformity in three planes: Lateral curvature, spinal rotation causes rib asymmetry, and thoracic hypokyphosis.
- Multifactorial causes: No apparent cause **(idiopathic scoliosis)**; genetic autosomal dominant trait; spinal trauma; concurrent neuromuscular conditions such as rheumatoid arthritis, dwarfism.
- X-ray confirms deformity.

Signs and Symptoms

- Most seen during preadolescent growth spurt by primary health-care provider or school-based screening.
- Scapular and hip heights are asymmetrical when child is viewed from behind; asymmetry and prominence of rib cage when bending forward.
- One breast may be larger; clothes do not fit well, such as uneven pants legs or crooked skirt hem.

Treatment

- Depends on extent, location, and type of curve.
- Orthotics such as Milwaukee brace or under arm/low-profile brace.
- Spinal fusion for curves greater than 40°.
- Exercises to prevent atrophy of spinal and abdominal muscles.

Nursing Care

- Teach purpose, function, application, and care of appliance.
- Check skin for irritation; skin care; pad skin under brace.
- Assist with clothing to disguise brace; encourage wearing brace for 16–23 hr daily for several yr.
- Support expression of feelings; role-play how to deal with reaction of others to brace.

Postoperative

- Assess VS, wound, neurovascular status of extremities.
- Maintain prescribed PCA pump or give analgesics routinely, because pain is intense 1st 48–72 hr.
- Maintain NGT and urinary catheter and assess bowel sounds and urinary output when removed due to risk for paralytic ileus and urinary retention.
- If anterior approach used, institute care related to thoracotomy.
- Encourage isometric exercises progressing to ambulation and ROM.

Juvenile Idiopathic Arthritis

- Infectious agent activates autoimmune inflammation; familial with female predominance between 1–3 and 8–10 yr of age.

- Results in chronic inflammation of synovium with joint effusion ultimately leading to erosion, destruction, fibrosis of articular cartilage, development of adhesions between joint surfaces, ankylosis of joints.
- Demonstrates remissions and exacerbations.

Signs and Symptoms

- Variable; one or more joints involved, joint swelling due to edema, joint effusion, synovial thickening, weakness and fatigue.
- Stiffness in a.m. and after inactivity and loss of motion due to muscle spasms and joint inflammation; spindle fingers with thick proximal joint and slender tip.
- Joints may be pain-free, tender, or painful.
- Laboratory results such as ↑ erythrocyte sedimentation rate; ↑ C-reactive protein; leukocytosis; presence of antinuclear antibodies; positive rheumatoid factor.
- Systemic arthritis: ↑ T; rash; intraocular inflammation **(uveitis)**; pericarditis; enlarged liver, spleen, lymph nodes.

Treatment

- Suppress inflammation and pain with NSAIDs; disease-modifying antirheumatic meds such as methotrexate and leflunomide; biologic agents such as etanercept and adalimumab.
- Corticosteroids used until other meds are effective or when other meds are ineffective.
- PT and OT to ↑ muscle strength; mobilize joints; prevent and correct deformities; splinting of knees, wrists, hands to ↓ pain and flexion deformities; surgery to improve joint position.

Nursing Care

Child

- Teach to take meds as prescribed even during remissions.
- Maintain functional alignment: Positioning, splints, firm mattress, periodic prone position, small pillow under head.
- Apply prescribed heat: 10-min warm tub bath in a.m.; warm packs to joints for 20 min.
- Encourage independence in ADLs; exercise program; incorporate play in the program such as throwing ball, swimming, or riding bike.
- Balance activity/rest.
- *During exacerbations:* Give meds to ↓ pain; rest joints; maintain functional alignment; encourage isometric not isotonic exercises; maintain contact with school and peers; support developing initiative and industry.

Parents

- Support coping with exacerbations, constant discomfort, risk of overindulgence, and seeking alternative therapies.

Infections and Infestations

Disorder and Etiology	Signs and Symptoms	Treatment	Specific Nursing Care
SCABIES			
• Scabies mite burrows into and multiplies in epidermis. • Transmitted by direct contact with infected person, rarely by fomites.	• Inflammatory response, intense itching. • Papules, vesicles, pustules usually involving hands, wrists, axillae, genitalia, and inner thighs, feet, ankles. • Mite appears as black dot at end of linear, grayish brown threadlike burrow.	• Permethrin 5% cream. • Antibiotics for secondary infection.	• Contact precautions. • Contacts treated because time between infestation and S&S is 1–2 mo. • Massage cream thoroughly into skin from head to under feet; keep on 8–14 hr; then shampoo and bathe. • Teach pruritus may take 2–3 wk to subside; contaminated linen and clothing must be washed and dried at high heat.
PEDICULOSIS (Lice)			
• Louse infests head, body, or pubic hair. • Spread by personal articles such as combs, hats, bedding.	• White eggs (nits) attach to base of hair shafts behind ears and at nape of neck. • Intense pruritus due to crawling insect and insect saliva.	• Pediculicide permethrin 1% cream rinse (Nix). • Nit removed with fine-tooth comb.	• Contact precautions. • Protect eyes and wear gloves during med application. • Remove visible nits with nit comb.

Continued

Disorder and Etiology	Signs and Symptoms	Treatment	Specific Nursing Care
PEDICULOSIS (Lice) (con't)			
	• Papules due to secondary infections.		• Teach contaminated linen and clothing must be washed and dried at high heat; vacuum rugs, floors, furniture; soak brushes, combs, hats, scarves in pediculicide for 1 hr.
IMPETIGO			
• Skin infection due to *Staphylococcus* or *Streptococcus* organisms; from autoinoculation or infected person. • Superimposed on eczema.	• Reddish macule becomes vesicular and ruptures, leaving superficial, moist erosion. • Lesions dry as honey-colored crusts; pruritus.	• Removal of undermined skin, crusts, and debris. • Topical application of bactericidal ointment. • Systemic antibiotic.	• Teach parents hand hygiene, contact isolation, preventing scratching, gently rubbing lesions to remove crusts before topical antibiotic.
RINGWORM			
• Fungal infection of skin. • ***Tinea capitis*** Scalp, hairline, neck. • ***Tinea cruris*** **(jock itch)** Inner thigh, crural fold, scrotum in men.	• Pruritus, characteristic lesions. • ***Tinea capitis*** Patchy, scaly areas of alopecia. • ***Tinea cruris*** Round, erythematous, scaling patch.	• Oral antifungal. • Local application of antifungal. • ***Tinea capitis*** Selenium shampoos.	• Teach personal hygiene. • Avoid pets, particularly cats. • Avoid sharing personal items such as combs and hats.

Disorder and Etiology	Signs and Symptoms	Treatment	Specific Nursing Care
RINGWORM (con't)			
• ***T. capitis*** and ***T. cruris*** Transmitted person-to-person, animal-to-person, via contaminated items. • ***Tinea pedis* (athlete's foot)** Between toes or plantar surface of feet; often transmitted in locker room.	• ***Tinea pedis*** Maceration, fissures, small vesicles.		• Wear plastic shoes in swimming areas and locker rooms. • Wear cotton socks and underwear, ventilated shoes, to ↓ heat and perspiration.

Viral Infections

Disorder and Etiology	Signs and Symptoms	Treatment	Specific Nursing Care
VERRUCA (WARTS)			
• Caused by human papillomavirus. • *V. plantaris*—plantar wart. • *V. vulgaris*—limited to epidermis (common wart).	• Gray or brown, elevated papules mostly on hands, face, soles of feet (plantar wart). • Unpredictable course; may disappear spontaneously.	• Removed by curettage, electrocautery, cryotherapy, caustic solutions. • Laser, duct tape occlusion, and garlic extract therapy.	• Teach to avoid skin-to-skin contact. • Encourage frequent hand hygiene. • Give prescribed meds.

Continued

Disorder and Etiology	Signs and Symptoms	Treatment	Specific Nursing Care
MOLLUSCUM CONTAGIOSUM			
• Pox virus. • Spread by skin-to-skin, fomite-to-skin, autoinoculation.	• May be asymptomatic; flesh-colored papules. • May spontaneously resolve.	• Caustic solutions: Salicylic acid, potassium hydroxide dissolve lesion over time. • Topical creams: Tretinoin, adapalene. • Surgical scraping, cryotherapy, laser therapy.	• Same as for VERRUCA (WARTS).
HERPES VIRUS **TYPE I–SIMPLEX OR TYPE II–GENITAL**			
• Transmitted via respiratory droplets, virus containing fluids such as saliva or cervical secretions (vaginal birth and sexual contact).	• Itching, burning vesicles near lips, nose, genitals, buttocks; forms crust, then exfoliates. • Spontaneous healing in 8–10 days; may be fatal in child with ↓ immunity.	***Herpes Virus—Type I and II*** • Topical or systemic antivirals; topical anesthetic. • Sunscreen to ↓ risk. ***Herpes Virus—Type II*** • Cesarean birth if mother has active genital lesions.	***Herpes Virus—Type I and II*** • Same as VERRUCA (WARTS). ***Herpes Virus—Type II*** • Encourage open communication with sexual partner(s) and to join a support group. • Teach to use a latex condom during every sexual contact; avoid intercourse during an outbreak.

Disorder and Etiology	Signs and Symptoms	Treatment	Specific Nursing Care
HERPES VIRUS TYPE I—SIMPLEX OR TYPE II—GENITAL (con't)			
			• *Pregnancy:* Instruct to tell primary health-care provider of diagnosis; antiviral late in pregnancy may prevent outbreak at term; cesarean advised during an outbreak.

Integumentary System Problems

Atopic Dermatitis (Eczema)

- Symmetrical cutaneous inflammation with erythema, papules, vesicles, pustules, scales, crusts, scabs; may be dry or have a weeping discharge; secondary infections common.
- Multifactorial causes: Genetics, stress, abnormal function of skin such as alterations in perspiration, peripheral vascular function, heat tolerance; environmental factors such as dry climate, exacerbations in fall and winter; IgE food sensitization; T-cell dysfunction resulting in allergy to dust, mold, animal hair, and chemicals.

Signs and Symptoms

- Characteristic lesions on cheeks, scalp, neck, flexor surface of arms and legs.
- Intense itching or burning, facial pallor, bluish discoloration beneath eyes **(allergic shiners)**. S&S of secondary infections. Diagnosis based on history and morphological findings.

Treatment

- Depends on cause; topical lotions to hydrate skin; colloid tub baths; phototherapy with ultraviolet light; avoid precipitating agent.
- Antihistamines; topical steroids; topical or systemic immunosuppressants; interferons; essential fatty acids; topical pimecrolimus; systemic antibiotics for skin infections.

Nursing Care

Child

- Hydrate skin: Short bath with mild soap such as Neutrogena or Dove and immediately lubricate moist skin (Eucerin, Aquaphor, Cetaphil).
- ↓ itching and scratching: Short nails filed to remove edges; cotton socks on hands and pinned to shirt; soft cotton fabrics; moderate environmental temperatures; teach S&S of secondary infection.
- Avoid irritants: Harsh soap, fabric softeners, bubble baths, excessive bathing, rough and woolen fabrics; double-rinse clothing after washing.
- Allergy-proof home: No rugs, drapes, down pillows, wool blankets; wet dust and vacuum when child is out of house.
- Hypoallergenic diet: Teach diet; introduce one food at a time.

Parents

- Cuddle child coping with itching; teach that condition is not communicable, scars generally will not occur if secondary infections are prevented.

Burns

For additional information, see Tab 6, Med Surg, Burns, p. 181.

Estimating Extent of Injury

- Total body surface area (TBSA) injured represented as a percentage of body surface.
- Modified rule of nines:
  - Head and neck are 18%.
  - Anterior trunk is 18%.
  - Posterior trunk is 18%.
  - Each arm is 9%.
  - Each leg is 14%.
  - For each yr of life after 2, 1% is deducted from head and 0.5% is added to each leg until adult percentages are reached.
- *Burn diagrams are more accurate for pediatrics:* Diagrams contain smaller body segments and less percentage for head and more for trunk and limbs as child ages.

Fluid Replacement Therapy

- Initiated for burns >15%–20% TBSA.
- Parkland formula often used.
- IVF to maintain urine output of 1–2 mL/kg for child weighing <30 kg and 30–50 mL/hr in older child.
- Urinary output, capillary refill, and sensorium are used to evaluate hydration status and fluid replacement needs.

Nursing Care

Child

- Medicate before painful procedures; explain treatments are not punishments.
- Provide age-appropriate support; allow choices whenever possible.
- Encourage expression of feelings; young children coping with separation anxiety and adolescents developing an identity are most affected.
- Assist coping with physical changes; compression bandages and splints; reactions of peers.
- Accept regression; use behavior modification to motivate.
- Teach age-appropriate fire safety information such as stop, drop, and roll if clothing is on fire; not playing with matches, outlets, or stoves.

Parents

- Support coping with critically ill child; guilt; helplessness; concerns for child's physical and emotional future.
- Explain multidisciplinary follow-up because scar tissue will require grafts, reconstructive surgery, PT & OT.

Poisoning

Chemical	Signs and Symptoms	Treatment	Nursing Care
HYDROCARBONS AND CORROSIVE CHEMICALS			
• **Hydrocarbons:** Kerosene, gasoline, turpentine, furniture polish, cleaning fluids. • **Corrosive chemicals:** Bleach, oven or drain cleaners, detergents, electric dishwasher granules.	• Coughing, gagging, N&V, lethargy, ↑ P, cyanosis, oral pain, dyspnea, altered LOC.	• Gastric lavage with endotracheal tube to prevent aspiration. • IVF, O_2, NPO. • Repeated dilations or surgery for esophageal stricture.	• Never induce vomiting. • Assess for clinical indicators of burns: Swollen lips, tongue, mucous membranes; painful oral cavity; hemoptysis; hematemesis. • Maintain patent airway, intubation may be necessary.

Continued

Chemical	Signs and Symptoms	Treatment	Nursing Care
LEAD (Plumbism)			
• Lead in paint, soil, dust, drinking water.	• Blood concentration >5 mcg/dL indicates unsafe level of lead. • Anemia, pallor, fatigue. • Lead line on teeth and long bones. • Joint pain, headache, lethargy, irritability, hyperactivity, insomnia, seizures.	• Chelation therapy when blood lead level nears 45 mcg/dL.	• Screen at 1–2 yr; routinely if high risk. • Eliminate source. • Ensure adequacy of urinary output before chelation therapy.
ACETAMINOPHEN			
• Most common med poisoning in children. • History of 150 mg/kg for several days.	• N&V, diaphoresis, $\downarrow$ urine output, pallor, weakness, bradycardia, liver failure, right upper quadrant pain, coagulation abnormalities, jaundice, confusion, and coma.	• Assess for S&S of liver failure. • Activated charcoal if ingestion ≤ 1 hr; if >1 hr, *N*-acetylcysteine in loading dose, then 17 maintenance doses. • Oral or IV fluids.	• Give prescribed antidote. • Teach med regimen. • Give prescribed oral and IV fluids.

Nursing Care for Children With Poisoning

Emergency Care

- Identify agent; stop exposure; do not induce vomiting—may redamage mucosa; prevent aspiration; flush eyes and skin with water if involved.
- Call American Association of Poison Control Centers for directions.
- Transport to hospital; bring evidence such as container and vomitus.

Acute Care

- Ensure airway; assess VS, hepatic and renal function; do not scold child or parent.

Prevention

- Teach child not to eat nonfood items **(pica)**; obey parent's safety rules.
- Teach to keep toxins/meds in locked cabinet; use childproof containers.

Legal and Ethical Issues Overview

- **Voluntary admission/commitment:** Client consents to admission; free to leave even against medical advice.
- **Emergency commitment:** Without client consent when a danger to self or others or is gravely disabled; assessed by two mental health professionals within 24 hr; probable cause hearing must take place within 4 to 5 days where convincing evidence must be produced to continue in- or outpatient treatment; rules vary by state.
- **Civil or judicial commitment:** Longer than emergency commitment to provide treatment (parens patriae: state power to protect or care for clients with disabilities or to protect public); rules vary by state; generally renewable in 90 days or 6 mo.
- **Right to least restrictive environment:** Restraints or seclusion cannot be used until less-restrictive interventions are tried 1st.
- **Confidentiality:** Health Insurance Portability and Accountability Act (HIPAA) of 1996 guarantees privacy and security of health information and enforcement standards; psychotherapy and substance use disorder treatment have additional privacy protection.
- **Competency:** Client capable of making decisions about treatment.
- **Informed consent:** Right to know risks and benefits to make decisions.
- **Reporting laws:** Nurses must report suspected child and elder abuse or neglect; warn a person and those able to protect a person about a threat made to kill the person even if it breaches confidentiality.

Nursing Care

- Know federal and state regulations and standards regarding legal issues because rules vary by state.
- Employ advocacy role.
- Inform and protect clients' rights, such as provide information for informed consent, accept right to refuse treatment or meds.
- Maintain confidentiality; consult with agency attorney before releasing information about client to others or secure signed release from client.
- Enact duty to warn clients' potential intended victims.
- Support least restrictive environment, including decreased use of chemical restraints; refer to The Joint Commission and federal and state standards.
- Know S&S of child, domestic partner, and elder abuse such as bruises, burns, injuries, inconsistent reporting, signs of sexual abuse; see Domestic Violence, p. 157.

Mental Health Assessment

- **Stressors:** Assess internal and external stressors.
- **Appearance:** Note grooming, hygiene, posture, eye contact, clothing. Is appearance congruent with developmental stage and age?
- **General attitude:** Is client cooperative or uncooperative; ingratiating, friendly, or distant; hostile, open or defensive, passive, resistive?
- **Activity and behavior:** Congruent with feelings? Note mannerisms, gestures, gait. Is client restless, agitated, or calm? Is activity hyperactive, aggressive, rigid, or relaxed? Are there tremors, tics?
- **Sensory and cognitive status:** Assess LOC; orientation to person, place, time; recall, recent and remote memory; confusion; ability to concentrate.
- **Thought processes:** Is thinking rapid, slow, or repetitious? How long is the client's attention span? Assess content: Is client delusional, suicidal, obsessive, paranoid, phobic, or expressing religiosity or magical thinking? How is the client's thinking disorganized? Assess for echolalia, tangentiality, confabulation, loose associations, concrete thinking, clang associations, referential thinking, circumstantiality, and neologisms.
- **Judgment and insight:** Assess decision-making, problem-solving, and coping ability. Can client manage activities of daily living? Does client understand the concepts of cause and effect?
- **Mood:** Is client emotionally labile, depressed, sad, happy, anxious, fearful, irritable, euphoric, guilty, despairing, apathetic, angry, ashamed, proud, relieved, content, confident, or bizarre?
- **Affect (ability to vary emotional expression):** Is client's affect congruent with mood or is it flat or inappropriate?
- **Speech:** Are volume and rate congruent with feelings and behavior? Is there pressured speech or aphasia?
- **Self-concept and self-esteem:** Does client make negative or positive statements about self? What is the extent of client's satisfaction with self and/or body image?
- **Perception:** Is client experiencing hallucinations, illusions, or depersonalization?
- **Impulse control:** Does client exhibit disinhibition, aggression, hyperactivity, hypersexuality, or inappropriate social behavior?
- **Potential for violence:** Are there signs of risk for violence such as depression, suicidal ideation, increased muscle tension, pacing, profanity, and verbal and/or physical threats?
- **Family and social systems:** What is client's attainment and maintenance of interpersonal relationships and extent of support system?
- **Spiritual status:** Note client's presence or absence of and comfort with beliefs, values, and religious affiliation.

Defense Mechanisms

Defense Mechanism	Example
Compensation: ↑ capabilities in one area to make up for deficiencies in another.	Nonathletic student joins debate team.
Denial: Ego unable to accept painful reality.	Client assumes false cheerfulness or fails to seek medical help when needed.
Displacement: Directing anger toward less-threatening substitute.	Client yells at a significant other after being diagnosed with cancer.
Intellectualization: Situation dealt with on cognitive, not emotional, level.	Client discusses all test results but avoids focusing on fears and feelings.
Projection: Attaching to others feelings that are unacceptable to self.	Preoperative client says to wife, "Don't be scared."
Rationalization: Attempt to logically justify or excuse unacceptable behaviors.	Parent of a latchkey 10-yr-old says, "He needs to learn to be self-sufficient."
Reaction formation: Opposite reaction to the way one feels.	A person does not like a neighbor but is overly friendly.
Regression: Retreat to an earlier, more comfortable developmental age.	Adolescent has a temper tantrum when told not to do something.
Repression: Unconscious blocking of unacceptable thoughts from the conscious mind.	A female adult has no recollection of her father's sexual abuse.
Suppression: Conscious blocking of thoughts from the mind.	Client states, "I'll worry about that after my test tomorrow."
Undoing: Action or words cancel previous action or words to decrease guilt.	A man gives a woman a gift after abusing her.
Freud's Theory of Psychosocial Development includes that the use of defense mechanisms protects ego integrity.	

Review of Mental Health Disorders

Neurocognitive Disorders

Level of Cognitive Dysfunction

- **Minor Neurocognitive Disorder**
  - Modest decline in ≥1 cognitive domain.
  - Deficits do not interfere with ability to be independent.
- **Major Neurocognitive Disorder (Dementia)**
  - Substantial decline in ≥1 cognitive domain.
  - Deficits interfere with ability to be independent in everyday activities.

Level of Severity

- *Mild:* Difficulty with instrumental ADL (housework, managing money).
- *Moderate:* Difficulty with basic ADL (dressing, bathing, eating).
- *Severe:* Fully dependent.

Neurocognitive Domains: Common Symptoms and Observations

Cognitive Domain	Minor Neurocognitive Disorder	Major Neurocognitive Disorder (Dementia)
Complex Attention	Tasks take longer; thinking is easier without external stimuli.	Easily distracted by external stimuli; unable to perform mental calculations or recall phone numbers just given.
Executive Function	Difficulty multitasking; fatigue from effort to organize, plan, and make decisions; unable to follow group conversations.	Abandons complex tasks; focuses on only one task at a time; must rely on others for decision making and planning ADL.
Learning and Memory	Repeats self occasionally; difficulty recalling recent events; relies on lists; needs reminders; loses track of bill paying.	Repeats self often even in same conversation; requires reminders to stay on task; cannot keep track of plans for ADL.
Language	Difficulty finding words; avoids names of acquaintances; uses incorrect particles of speech; substitutes general for specific terms.	Significant difficulties with expressive or receptive language; forgets names of family members; echolalia and automatic speech precede mutism.

Neurocognitive Domains: Common Symptoms and Observations—cont'd

Cognitive Domain	Minor Neurocognitive Disorder	Major Neurocognitive Disorder (Dementia)
Perceptual-Motor	Gets lost; less precise in parking; ↑ effort required for motor tasks such as assembly, sewing, carpentry.	Significant difficulties with familiar activities or navigating in familiar environments; more confused at dusk **(sundowning)**.
Social Cognition	Difficulty recognizing social cues; ↓ empathy and inhibition; apathetic; ↑ extraversion or introversion; restlessness.	Behavior outside of acceptable norms; insensitive to standards of modesty or political, religious, or sexual conversations; acts without regard to others; makes decisions disregarding safety; lacks insight into behavior.

- A diagnosis of minor or major neurocognitive disorder must also specify etiology (Alzheimer disease, vascular disease, traumatic brain injury, substance use, Parkinson disease).
- Additional behaviors associated with neurocognitive disorders:
  - *Agnosia:* Fails to recognize words or objects.
  - *Aphasia:* Exhibits disturbances in language.
  - *Apraxia:* Displays decreased motor activity.
  - *Confabulation:* Fills in memory gaps with invented facts.
  - *Disinhibition:* Acting on thoughts or feelings without social control.
  - *Dysphagia:* Difficulty swallowing.
  - *Neologisms:* Invents words that have no common meaning.
  - *Perseveration:* Repeats same idea in response to different stimuli.
  - *Sundowning:* Confusion or irritation at the end of the day.
- Alzheimer disease:
  - Most common cause of dementia in older adults.
  - S&S progress and worsen over time; varies among people.
  - Brain contains abnormal clumps (amyloid plaques) and tangled bundles of fibers (neurofibrillary tangles); initially in hippocampus and then extends to other brain areas; brain tissue shrinks.
  - See Nursing Care for Clients With Decreased Cognition, p. 163.

Eating Disorders

Signs and Symptoms

	Behavioral	Physical	Psychological
Anorexia	• Self-starvation. • Rituals regarding food, eating. • Weight loss. • Behaviors to ↓ weight: Purging, exercise, use of laxatives, enemas, and diuretics.	• Weight loss 15% below ideal. • Cachexia (sunken eyes, protruding bones, dry skin). • Amenorrhea. • ↓ pulse and body T. • Lanugo on face. • Constipation. • Sensitivity to cold.	• Appears fat to self. • Intense, irrational fear of being fat. • Preoccupation with cooking, food, nutrition. • Delayed psychosexual development. • Perfectionist, high achiever.
Bulimia	• Repetitive bingeing and purging. • Behaviors to ↓ weight: Purging, exercise, use of laxatives, enemas, and diuretics. • Fasts to compensate for bingeing.	• Weight usually is normal; may be higher or lower. • F&E imbalances such as hypokalemia, metabolic alkalosis, dehydration. • Lack of control over eating during bingeing. • Menstrual irregularities. • Dental caries, loss of dental enamel. • Hypotension, cardiac dysrhythmias. • Constipation or diarrhea. • GERD, parotid enlargement.	• Excessive concern about weight, shape, proportions. • Depression, shame, self-contempt follow bingeing. • Mood swings, irritability. • Impulsive, extrovert.

See Nursing Care for Clients With Eating Disorders, p. 163.

Anxiety Disorders

Generalized Anxiety

- Excessive anxiety for 6 mo; hypervigilance; difficult to control worry.
- Three or more of the following S&S:
  - Restlessness
  - Irritability
  - Easily fatigued
  - Sleep disturbance
  - Increased muscle tension
  - Decreased concentration

Panic Disorder

- **Panic attack:** Abrupt onset of intense fear that peaks within minutes; recurrent unexpected attacks.
- Exhibit ≥4 of the S&S related to perception and physiological responses associated with panic in the chart Levels of Anxiety and Related S&S, p. 146.
- One of the attacks followed by ≥1 mo of ≥1 of the following:
  - Persistent concern about having more panic attacks.
  - Worry about implications of an attack or its consequences.
  - Significant change in behavior related to attacks.

Posttraumatic Stress Disorder (PTSD)

- Self or significant other experienced a traumatic event in which severe physical harm occurred or was threatened.
- S&S usually occur within 3 mo of the event and persist beyond 1 mo; may persist for life.
- S&S associated with PTSD
  - *Re-experiencing the terrifying event:* Spontaneous intrusive memories, recurrent dreams, flashbacks; intense, prolonged psychological stress.
  - *Heightened arousal:* Hypervigilant, aggressive, self-destructive behaviors; ↓ concentration; exaggerated startle response; sleep disturbances.
  - *Avoidance:* Efforts to avoid thoughts, feelings, or external reminders of the traumatic event.
  - *Negative thoughts, mood, or feelings:* Distorted sense of blame of self or others, estrangement from others, ↓ interest in activities, unable to recall important aspects of the event.

Levels of Anxiety and Related S&S

Factor	Mild	Moderate	Severe	Panic
Perception	Broad, alert.	Narrowed, focused.	Greatly narrowed, selective attention.	Feeling of unreality or depersonalization, fear of losing control, fear of dying.
Motor activity	Slight muscle tension.	↑ muscle tension, tremors.	Extreme muscle tension, ↑ motor activity.	Erratic behavior, combative or withdrawn.
Communication	Questioning.	Pitch changes, voice tremors.	Difficulty communicating.	May be incoherent.
Mood	Relaxed, calm.	Energized, nervous.	Irritable, extremely upset.	Panicky, angry, terrified.
Physiological responses	Normal VS.	Slight ↑ in pulse and respirations.	Fight or flight response: ↑ VS, dilated pupils, hyperventilation, headache, diaphoresis, nausea, diarrhea, urgency, frequency.	Palpitations, diaphoresis, trembling, SOB, feeling of choking, chest pain, nausea or abdominal distress, lightheadedness, chills or heat sensations, paresthesias.
Learning	Enhanced, uses learning to adapt.	Impaired, focuses on one issue, selective attention.	Greatly diminished, improbable, ↓ concentration, ↑ distractibility.	Impossible, unable to learn.

See Nursing Care for Clients Who Are Anxious, p. 162.

Dissociative Disorders

Disorder	Description
Dissociative identity	Coexistence of two or more distinct personalities within one person.
Depersonalization and Derealization	Persistent and recurrent feelings of detachment from one's body concerning thoughts, feelings, sensations, or actions **(depersonalization)**; feelings of unreality or detachment concerning surroundings **(derealization)**.
Dissociative amnesia	Inability to remember previous personal information, usually of a stressful or traumatic nature.

Bipolar and Depressive Disorders

Disorder	Signs and Symptoms
Bipolar I and II Disorder Triggers: Bereavement, financial ruin, natural disasters, serious illness or disability.	
Bipolar I Disorder	Experience at least 1 manic episode that may be preceded by or followed by hypomanic or major depressive episodes. **Manic episode:** Elevated, expansive and irritable mood with changes in energy and activity levels that last for at least 1 wk plus ≥3 of the following: Grandiosity, ↓ need for sleep, more talkative, flight of ideas, distractibility, psychomotor agitation, ↑ pleasurable activities with negative consequences; S&S cause severe impairment of functioning, possibly requiring hospitalization. **Hypomanic episode:** Same S&S as manic episode but ↓ severe; lasts 4 days; usually does not require hospitalization. **Major depressive episode:** Depressed mood or loss of interest or pleasure for at least 2 wk plus ≥5 of the following: Depressed mood, ↓ interest in activities, ↑↓ weight, ↑↓ appetite, ↓↑ sleep, psychomotor agitation or retardation, fatigue, feelings of worthlessness or inappropriate guilt. Causes social/occupational impairment, psychotic features, suicidal ideation, and potential for hospitalization.

Continued

Disorder	Signs and Symptoms
Bipolar II Disorder	Experience at least 1 hypomanic episode and 1 major depressive episode.
Cyclothymic Disorder	Mood cycling from moderate depression to hypomania lasting 2 yr; does not meet criteria for bipolar I or II.
Major Depressive Disorder	Depressed mood or ↓ pleasure **(anhedonia)** for ≥2 wk plus ≥4 of the following: ↑↓ weight, ↑↓ sleep, psychomotor agitation or retardation, fatigue, feelings of worthlessness or inappropriate guilt, ↓ concentration, recurrent thoughts of death or suicide. *Seasonal affective disorder:* Depression with a seasonal pattern, usually winter. *Postpartum depression:* Depression during pregnancy or within 4 wk after birth (perinatal onset); also associated with bipolar disorders. *Postpartum psychosis:* Depression with psychotic features during postpartum period; also associated with bipolar disorders.
Persistent Depressive Disorder (Dysthymia)	Depressed mood for most of the day for at least 2 yr plus ≥2 of the following: ↑↓ appetite, ↑↓ sleep, fatigue, ↓ self-esteem, ↓ concentration, hopelessness.
See Nursing Care for Clients Who Are Hyperactive, p. 164. See Nursing Care for Clients Who Are Suicidal, p. 165. See Nursing Care for Clients Who Are Withdrawn, p. 166.	

Personality Disorders

- Enduring pattern of behavior that deviates from individual's culture.
- Behavior is pervasive, inflexible, stable over time.
- Onset in adolescence or young adulthood.
- Behavior leads to distress or impairment.
- Nursing Care: See Nursing Care for Clients With a Personality Disorder, p. 165.

	Cluster A (Odd, eccentric behavior)
Paranoid	Suspicious without justification, particularly fidelity of sexual partner; feels exploited, harmed, or deceived; bears grudges; reacts with anger to misperceived attacks by others.
Schizoid	Loner; blunted affect; emotionally cold and detached; indifferent to others.
Schizotypal	Eccentric behavior, appearance, speech; inappropriate affect; paranoid ideation; magical thinking; excessive social anxiety.
	Cluster B (Dramatic, emotional, erratic behavior)
Borderline personality	Unstable relationships; impulsive; intense mood swings; identity disturbance; self-destructive behavior; inappropriate, intense anger; recurrent self-mutilating and/or suicidal behaviors.
Antisocial personality	Fails to conform to social norms; exploits others without guilt; deceitful, impulsive, aggressive, irresponsible; disregards safety of self and others.
Histrionic personality	Rapidly shifting, shallow expression of emotions; dramatic; must be center of attention; seductive or provocative behavior; easily influenced by others.
Narcissistic personality	Grandiosity; need for attention and admiration; egocentric; arrogant; sense of entitlement; exploits others; lacks empathy.
	Cluster C (Anxious, fearful behavior)
Avoidant personality	Socially inept; feelings of inadequacy and hypersensitivity; avoids significant interpersonal contact; fear of embarrassment; hurt by criticism.
Dependent personality	Dependent; submissive; indecisive; decreased self-concept; fears rejection; fears being left to care for self.
Obsessive-compulsive	Preoccupied with orderliness, perfectionism, and mental and interpersonal control; inflexible; stubborn; reluctant to delegate; miserly.
See Nursing Care for Clients With a Personality Disorder, p. 165.	

Neurodevelopmental Disorders

Autism Spectrum Disorder

- Spectrum refers to variety in impairments in language, interpersonal interactions, and intellectual abilities; can be mild, allowing self-sufficiency, to major, requiring complete dependence on others.
- First evident in early childhood but may not fully manifest until social demands exceed abilities.
- Persistent deficit in communication and social interaction (deficits in social–emotional reciprocity, verbal and nonverbal communication, and developing, maintaining, and understanding relationships).
- Restricted, repetitive patterns of behavior, interests, or activities (repetitive words or motor movements **(perseveration)**, inflexible routines, ritualized patterns of verbal/nonverbal behavior, fixated interests, hyper- or hyporeactivity to sensory input, fixation with lights or movement, adverse response to sounds, textures, or smells).
- Asperger was merged under autism spectrum disorder in DSM 5.
- *Treatment:* There is no cure; maximize functional abilities—behavioral, communication, educational, and family therapies.

Attention Deficit Hyperactivity Disorder

- *Persistent inattention:* Carelessness; easily distracted; forgetful; loses things; does not finish tasks; ↓ concentration; ↓ organization; avoids tasks that require mental effort; appears not to listen when spoken to directly.
- *Hyperactivity and impulsivity:* Runs, climbs, talks, fidgets excessively; leaves seat often when expected to sit; on the go constantly; interrupts others; ↓ ability to wait for turn.
- Usually identified between 3–12 yr of age; behavior interferes with functioning in at least 2 settings such as social, academic, work.
- *Treatment:* CNS stimulants, nonstimulant norepinephrine reuptake inhibitors.

Intellectual Disability

- No characteristic pathology; multifactorial causes, for example:
  - Genetic (Down and fragile X syndromes, PKU).
  - Perinatal (alcohol and drug use, infection, inadequate folic acid, prematurity, anoxia).
  - Acquired (meningitis, lead poisoning, measles, head trauma, chronic social deprivation).
- Deficits in intellectual functions: Reasoning, planning, abstract thinking, judgment, academic learning, learning from experience, problem solving.
- Deficits in ability to meet developmental and sociocultural standards to be independent and socially responsible.
- Level of severity defined on basis of adaptive functioning, not IQ scores.

Severity Level	Conceptual Domain	Social Domain	Practical Domain
Mild	Difficulty in learning academic skills (reading, writing, math, time, money), ↓ abstract thinking, concrete approach to problems.	Immature, ↓ perception of social cues, uses concrete language, ↓ ability to regulate emotions, gullible.	Cares for personal needs (eating, dressing, bathing), needs assistance with complex ADL (shopping, banking, transportation), holds jobs that do not require conceptual skills.
Moderate	Academic development at elementary level, partial or total support needed to complete conceptual tasks.	Uses spoken language that is less complex than peers, ↓ social and decision-making skills, requires significant social and communicative support.	Cares for personal needs after extensive teaching, needs assistance with complex ADL, holds job with significant support, maladaptive behavior may cause social problems.
Severe	Conceptual skills limited (written language, time, numbers, money), requires extensive support for problem solving.	Understands simple language and gestures; uses limited vocabulary, single words, phrases; focuses on the present; derives pleasure in relationships with family and friends.	Requires support for all ADL and supervision at all times, cannot make responsible decisions regarding well-being of self or others, requires long-term teaching and continuous support for skill acquisition.
Profound	Conceptual skill involves the physical, rather than the symbolic, world; motor and sensory impairments may prevent functional use of objects.	May understand simple words or gestures, expresses desires and emotions through nonverbal communication, enjoys relationship with familiar others, sensory and physical impairments prevent many social activities.	Depends on others for all ADL, simple actions with objects may be basis for participation, sensory and physical impairments are barriers to participation beyond watching, maladaptive behavior is present in significant minority.

Treatment

- Early identification; early intervention programs.
- Individualized education program; vocational programs, PT, OT.
- Placement in day care, group home, assistive living or long-term care facility.

Nursing Care

Child

- Use simple, concrete communication and a variety of senses.
- Teach tasks step-by-step while slowly removing assistance **(fading)**.
- Give positive reinforcement for desired behavior **(shaping)**.
- Role-play social behaviors; support independence with ADL; base play on developmental, not chronological, age.
- Encourage peer groups such as scouting and Special Olympics.
- Explore appropriate sexuality issues with child, adolescent, and parents such as code of conduct, protection from sexual abuse, contraception, sterilization.

Parents

- Support coping with diagnosis; encourage use of periodic respite programs.
- Support exploration of resources and decisions concerning temporary or permanent placement.

Gender Dysphoria and Paraphilic Disorders

Gender dysphoria	**Children** • Strong desire to be of the other gender. • Preference for simulating clothing of other gender, cross-gender role in fantasy play, toys/activities typical of other gender, playmates of other gender. • Dislike of one's sexual anatomy; strong desire for sex characteristics of other gender. **Adolescents and Adults** • Strong desire to be the other gender and be treated as the other gender. • Strong desire to be rid of one's primary/secondary sex characteristics and to have the sex characteristics of the other gender. • Strong conviction that one has the typical feelings and reactions of the other gender.

Paraphilic disorders	• Persistent, troubling fantasies, urges, or behaviors >6 mo. • Causes distress or impairment to the individual performing the behavior or where the individual's sexual behavior has involved risk of, or actual harm to, an unwilling person or person unable to give legal consent. • Paraphilic disorders related to sexual arousal: **Pedophilic:** Sexual activity with a child. **Exhibitionistic:** Genital exposure to an unsuspecting person. **Frotteuristic:** Touching or rubbing against a nonconsenting person. **Fetishistic:** Use of a nonliving object or specific focus on a nongenital body part(s). **Transvestic:** Wearing clothing of opposite gender (cross-dressing). **Voyeuristic:** Watching unsuspecting nakedness or sexual activity. **Sexual sadism:** Inflicting physical or psychological suffering on another. **Sexual masochism:** Self-induced humiliation and/or suffering.

Schizophrenia

- Mental disorder characterized by disturbances in form and content of thought, mood, affect, behavior, and sense of self.
- Two or more of the following S&S for 6 mo: Delusions, hallucinations, disorganized speech, grossly disorganized or catatonic behavior, negative symptoms.

Positive Symptoms: Type I

- **Delusion:** Fixed false belief despite evidence to the contrary.
- **Hallucination:** False sensory perception without external stimulus; person sees, hears, smells, tastes, or feels something that is not there.
- Excess or distortion of normal functions (see Disorganized Thinking and Disorganized Behavior, p. 154).

Negative Symptoms: Type II

- Decrease or loss of normal functions.
- **Affective flattening:** ↓ in range and intensity of emotion.
- **Alogia:** ↓ fluency and productivity of thoughts and speech.
- **Ambivalence:** Indecisive because of strong opposing feelings.
- **Anhedonia:** Inability to experience pleasure.
- **Avolition:** Unable to initiate/persist in goal-directed behavior.

Disorganized Thinking

- **Concrete thinking:** Lack of abstraction.
- **Circumstantiality:** Detailed, long discussion about a topic.
- **Clang association:** Repetition of similar-sounding words.
- **Echolalia:** Parrotlike repetition of another's words.
- **Flight of ideas:** Rapid, repeated change in topics.
- **Ideas of reference:** Remarks unrelated to the individual are interpreted personally by the individual.
- **Loose associations:** Decreased connectedness of thoughts and topics.
- **Neologisms:** Made-up words with no common meaning.
- **Pressured speech:** Rapid, forced speech.
- **Tangentiality:** Logical digression from original discussion.

Disorganized Behavior

- **Agitation:** Restlessness with increased emotions/tension.
- **Aggression:** Hostility with potential for verbal or physical violence.
- **Psychomotor disturbances**
  - **Stereotypy:** Repetitive, purposeless activity peculiar to client.
  - **Echopraxia:** Involuntary imitation of another's gestures.
  - **Waxy flexibility:** Fixed posturing for extended periods.
- **Regressed behavior:** Childlike, immature behavior.
- **Hypervigilance:** Sustained increased attention to external stimuli.

Nursing Care

- See Nursing Care for Clients With Delusions or Hallucinations, p. 162.
- See Nursing Care for Clients With Paranoia, p. 165.
- See Nursing Care for Clients Who Are Withdrawn, p. 166.

Somatic Symptom Disorder and Related Disorders

Disorder	Description
Somatic Symptom Disorder	Somatic symptoms without medical explanation; suffering is authentic, even though it is not medically explained.
Illness Anxiety Disorder (Formerly Hypochondriasis)	Abnormal concern about perceived physical symptoms and health despite minor symptoms or absence of illness.
Conversion Disorder	Altered voluntary motor or sensory function not explained by neurological disease.
Factitious Disorder Imposed on Self (Formerly Munchausen Syndrome)	Exaggeration or falsification of one's own physical or psychological S&S; self-induction of disease or injury; motive usually is need for comfort and attention.
Factitious Disorder Imposed on Another (Formerly Munchausen Syndrome by Proxy)	Individual fabricates S&S or causes disease or injury in another person, usually a child or vulnerable older adult (considered child or elder abuse); motive is sympathy and attention.

Obsessive-Compulsive and Related Disorders

Disorder	Description
Body Dysmorphic Disorder	Preoccupation with perceived flaw in appearance; may seek multiple plastic surgeries; causes significant distress and hinders social and occupational functioning.
Hoarding Disorder	Persistent difficulty discarding possessions regardless of value congesting active living areas; causes significant distress and interferes with safety and health.
Obsessive-Compulsive Disorder	**Obsession**: Recurrent, persistent thoughts, urges, or images that enter the mind causing anxiety and distress; may be intrusive and unwanted. **Compulsion**: Repetitive behavior (handwashing, rechecking) or mental acts (counting, repeating words silently); person feels compelled to perform repeated act in an attempt to ↓ anxiety or distress; they are excessive and time consuming.

See Nursing Care for Clients With Obsessive-Compulsive Disorder, p. 164.

Substance Use Disorders

Common Factors Related to Substance Use Disorders

- **Dependence**: Results from repeated substance use that causes S&S of withdrawal upon stopping the substance.
- **Intoxication**: Reversible substance-specific syndrome due to recent use; causes disturbances in cognition, perception, affect, judgment, behavior, and LOC.
- **Tolerance**: Increased dose needed for desired result.
- **Polysubstance use**: Use of two or more substances.
- **Potentiation**: Two or more substances produce effect more than sum of each.
- **Withdrawal**: Substance-specific syndrome due to decreased or cessation of intake.
- **Criteria for substance use disorder**:
  - *Impaired control:* Substance taken in ↑ amounts over a longer period of time than intended, unable to ↓ or stop use, intense craving for the substance, life revolves around substance.
  - *Social impairment:* Failure to fulfill life roles, persistent interpersonal problems, withdrawal from family activities, and ↓ social, occupational, or recreational activities.
  - *Risky use of substance:* Use results in hazardous activities, persistent use despite negative consequences.
  - *Pharmacological criteria:* Develops tolerance, experiences withdrawal when substance is discontinued.
  - See Nursing Care for Clients With Substance Use Disorders, p. 161.

Stimulant Use Disorder (Amphetamines, Cocaine)

- **S&S**: Euphoria, initial CNS stimulation, then depression, insomnia, ↓ appetite, dilated pupils, tremors, paranoia, aggressiveness.
- **Withdrawal**: Psychomotor retardation or agitation; dysphoria; fatigue and insomnia or hypersomnia; cravings; increased appetite; vivid, unpleasant dreams.

Sedative, Hypnotic, or Anxiolytic Use Disorder

- **S&S**: ↓ VS, disinhibition, impaired cognition, incoordination, slurred speech.
- **Withdrawal**: N&V; insomnia; anxiety; psychomotor agitation; transient visual, auditory, or tactile illusions or hallucinations; seizures.

Alcohol Use Disorder

- **S&S**: Decreased perception, coordination, and memory; slurring speech; disinhibition; aggression; blackouts.
- **Korsakoff psychosis:** Delirium, confabulation, illusions, decreased short/long-term memory, hallucinations.

- **Wernicke encephalopathy:** Neurological abnormalities such as oculomotor dysfunction, confusion, and ataxia due to ↓ thiamine.
- **Withdrawal:** Begins in 12 hr, peaks in 48–72 hr, improves by 4th to 5th day; N&V, ↑ VS, diaphoresis, anxiety, psychomotor agitation, insomnia, illusions, hallucinations, tremors; withdrawal delirium **(delirium tremens)** may occur as early as 2nd but as late as 14th day and lasts 2–3 days.

Assessment of Risk for Alcohol Misuse

	CAGE Questionnaire
C	Have you ever felt that you should Cut down on your drinking?
A	Have people Annoyed you by criticizing your drinking?
G	Have you ever felt Guilty about your drinking?
E	Have you ever had a drink in the morning as an Eye-opener?
Award 1 point for each question answered with a YES. 0–1 low risk of problem drinking; 2–3 high suspicion for alcoholism; 4 diagnostic for alcoholism.	

Opioid Use Disorder (Heroin, Codeine, Oxycodone)

- **S&S:** Euphoria; sedation; constricted pupils; constipation; decreased libido, memory, and concentration; slurred speech.
- **Withdrawal:** Dysphoric mood, rhinorrhea, watery eyes, dilated pupils, yawning, N&V, diarrhea, diaphoresis, muscle aches, insomnia, fever.

Other Misused Substances

- Tobacco; caffeine; hallucinogens (phencyclidine [angel dust, Sernyl], lysergic acid diethylamide [LSD]); cannabis (marijuana, hashish); inhalants (glue, lighter fluid).
- Gambling is viewed as a behavioral addiction.

Domestic Violence

Cycle of Battering

- Pattern of violence used to maintain power and control over another; abuser may be either gender, mostly male.
- Behaviors divided into 3 phases that vary in time and intensity.

Cycle of Battering

Phase	Abuser	Victim
Tension-Building Phase	Tolerance for frustration ↓, angry with little provocation, minor battering may occur.	Becomes compliant and anticipates abuser's needs in an effort to ↓ anger, accepts abuse, rationalizes abuser's behavior.
Acute Battering Incident	Begins with justification for behavior, causes traumatic emotional or physical injury, minimizes severity of abuse.	Accepts abuse, may fight back, tries to find safe place to hide.
Calm, Loving, Respite (Honeymoon) Phase	Begs forgiveness, becomes kind, loving, charming, and remorseful.	Perceives relationship based on these idealized behaviors, hopeful that violence will stop, remains due to fear of retaliation to self or children, financial dependence, lack of support, religious reasons.

Types of Abuse and Neglect

- *Physical abuse:* Threatening or inflicting nonaccidental physical harm to another.
- *Sexual abuse:* Any sexual act involving another without the person's consent; verbally undermining sexuality.
- *Psychological abuse:* Verbal or nonverbal acts that have reasonable potential to cause significant emotional harm to another.
- *Neglect/maltreatment:* Any act by omission or commission that deprives another of basic age-appropriate needs that has reasonable potential to result in physical or emotional harm.

Signs and Symptoms of Abuse and Neglect

Signs and Symptoms Common to All Types of Abuse and Neglect

- Injuries, bruises, fractures, burns; injuries at various stages of recovery; untreated medical or dental problems.
- Injuries inconsistent with stated cause; abuser shows little concern for victim.
- Victim expresses feelings of helplessness, guilt, depression, low self-esteem.

Signs and Symptoms Specific to Child Abuse and Neglect

Child

- Changes in behavior: Regression, aggression, anger, hyperactivity, depression.
- Delayed growth, inadequate hygiene, inadequate food or clothing.
- Fear of people or places, reluctance to leave school, frequent absences from school, ↓ academic performance.
- Vaginal or penile discharge, bruising or itching in genital area, recurrent UTI, play that recreates sexual abuse.

Abuser

- Blames or belittles child; uses harsh discipline.
- Has unrealistic expectation of age-appropriate behavior or abilities of child.

Signs and Symptoms Specific to Elder Abuse and Neglect

- Chafing at ankles or wrists indicating use of restraints.
- Physical or cognitive impairment; withdrawn, combative.
- Dependent on caregiver.

Signs and Symptoms Specific to Domestic Partner Abuse and Neglect

- Multiple injuries involving the nose, eyes, teeth, breasts, genitalia.
- Verbalizes seemingly believable reasons for injuries.
- Isolates self from others until injuries heal.

Nursing Care for Victims Who Are Abused and Neglected

- Legal implications for nurses
  - Notify appropriate authorities of suspected abuse or neglect of child, older adult, or adult with intellectual disabilities.
  - Follow local laws concerning reporting of domestic partner violence; an adult rape victim must be person to report rape to authorities.
  - Have a child protective services counselor, rape counselor, or sexual assault nurse examiner present as indicated.
- Provide privacy when interviewing victim; ensure interview is out of sight and hearing of suspected abuser.
- Keep victim in a safe environment; refer or transfer child/adult to agencies that provide a safe haven or other community services.
- Teach how to maintain personal safety
  - Seek medical care when necessary; take pictures of abuse.
  - Keep a journal of abuse not accessible to abuser.
  - File a police report; obtain an order of protection.
  - Design a safety plan (pack bag with money/credit cards, identification, legal papers, meds, clothing; memorize emergency phone numbers—police, shelters; put 911 on speed dial; arrange a code word with a trusted adult who can be called in an emergency; prearrange a safe haven).

Nursing Care of Clients With Dysfunctional Behavior Patterns

General Nursing Care for All Clients

- Maintain safe, supportive, nonjudgmental environment.
- Recognize all behavior has meaning.
- Encourage expression of feelings; do not deny or approve.
- Accept and respect clients as individuals; provide choices when able.
- Set simple, fair, consistent expectations and limits about behavior; address inappropriate behavior immediately.
- Help client to test new interpersonal skills.
- Assist with ADL as necessary.
- Encourage activities that involve client in recovery.
- Teach client and family members about prescribed meds; assess physical, emotional, and behavioral responses.

Nursing Care for Clients With Substance Use Disorders

- Use screening tools to assess risk; assess for S&S of specific addiction.
- Obtain urine and blood specimens for prescribed laboratory tests to monitor for presence of substance.
- Provide physical and emotional support while client is in withdrawal.
- Limit noise and light to decrease hallucinations and illusions due to withdrawal.
- Provide and encourage maintenance of a substance-free setting.
- Accept hostility without reprisal; set realistic limits to decrease manipulation and/or aggression.
- Expect client to assume responsibility for own behavior.
- Encourage client and family members to attend self-help groups and/or rehabilitation program.
- Help family members to identify and change enabling behaviors.
- Administer prescribed chlordiazepoxide during withdrawal from alcohol; see Anxiolytics, Sedatives, and Hypnotics, p. 274 and Opioid (Narcotic) Antagonists, p. 263 in MedsTab.

Nursing Care for Clients Who Are Aggressive

- Hostile verbal, symbolic, or physical behavior that intimidates others.
- Associated with substance use disorders, conduct disorders, mania, delirium, dementia, paranoia.
- Assign to a single room; use nonthreatening body language and calm approach; respect personal space; do not touch.
- Provide ongoing surveillance; position self near an escape route; know where colleagues are if help is needed.
- Remove potentially violent or violent client from vicinity of others.
- Anticipate needs to decrease stress that may cause anger.
- Assess for frustration, irritation, anger, distorted thinking that may precede violence.
- Assist to express anger in acceptable ways such as words, writing list of grievances, physical exercise, assertiveness; provide positive reinforcement for acceptable behavior.
- Teach to interrupt aggressive patterns such as count to 10 or remove self.
- See Antipsychotic Agents in MedsTab, p. 277.

Nursing Care for Clients Who Are Anxious

- Anxiety ranges from feelings of apprehension to doom; response to a perceived threat to physiological, emotional, or social integrity.
- Associated with phobias and anxiety, obsessive-compulsive, dissociative, and somatoform disorders.
- Assess level of anxiety; see Levels of Anxiety and Related S&S, p. 146.
- Provide single room; decrease environmental stimuli.
- Acknowledge feelings about phobic object or situation.
- Recognize somatic complaints but do not call attention to them.
- Assist to identify and avoid anxiety-producing situations.
- Assist with relaxation techniques to decrease anxiety.
- Postpone teaching when anxiety reaches severe or panic levels.
- Stay with client during a panic attack; provide for safety.
- Intervene when acting-out impulses may harm self or others.
- See Anxiolytics, Sedatives, and Hypnotics in Meds Tab, p. 274.

Nursing Care for Clients With Delusions or Hallucinations

- **Delusion**: Fixed false belief that is resistant to conflicting evidence.
  - Types: grandiosity, persecution, control, religiosity, erotomanic, somatic, ideas of reference, thought broadcasting, withdrawal, and insertion.
- **Hallucination**: False sensory perception without external stimulus; person sees (visual), hears (auditory), smells (olfactory), tastes (gustatory), or feels (tactile) something that is not there or is told to harm self or others (command).
- Associated with schizophrenia; depression with psychotic features; drug withdrawal; delirium; and bipolar, obsessive-compulsive, and body dysmorphic disorders.
- Recognize and accept delusions and hallucinations are real and frightening to client; stay with client because isolation will ↑ hallucinations.
- Identify commands of violence that may result in harm to self or others.
- Distract client from delusions that may precipitate violence.
- Point out reality, but do not reason, argue, challenge client.
- Focus on meaning and feelings rather than content.
- Praise reality-based perceptions.
- Identify factors that may exacerbate sensory and perceptual disturbances such as reflective glare, TV screens, and lights.
- Teach self-coping for delusions such as recreational and diversionary activities.

- Teach self-coping for hallucinations such as exercise, listening to music, saying "stop, go away!"; engage in structured activities.
- See Antipsychotic Agents in Meds Tab, p. 277.

Nursing Care for Clients With Decreased Cognition

- Progressive disturbance in cognitive and functional abilities.
- Associated with vascular dementia and Alzheimer, Parkinson, Creutzfeldt-Jakob, and Pick diseases.
- Provide a safe, nonstimulating, familiar environment with consistent routines and caregiver.
- Use a calm, unhurried, nondemanding approach.
- Consider client mood and easy distractibility when planning care.
- Reorient to time, place, person; use simple language and visual clues.
- Promote independence; assist with ADL.
- Encourage reminiscing about earlier yr.
- Identify events that increase agitation such as environmental stimuli, altered routines, strangers, increased expectations, "lost" items.
- Involve in simple, repetitive tasks and one-on-one activities.
- Shut shades and keep lights on if client experiences sundowning.
- Ensure safety of client who wanders (doors with alarms, GPS bracelet, continuous observation).
- Promote involvement in therapy such as music, pet, and current events.
- Support primary caregivers and encourage periodic respite.
- See Medications for Neurocognitive Disorders, Particularly Alzheimer Disease, in Meds Tab, p. 269.

Nursing Care for Clients With Eating Disorders

- Preoccupation with weight involving ↑ or ↓ intake of food with weight loss behaviors such as purging, exercise, and abuse of laxatives or diuretics.
- Associated with anorexia and bulimia.
- Assist with contract for behavior-modification program such as eating and weight goals with consequences for goal attainment or failure.
- Observe for 1 hr after eating to prevent purging.
- Assess for F&E imbalances.
- Maintain matter-of-fact approach, shift focus from food, eating, and exercise to emotional issues.
- Provide and encourage intake of nutrient-dense foods.
- Support therapeutic interactions with individuals, groups, and family members.

- Identify issues of ↓ self-esteem, identity disturbance, family dysfunction.
- Provide prescribed IV and/or tube feedings for client with anorexia.
- Administer prescribed meds; usually fluoxetine (Prozac) for bulimia and olanzapine (Zyprexa) for anorexia.

Nursing Care for Clients Who Are Hyperactive

- Increased motor activity and speech, impulsivity, inattention, and expansive and/or irritable mood.
- Associated with attention deficit hyperactivity disorder, bipolar disorder (manic and hypomanic episodes).
- Provide a safe, nonstimulating environment.
- Approach in a calm, nonargumentative manner.
- Channel hyperactivity into safe, controlled activities.
- Use easy distractibility to redirect inappropriate behavior.
- Keep activities simple, repetitive, and of short duration.
- Use rewards such as tokens and praise to reinforce appropriate behavior.
- Balance energy expenditure and rest.
- Provide high-protein, high-calorie, and handheld foods.
- See Medications for Attention Deficit Hyperactivity in Meds Tab, p. 279.

Nursing Care for Clients With Obsessive-Compulsive Disorder

- **Obsession:** Recurrent, persistent thoughts, urges, or images that enter the mind; may be intrusive and unwanted.
- **Compulsion:** Repetitive behavior (handwashing, rechecking) or mental acts (counting, repeating words silently) that person feels compelled to perform in an attempt to ↓ anxiety or distress; they are excessive and time consuming.
- Know client may realize the ritual is not rational but cannot control it.
- Allow performance of ritual until client develops other defenses.
- Intervene when acting-out impulses may result in harm to self or others.
- Limit time and frequency of ritual after other defenses develop.
- Reduce stress of decision making to decrease anxiety.
- Assist to identify and avoid anxiety-producing situations.
- Help to identify and use positive anxiety-reducing behaviors.
- See Antidepressants in Meds Tab, p. 275.

Nursing Care for Clients With Paranoia

- Suspicious thinking that is persecutory such as being harassed, poisoned, or judged critically.
- Associated with paranoid personality disorder; paranoia associated with schizophrenia.
- Respect personal space; do not touch.
- Use nonthreatening body language; be calm and reassuring.
- Provide environment and activities that do not challenge security.
- Recognize and accept that delusions are real and frightening to client.
- Identify presence of dangerous command hallucinations.
- Point out reality but do not directly challenge delusions.
- Praise reality-based perceptions.
- See Antipsychotic Agents in Meds Tab, p. 277.

Nursing Care for Clients With a Personality Disorder

- Persistent, pervasive, inflexible pattern of inner experience or behavior that deviates markedly from the norm.
  - **Cluster A:** Paranoid, schizoid, schizotypal.
  - **Cluster B:** Borderline, antisocial, histrionic, narcissistic.
  - **Cluster C:** Avoidant, dependent, obsessive-compulsive.
- Recognize development of trust will take time.
- Assess level of dependence and independence.
- Support decision making and independence.
- Involve client in activities that ↑ self-esteem.
- Engage in social skills training specific to the disorder.
- Cluster A: See Nursing Care for Clients With Paranoia, p. 165.
- Cluster B: See Nursing Care for Clients Who Are Hyperactive, p. 164, and Nursing Care for Clients Who Are Aggressive, p. 161.
- Cluster C: See Nursing Care for Clients Who Are Withdrawn, p. 166, and Nursing Care for Clients With Obsessive-Compulsive Disorder, p. 164.

Nursing Care for Clients Who Are Suicidal

- Increased risk is associated with bipolar and depressive disorders; command hallucinations; young adults and adolescents; single older adults; higher incidence with men; stress and loss; social isolation; substance use disorders; hopelessness or helplessness; serious illness; sexual identity crisis; and physical or emotional abuse.

- **Levels of suicidal behavior**
  - **Suicidal ideation:** Thoughts of suicide or self-injurious acts expressed verbally or symbolically.
  - **Suicide threat:** Expression of intent to commit suicide without action.
  - **Suicide gesture:** Self-directed act that results in minor injury.
  - **Suicidal attempt:** Self-directed act that may result in minor or major injury by person who intended to die.
  - **Suicide:** Self-inflicted death.
- Ask client if there is a suicide plan, and identify if the client has the means to carry it out.
- Provide constant observation and safe environment such as no sharps, shoelaces, or cords; assign to a two-bedded room.
- Identify if client is giving away possessions or putting affairs in order.
- Identify what precipitated or contributed to suicide crisis.
- Focus on client's strengths rather than weaknesses.
- Encourage exploration of consequences if suicide attempt is unsuccessful, impact on others if successful, feelings about death, and reasons for living.
- Assist with problem solving; prioritize problems; focus on one at a time.
- Assist client to write a list of support systems and community resources and how to ask for help.
- Ensure family members are aware of the need to maintain safety, as most suicides occur within 90 days after release from the hospital.
- See Antidepressants in Meds Tab, p. 275.

Nursing Care for Clients Who Are Withdrawn

- Client retreats from people and reality.
- Associated with autism, major depression, anxiety, schizophrenia, bipolar disorder depressive episode, avoidant and dependent personality disorders.
- Assess risk for suicide especially as depression and energy lift.
- Accept feelings of worthlessness as real.
- Sit quietly next to client, then encourage one-on-one interaction.
- Spend time with client to support worthiness; provide realistic praise.
- Accept but do not reward dependence; provide simple choices.
- Minimize isolation; involve in simple, repetitive activities.
- Assist to identify and replace self-deprecating thoughts with positive thoughts through cognitive restructuring.
- See Antidepressants, p. 275 and Antipsychotic Agents, p. 277 in Meds Tab.

Therapeutic Modalities

Nurse

- Therapeutic use of self to diagnose and treat human responses to actual or potential mental health problems.
- **Nursing care:** Engage in activities such as health promotion; intake screening and evaluation; case management; support of self-care activities; psychobiological interventions; teaching; counseling; crisis intervention; milieu therapy; psychosocial rehabilitation.

Individual Psychotherapy

- Client and therapist enter into a therapeutic relationship.
- **Nursing care:** Assist to clarify perceptions; identify feelings; make connections among thoughts, feelings, and events; ↑ insight.

Family Therapy

- Family treated as a unit; focuses on dynamics to attain and maintain balance and harmony.
- **Nursing care:** Help establish boundaries; assess hierarchy and subsystems; ↑ communication; ↑ interpersonal skills; promote family cohesion and flexibility (see Group Therapy, on next page).

Self-Help Groups

- Participants have common beliefs, values, and behaviors.
- Must desire to change behavior; receive and give assistance to peers; leadership is shared by peers; lifelong process.
- **Nursing care:** Refer to appropriate group.

Behavioral Therapy

- Reward acceptable behaviors so they are reinforced **(operant conditioning)**; based on fact that *behavior has consequences*; clients are active participants.
- **Nursing care:** Establish behavioral contract with goals and consequences; set firm, consistent limits on unacceptable behavior; and reward acceptable behavior and achievement of goals **(token economy)**.

Group Therapy

- People share thoughts and feelings and help each other examine common issues and concerns.
- **Nursing care:** Refer to an appropriate group.

Stages of Group Process

Stage	Characteristics	Nursing Care
Beginning	Polite behavior initially; concerned with role and place in group; conflict dominates the end of this stage.	Provide orientation, set boundaries, help identify purpose and tasks.
Working	Develop rules, rituals, behavioral norms; develop cooperative relationships; share ideas, experiences, feelings; focus on present.	Provide structure, model acceptance, facilitate interaction, promote task accomplishment.
Termination	Begin to grieve termination of group; attempt to reestablish self as individual; may attempt to raise new concerns.	Promote summary of group work, resist introduction of new topics, facilitate closure.

Light Therapy (Phototherapy)

- Exposure to bright full-spectrum fluorescent lamps suppresses melatonin production and normalizes disturbance in circadian rhythms; used for depressed clients with a seasonal pattern, usually winter; given from 30 min to 2–5 hr daily; depression begins to lift within 1–4 days; full effect in 2 wk; maintained with daily sessions of 30 min.
- **Nursing care**
  - Ensure assessment for preexisting eye problems; teach importance of arising before 8:00 a.m., sitting 3 feet from lights, engaging in other activities permitted but glancing at light every few min.
  - Assess for side effects such as eyestrain, headache, insomnia, irritability.

Electroconvulsive Therapy (ECT)

- Short-acting barbiturate and muscle relaxant given before a brief electrical current is passed through brain to produce a generalized seizure; alters brain chemistry to improve mood; 2–3 treatments a wk for 3–4 wk.
- Still used for severe depression, severe mania, catatonia, agitation and aggression in clients with dementia.
- **Nursing care before ECT:** Witness informed consent; allay concerns; reassure that memory returns in 6–9 mo and procedure is not painful; ensure ECG, physical exam, and lab work are done, no food and fluid after midnight, empty bladder; remove jewelry, dental appliances, and nail polish.
- **Nursing care during and after ECT:** Assess VS before, during, and after ECT; insert mouth guard; preoxygenate before and maintain O_2 after ECT; prevent harm during seizure; ensure patent airway after seizure; assess for side effects when client awakens 10–15 min after ECT such as headache, muscle aches, confusion, and disorientation; usually disappear within 1 hr.

Seclusion and Restraint

- See Nursing Care for Clients in Seclusion or Restraints in Basics Tab, p. 22.
- **Nursing care**
  - Use less-restrictive interventions 1st; ensure restraint is not done for convenience, retaliation, coercion, or discipline.
  - When used in an emergency, a primary health-care provider must perform face-to-face evaluation (1-hr rule); continuous in-person observation of client for duration of use.
  - When seclusion only is used, audio and video equipment permitted after 1st hr; family must be notified.

Activity Therapy

- Therapeutic, expressive activity to ↓ pathology and ↑ mental and emotional health; ↑ awareness of feelings, behaviors, thoughts, and sensations.
- **Nursing care**
  - Determine level of functioning; provide a variety of groups such as recreation, art, music, dance, movement, and pet therapy; support efforts.
  - Children benefit from play because they are less able to verbalize thoughts and feelings.
  - Clients with cognitive impairments do better in less challenging, low-functioning groups.

Crisis Intervention

- Assist to return to previous level of functioning; develop more constructive coping skills; short-term, goal-directed care.
- **Crisis:** Positive or negative sudden stressful experience perceived as threatening when usual coping does not maintain integrity; lasts from hr to a few wk.
- **Phases of a crisis**
  - *Phase I:* Stressful event causes anxiety, usual strategies used to cope, crisis resolves or anxiety ↑.
  - *Phase II:* New strategies are tried, crisis resolves or strategies are ineffective and anxiety ↑.
  - *Phase III:* All internal and external resources are called on, crisis resolves or anxiety ↑.
  - *Phase IV:* Anxiety ↑ to beyond ability to cope (panic), cognitive functions disorganized, emotions are labile, behavior reflects psychotic thinking.
- Influencing factors: Include individual's perception, personal coping mechanisms, and situational support.
- **Types of crises**
  - *Maturational and developmental (internal):* Related to life events such as adolescence, completing school, marriage, childbirth, menopause and climacteric, retirement, and aging.
  - *Situational (external):* Related to unexpected situations such as relocation, loss of job, environmental disasters, and health problem.
  - *Adventitious:* Related to disasters such as floods, earthquakes, war, and terrorist attacks.
- **Nursing care**
  - Assume a calm, controlled presence and avoid overwhelming client.
  - Have client describe event; support when confronting reality; encourage expression of feelings; clarify fantasies with facts.
  - Explore strengths, weaknesses, and support systems.
  - Assist with problem solving and developing new coping strategies; refer to community resources.

Psychopharmacology

- Drugs that affect emotion, behavior, and cognition: Anxiolytics, sedatives, and hypnotics; antidepressants; antipsychotic agents; antimanic and mood stabilizing agents; meds for attention deficit hyperactivity disorder.
- **Nursing care:** See Meds Tab for sections addressing each of the drug classifications indicated above and for Nontherapeutic Effects of Psychotropic Meds.

Care of Clients With Cancer

ancer (Ca) is the mutation of cellular DNA resulting in abnormal cells that vade other tissue by direct extension or metastasis via lymph or blood.

ypes

denocarcinoma (glandular), carcinoma (epithelial), glioma (central nervous ystem), leukemia (blood forming), lymphoma (lymphatic), melanoma (pig-nented), myeloma (plasma of bone marrow), sarcoma (soft tissue, muscle, ascular, synovial).

isk Factors

ienetics, microbiological agents (herpes simplex virus/cervical Ca), physical gents (sun exposure/skin Ca), hormones (estrogen/breast Ca), chemical agents smoking/lung Ca), diet (↑ fat/colon Ca), ↓ immune response (AIDS/Kaposi arcoma).

Early Detection

- See CAUTION in Basics Tab, p. 7.
- Screening:
  - Cervical Pap test—every 3 yr ages 24–29, every 3–5 yr ages 30–65, unnecessary after 65 yr if negative for 10 yr;
  - Mammogram—yearly ages 40–44 yr if desired, yearly 45–54 yr, every 2 yr 55 and older;
  - Flexible sigmoidoscopy every 5 yr OR colonoscopy every 10 yr at 50 yr of age;
  - Prostate—screening on individual basis.

Staging

Staging helps determine treatment and prognosis; see TNM Staging.

TNM Staging

Size of Tumor (T)	Nodal Involvement (N)	Metastasis (M)
TX: Not assessable. TO: No evidence of tumor. Tis: In situ. T1–4: Increasing tumor size.	NX: Not assessable. NO: No metastasis to regional nodes. N1–3: Increasing regional node involvement.	MX: Not assessable. MO: No metastasis. M1: Metastasis.

General Nursing Care for Clients With Cancer

- Teach healthy lifestyle (no smoking, weight control, ↓ fat in diet, ↑ intake of cruciferous vegetables and carotenoids, ↓ sun exposure).
- Encourage routine screening; refer to American Cancer Society.
- Support pain management.
- Support advance directives (living will, health-care proxy), decision for palliative/hospice care.
- Document client status and nursing interventions; notify primary health-care provider if infection, bleeding, F&E imbalances, tumor lysis syndrome, nephrotoxicity, hepatotoxicity, or cardiotoxicity occur.

Nursing Care for Clients With Cancer or Experiencing Nontherapeutic Effects of Antineoplastic Therapies

- See Antineoplastics and Related Medications in Meds Tab, p. 248.

Anorexia

- Obtain a calorie count, weigh weekly.
- Plan small frequent, bland meals; support food preferences.
- Increase protein and calories, provide supplements between meals.

Nausea and Vomiting

- Assess for S&S of F&E imbalances; monitor I&O.
- Prevent aspiration.
- Provide adequate hydration.
- Hold food and fluids 4–6 hr before chemotherapy that causes N&V.
- Give prescribed antiemetic, usually via IV 30–45 min before and for 24 hr after caustic med.

Inflammation of Oral Mucosa (Stomatitis)

- Assess mucous membranes, gag reflex, ability to chew or swallow.
- Avoid extreme temperature of food/fluid and spicy foods/fluids.
- Provide prescribed puree/fluid diet.
- Rinse mouth with normal saline every 2 hr; provide popsicles for moisture.
- Use sponge toothbrush, avoid mouthwash, remove dentures except when eating.
- Give prescribed topical antiseptics/analgesics (swish and spit, or swish and swallow).

Rectal Sores or Bleeding

- Assess for occult or frank blood in stool.
- Apply prescribed topical ointments/warm compresses to rectum.
- Avoid suppositories and taking rectal temps.

Alopecia

- Assess self-esteem, provide emotional support.
- Explain that hair eventually will grow back but may be a different color/texture.
- Use mild shampoo and wide-tooth comb, minimize combing, avoid hair dryers and curling irons, wear hat in sun.
- Encourage purchase of a wig and cutting hair before hair loss.

Diarrhea

- Assess perianal skin; S&S of F&E imbalances.
- Provide perianal skin care; use barrier ointment.
- Give prescribed antidiarrheals.

Fatigue

- Assess activity tolerance.
- Balance activity/rest; organize activities to provide uninterrupted rest.
- Encourage delegation of responsibilities to conserve energy.

Decreased Platelets (Thrombocytopenia)

- Assess for S&S of bleeding: Ecchymosis, petechiae, hematuria, melena, hematemesis, hemoptysis, bleeding from gums or venipuncture sites, ↓ platelets, ↓ Hct, ↓ Hb.
- Avoid taking rectal T, use electric razor, use emery board for nail care.
- Use largest gauge needle for injections, compress site for 5–10 min.
- Avoid aspirin, NSAIDs, alcohol.
- Administer prescribed platelets.

Decreased Leukocytes (↓ White Blood Cells [WBC], Neutropenia)

- Assess for S&S of infection (↑ T, chills, diaphoresis); monitor WBC count.
- Provide neutropenic precautions when WBC ≤1,000/mm³: Private room; eliminate fresh fruits, vegetables, flowers/potted plants; avoid people with infections.
- Obtain specimen for C&S before initiating prescribed antibiotic.
- Provide care for sites of potential microbial growth (IV and catheter sites, wounds, skin folds, perineum, oral cavity).
- Give prescribed meds to ↑ WBC such as filgrastim, pegfilgrastim.

Decreased Red Blood Cells (RBC)

- Monitor RBC, Hb, Hct.
- Assess for tachycardia, pallor, fatigue; encourage rest.
- Give prescribed epoetin and blood products to ↑ RBC.

Nephrotoxicity

- Monitor BUN, creatinine, creatinine clearance, F&E, I&O.
- Provide 2–3 L of fluid daily.

- Assess for S&S of gout; give prescribed allopurinol to prevent uric acid crystals.

Cardiotoxicity

- Assess for dyspnea, crackles, ↑ R, peripheral edema, ↑ weight.
- Assess for tachycardia, dysrhythmias.

Hepatotoxicity

- Assess for N&V, malaise, bruising, bleeding, jaundice.
- Monitor liver function test results.

Tissue Necrosis from Extravasation of a Vesicant

- Ensure IV is in vein and patent.
- Assess for infiltration or inflammation of IV site.
- Discontinue, restart in another vein if indicated; elevate extremity for 24 hr; apply ice or warm compresses as per protocol.

Tumor Lysis Syndrome

- Assess for hyperkalemia, hypocalcemia, hyperphosphatemia, hyperuricemia (destroyed tumor cells release excessive intracellular metabolites).
- Administer prescribed IV fluids, sodium polystyrene sulfonate to ↓ potassium level, allopurinol to ↓ uric acid level, phosphate-binding gels to ↓ phosphate level.

Renal and Urinary Tract Disorders

Urinary Tract Infections (UTI)

Lower UTI: Urethritis, Cystitis

Ascending pathogens such as *E. coli* cause inflammation of the urethra **(urethritis)** and inflammation of the bladder **(cystitis)**; may lead to bacterial sepsis and kidney failure.

Risk Factors

- Catheterization, female gender, incontinence, ↑ age, DM.

Signs and Symptoms

- Frequency, urgency, burning.
- Bacteria, RBC, and WBC in urine; ↑ serum WBC.

Treatment

- Urine and blood cultures prn.
- Antibiotics, antispasmodics, urinary tract antiseptics, sulfonamides, urinary tract analgesic such as phenazopyridine.
- Sepsis requires IV fluid replacement, antibiotics, nutritional support.

Nursing Care

- Assess for S&S, C&S to determine appropriate antibiotic, ↑ fluids to 3–4 L daily, encourage to empty bladder every 3–4 hr, provide perineal care.
- Maintain indwelling catheter: Surgical asepsis during insertion, closed system, secure to leg to prevent trauma to urethra, keep collection bag lower than bladder.

Upper UTI: Pyelonephritis

Urine reflux from bladder into ureters **(ureterovesical reflux)** or obstruction causes inflammation of renal pelvis; may cause bacterial sepsis and kidney failure.

Risk Factors

- Calculi, stricture, enlarged prostate, incompetent ureterovesical valve.

Signs and Symptoms

- ↑ T, chills, N&V.
- Tender costovertebral angle **(flank pain)**.

Treatment and Nursing Care

- See Treatment and Nursing Care under Lower UTI, p. 174–175.

Upper UTI: Glomerulonephritis

Infections elsewhere in the body precipitate inflammation of glomerular capillaries; may lead to bacterial sepsis and kidney failure.

Risk Factors

- Beta-hemolytic streptococcal throat infection.
- Bacterial, viral, or parasitic infection elsewhere in the body.
- Exogenous antigens such as meds.

Signs and Symptoms

- Hematuria, proteinuria, ↓ urination.

Treatment and Nursing Care

- See Treatment and Nursing Care under Lower UTI, p. 174–175.

Prostate Disorders: Benign Prostatic Hyperplasia (BPH) and Prostate Cancer

BPH

Enlarged prostate → urethral constriction → urinary retention → ↑ risk for UTI, hydronephrosis, and hydroureter.

Prostate Cancer

Cancerous cells in prostate; may metastasize to pelvis, bone, lymph nodes, liver.

Risk Factors

- ↑ age, familial history, African heritage, ↑ intake of red meat, smoking.

Signs and Symptoms

- Frequency, urgency, ↓ stream, hesitancy, nocturia, retention, sexual dysfunction.
- *Prostate cancer:* Prostatic-specific antigen (PSA) >2 ng/mL; confirmed by biopsy; Gleason scale grades tumor cells from 1 to 5, predicts level of aggressiveness.
- *Bony metastasis:* Back/hip pain, ↓ weight, fatigue, anemia, ↑ alkaline phosphatase.

Treatment

- *BPH:* Alpha blockers (terazosin) to ↓ urgency, frequency, nocturia; antiandrogens (finasteride) to ↓ prostate size and urinary S&S; heat; lasers; surgery (transurethral resection of prostate, suprapubic prostatectomy).
- *Cancer:* Radical prostatectomy, orchiectomy, radiation; leuprolide or goserelin to ↓ testosterone; antiandrogens—flutamide, bicalutamide.

Nursing Care

- Assess for S&S; provide indwelling catheter care; give prescribed meds.
- Provide postoperative care
  - Traction on catheter balloon if present to ↓ bleeding.
  - Continuous bladder irrigation: Three-way catheter to maintain patency.
  - Discuss concerns about sexual dysfunction, urine dribbling.
- Meds for prostate cancer: Teach—bone pain will ↓ in time with meds to ↓ testosterone; antiandrogens—report hepatotoxicity to primary health-care provider.

Urolithiasis (Kidney Stones, Calculi)

- Urinary stasis or chemical environment that → precipitation and crystallization of minerals; stones form that obstruct the ureter, resulting in hydroureter and hydronephrosis; stones can recur.
- Components of calculi vary: Calcium with phosphorus or oxalate (75%); uric acid (10%); struvite (15%); cystine (1%).

Risk Factors

- 30–50 yr, male, dehydration, diet with ↑ dairy and vitamin D.
- UTIs → struvite calculi, hyperparathyroidism → calcium calculi, gout and myeloprolific disease increase uric acid → uric acid calculi.

Signs and Symptoms

- Pain, depending on stone location; may have little or no pain ranging to severe pain radiating from flank to bladder or genitals.
- N&V, hematuria, pallor, diaphoresis, UTI.

Treatment

- Opioids, NSAIDs.
- Calcium stones: Ammonium chloride to acidify urine, thiazide diuretics.
- Uric acid stones: Allopurinol to ↑ urine pH and ↓ uric acid level.
- Lithotripsy: Extracorporeal shock wave, percutaneous ultrasonic, or laser.
- Diet based on stone composition, hydration.

Nursing Care

- Assess for S&S, strain urine, ↑ fluids to 3–4 L daily, control pain.
- Calcium stones: Acid ash diet with ↓ dairy, protein, and Na intake.
- Uric acid stones: Alkaline ash diet with ↓ purine (organ meat) intake.
- Oxalate stones: ↓ tea, spinach, nuts, chocolate, and rhubarb intake.

Kidney Failure

Acute Kidney Failure	End Stage Renal Disease (ESRD)
• ↓ glomerular filtration rate due to ↓ kidney perfusion, tubular or glomeruli damage, obstruction. • Moves from <100 mL **(anuria)** or <400 mL **(oliguria)** to ↑ urine output **(diuresis)**. • Progresses to recovery or ESRD. • **Risk factors:** Hemorrhage; septic shock; ↓ cardiac output; myoglobinuria due to burns or crushing injury; nephrotoxic agents; transfusion reaction; calculi; BPH; infections.	• Progressive, irreversible ↓ nephron function → uremia, retention of water, potassium, and phosphorus. • Metabolic acidosis due to inability to excrete ammonia and reabsorb bicarbonate. • **Risk factors:** DM; ↑ BP; chronic infections (pyelonephritis, glomerulonephritis); polycystic kidney disease; nephrotoxic agents (aminoglycosides, lead, mercury, NSAIDs).

Signs and Symptoms

- ↓ urine output, ↑ BUN, ↑ creatinine, ↑ K, ↑ phosphate, ↓ calcium.
- *Metabolic acidosis:* ↓ pH, ↓ HCO_3, ↓ CO_2, ↑ BP, Kussmaul respirations, proteinuria, lethargy, confusion, headache, seizures, nausea, anemia due to ↓ erythropoietin, fluid excess (dyspnea, crackles, ↑ P, ↑ R, distended neck veins).

Treatment

- Epoetin alfa, calcium carbonate, antihypertensives.
- ↓ fluid, sodium, potassium intake; ↓ dietary protein to ↓ nitrogenous wastes.
- Hemo- or peritoneal dialysis; hemofiltration.
- ESRD: Renal transplant with immunosuppressives to prevent rejection.

Nursing Care

- Assess for S&S and adherence to diet; weigh before and after dialysis.
- *Hemodialysis:* Assess patency of graft/fistula if present (auscultate bruit, palpate thrill); avoid trauma to arm (no injections, IV, BP).
- *Assess for complications of hemodialysis:* ↓ BP, air embolism, dysrhythmias, atherosclerosis.
- *Peritoneal dialysis:* Instill and drain dialysate via gravity, assess for dyspnea (if present may need to drain fluid), periodically alternate client position.
- *Assess for complications of peritoneal dialysis:* Peritonitis, ↑ triglycerides, dyspnea, and hernias due to ↑ abdominal pressure.
- *Kidney transplant:* Explain need for lifelong immunosuppressive drugs → ↑ infection.
- *Assess for S&S of rejection:* Oliguria, ↑ T, ↑ creatinine, flank pain.

Fluid, Electrolyte, and Acid–Base Disturbances

Common Fluid Imbalances

Deficient Fluid Volume	Excess Fluid Volume
• **Hypovolemia**: Proportional loss of extracellular fluid volume and electrolytes. • **Dehydration**: Loss of only water with ↑ Na related to causes. • **Causes**: N&V, diarrhea, GI suction, sweating, ↓ fluid intake, diuretics, adrenal insufficiency. • **S&S**: ↓ weight, ↓ turgor, dry skin, muscle weakness/cramps, thirst, oliguria, postural hypotension, ↑ T, ↑ P, ↑ Hct, ↑ BUN, ↑ specific gravity. • **Nursing care**: Assess for S&S; ↑ oral fluids; give prescribed isotonic/hypotonic IV fluids, prescribed prn antiemetics or antidiarrheals.	• **Hypervolemia**: ↑ extracellular fluid volume. • **Causes**: Heart or renal failure, cirrhosis, ↑ Na, excess IV fluids, ↓ albumin, ↑ aldosterone secretion. • **Syndrome of inappropriate antidiuretic hormone (SIADH)**: ↑ ADH → water retention and ↓ Na due to disorders of CNS and lungs, infections, malignant tumors. • **S&S**: ↑ T, ↑ P, ↑ BP, edema, ascites, crackles, jugular vein distention, ↓ Hct, ↓ BUN. • **Nursing care**: Assess for S&S; teach ↓ Na diet, fluid restriction, Na content of over-the-counter meds; give prescribed diuretics and potassium supplements.

Common Electrolyte Imbalances

Hypokalemia	Hyperkalemia
• Potassium (K) <3.5 mEq/L. • **Causes:** Vomiting; diarrhea; gastric suction; diuretics; corticosteroids; diabetic ketoacidosis **(osmotic diuresis)**; starvation. • **S&S:** Muscle weakness, fatigue, N&V, ↓ GI motility, ↓ reflexes, abdominal distention, dysrhythmias, elevated U wave and flattened T wave on ECG. • **Nursing care:** Assess for S&S, teach about foods high in potassium (melon, apricots, bananas, milk, meat, citrus, grains). • **Meds:** Give prescribed IV or oral potassium supplements; if client is taking digoxin, assess for digoxin toxicity because hypokalemia increases this risk.	• Potassium (K) >5 mEq/L. • **Causes:** Kidney disease, burns, crushing injury, metabolic acidosis, adrenal insufficiency, excess potassium supplements. • **S&S:** Dysrhythmias; peaked T waves, flattened P waves, and wide QRS complexes on ECG; muscle weakness; flaccid paralysis; intestinal colic; diarrhea. • **Nursing care:** Assess for S&S; avoid salt substitutes and potassium-sparing diuretics with renal disease. • **Meds:** Give prescribed calcium gluconate IV to ↓ risk of cardiac dysrrhythmias; regular insulin with glucose and exchange resin (Kayexalate) to ↓ serum potassium level.

Hyponatremia	Hypernatremia
• Sodium (Na) <135 mEq/L. • **Causes:** Vomiting, diarrhea, gastric suction, sweating, excess intake of Na-free fluids, diuretics, renal disease, adrenal insufficiency, SIADH. • **S&S:** Muscle cramps; weakness; papilledema, headache, confusion, seizures due to ↑ ICP. • **Nursing care:** Assess for S&S; ↑ Na intake, give IVF (usually normal saline), ↓ fluids to 800 mL/daily as prescribed.	• Sodium (Na) >145 mEq/L. • **Causes:** Diarrhea, ↓ fluid intake, heat stroke, excess Na intake (near drowning in ocean, sodium bicarbonate, hypertonic NaCl). • **S&S:** Thirst; ↑ T; ↑ P; ↑ BP; dry, sticky mucous membranes; N&V; ↑ reflexes; restlessness; seizures. • **Nursing care:** Assess for S&S; give prescribed IVF (D_5W, hypotonic solution) and diuretics.

Continued

Hypocalcemia	Hypercalcemia
• Calcium <8.5 mEq/L. • **Causes**: Hypoparathyroidism, renal failure, malabsorption, ↓ albumin, ↓ vitamin D, alkalosis, pancreatitis, meds (loop diuretics, steroids, some antineoplastics, isoniazid [INH]). • **S&S**: Paresthesias, tetany, facial nerve twitching **(Chvostek sign)**, carpopedal spasm **(Trousseau sign)**, ↑ ST segment on ECG; confusion, seizures. • **Nursing care**: Assess for S&S; give prescribed calcium and vitamin D supplements; teach high-calcium foods (milk, salmon, green leafy vegetables, sardines).	• Calcium >10.5 mEq/L. • **Causes**: Immobility, bone cancer, hyperparathyroidism, meds (thiazide diuretics, lithium, excess calcium or vitamin D supplements). • **S&S**: Deep bone pain, flank pain due to renal calculi, constipation, vomiting, ↓ reflexes, ↑ urine calcium **(Sulkowitch test)**, osteoporosis, ↑ hyperparathyroid hormone (PTH) levels, ↓ PTH levels (with malignancy). • **Nursing care**: Assess for S&S; ↑ fluids; ↑ fiber; give prescribed IVF and meds (calcitonin, loop diuretic, bisphosphonate) to ↓ serum calcium levels.

Common Acid–Base Imbalances

Metabolic Acidosis	Metabolic Alkalosis
• Serum pH <7.35 and bicarbonate (HCO_3) <22 mEq/L. • **Causes:** ↑ acid (aspirin poisoning, lactic or ketoacidosis, uremia); ↓ HCO_3 (diarrhea, chlorides, diuretics); hypoproteinemia. • **S&S**: Headache, confusion, weakness, fruity breath, ↑ rate and ↑ depth of respirations **(Kussmaul respirations)**, N&V, dysrhythmias, coma. • **Nursing care:** Assess for S&S, give prescribed sodium bicarbonate, supportive care for underlying problem.	• Serum pH >7.45 and bicarbonate (HCO_3) >26 mEq/L. • **Causes**: Loss of acidic gastric secretions (vomiting, gastric suction), thiazide and loop diuretics, ↑ intake of sodium bicarbonate. • **S&S**: Paresthesias, muscle hypertonicity, tremors, ↓ rate and ↓ depth of respirations, dizziness, confusion, coma. • **Nursing care**: Assess for S&S; give prescribed NaCl fluids, KCl replacement, and H_2 antagonists.

Respiratory Acidosis	Respiratory Alkalosis
• Serum pH <7.35 and $Paco_2$ >45 mm Hg. • **Causes:** ↓ ventilation and CO_2 retention from pulmonary edema, pneumonia, acute respiratory distress syndrome, narcotic overdose, aspiration, emphysema, obstructed airway, neuromuscular disease, apnea. • **S&S**: SOB, ↑ P, ↑ R, ↑ BP, restlessness, disorientation, cyanosis, coma. • **Nursing care:** Assess for S&S; care for underlying cause (antibiotics, bronchodilators, thrombolytics); ↑ oxygenation (suction airway, Fowler position, mechanical ventilation).	• Serum pH >7.45 and $Paco_2$ <35 mm Hg. • **Causes:** Blowing off CO_2 due to hyperventilation or excess mechanical ventilation. • **S&S:** Deep, rapid breathing; ↑ P; paresthesias; light-headedness; dysrhythmias; ↓ LOC. • **Nursing care:** Assess for S&S; teach to breathe slowly; give prescribed sedative; ↓ rate and/or depth of ventilator settings as prescribed.

Integumentary Disorders

Burns

Thermal, electrical, or chemical trauma → tissue destruction; intensity and duration of heat determine depth of destruction; prognosis depends on location and % of total body surface area (TBSA) involved.

Extent of Burn

- *Rule of nines:* Body divided into sections by % to quickly assess TBSA involved; head and neck (9%), each arm (9%), anterior trunk (18%), posterior trunk (18%), each leg (18%), perineum (1%).
  - *Minor:* <15% TBSA; face, hands, feet, and genitals not involved.
  - *Moderate:* Partial thickness 15%–25% or full thickness <10%.
  - *Major:* Partial thickness >25%; full thickness >10%; burns of face, hands, feet, or genitals, other complications.

Depth of Burn

- *Partial-thickness (superficial):* Includes epidermis; may include top layer of dermis; erythema; pain; blanching with pressure.
- *Partial-thickness (deep):* Includes deeper layer of dermis; erythema; hypersensitive to touch/air; moderate to severe pain; moist blebs; blisters.
- *Full-thickness:* Extends through dermis and may involve underlying tissue; pale, white, or brown charred appearance **(eschar)**; edema; absence of pain in burned tissue but severe pain in surrounding tissue; burn odor.
- *Inhalation injury:* Facial burns, singed nostril hair, sooty sputum, voice change, blisters in mouth or throat, dyspnea.

Signs and Symptoms

- *Immediate resuscitative phase—first 48 hr:* Shock from pain and hypovolemia; fluid shift to interstitial and 3rd spaces; edema; adynamic ileus; shivering related to heat loss, anxiety, pain; altered mental state (hypoxia due to smoke inhalation, pain meds); ↑ Hct; ↓ WBC.
- *Acute phase—wk or mo until burn heals:* ↓ edema; necrotic tissue sloughs; granulation occurs in partial-thickness burns.
- *Rehabilitation phase—2 wk to several mo:* Flat, pink new skin becomes raised and hyperemic in 4–6 wk → altered contour and joint flexion and fixation **(contracture)** if not prevented; pain replaced by itchiness; mature healing of skin may take 6 mo to 2 yr.

Treatment

At Scene of Burn

- Extinguishing of flames.
- Maintenance of airway, breathing, circulation.
- First aid to prevent shock and respiratory distress.
- Application of cool water briefly to ↓ trauma and pain (avoid ice because it ↑ damage); sustained flushing of skin/eyes if chemical burn.
- Removal of clothing and jewelry to prevent constriction as edema progresses; leave adherent clothing because removal will ↑ tissue damage and pain.
- Burn covered with sterile/clean dressing (no ointments).

In Hospital

- May require intubation, O_2, mechanical ventilation.
- Assessment of extent and depth of burns; hemodynamic monitoring; ECG for electrical burns.
- Fluid replacement using an established formula (1/2 of fluids in 1st 8 hr and other 1/2 over next 16 hr).
- Prevention of electrolyte imbalance (hyper/hypokalemia and hyper/hyponatremia).
- IV opioids to ↓ pain; antisecretories to prevent Curling ulcer; tetanus toxoid; topical and systemic antibiotics.

- Operative debridement of full-thickness burns and temporary or permanent skin grafting; ReCell—a solution created from client's skin—is sprayed onto treatment area in clinical trials in U.S.
- Wound care; pressure garments to ↓ scars, splints to ↓ contractures.
- ↑ calorie and protein intake; vitamins and iron.

During Rehabilitation

- PT, OT, vocational education.
- Reconstruction surgery (cosmetic, functional).
- Counseling to manage ↓ function, disfigurement, economic burden, and return to work.

Nursing Care

Immediate Resuscitative Phase

- Maintain respirations and patent airway (suction, endotracheal tube, mechanical ventilator); place in Fowler position.
- Assess arterial blood gases, O_2 sat, breath sounds.
- Assess fluid shift from intravascular to interstitial space.
- Assess hourly urine output and for S&S of hyperkalemia.
- Encourage coughing and deep breathing; teach use of incentive spirometer.

Acute Phase

- Assess fluid shift from interstitial to intravascular space; assess for S&S of hypokalemia.

Rehabilitation Phase

- Continue assessing for infection and providing nutritional support until skin coverage is achieved.
- Protect new skin from injury; teach self-care and wound care.
- Reassure appearance will improve over time; refer to support group.

All Phases

- *Maintain fluid balance:* Assess for S&S of fluid shifts and edema; monitor daily weight, I&O, hemodynamic status; give prescribed oral fluids.
- *Maintain circulation:* Provide prescribed intravenous F&E and colloids; ensure urinary output ≥30–50 mL/hr, systolic BP ≥100 mm Hg, P ≤120 bpm.
- *Prevent infection:* Assess for S&S of infection (↑ T, ↑ WBC, wound bed and donor sites for purulent drainage, edema, and redness); use contact precautions; give prescribed systemic/topical antimicrobials/antibiotics; provide prescribed surgical aseptic wound care.
- *Manage pain:* Give pain meds before procedures and routinely; use distraction; teach imagery; use lifting sheet; keep room temperature 80°–85°F, humidity >40%; prevent drafts.
- *Maintain nutrition:* NPO initially; tube feedings or parenteral nutrition; high-calorie, high-protein diet with supplements when prescribed.

- *Provide emotional support:* Address fear, grief, altered role, body image; explain that edema will subside in 2–4 days; explain all care.
- *Maintain bowel function:* Gastric decompression (↓ N&V, aspiration, ileus formation); assess bowel function (bowel sounds, stool).
- *Ongoing care:* Assist with hydrotherapy, debridement, grafting; plan for rest; maintain mobility and prevent contractures (positioning, splints, ambulation, ROM); teach use of pressure garments and skin lubrication; ↑ self-care activities when able.

Hormonal Disorders

Addison Disease

- Adrenocortical disorder exhibited by ↓ secretion of adrenocortical hormones (glucocorticoids, mineralocorticoids, and androgens), which → ↓ stress response.
- Causes: Surgical removal of adrenal glands, autoimmune or idiopathic causes, abrupt cessation of steroid therapy, infection.

Signs and Symptoms

- Dehydration, ↓ serum glucose, weakness, diarrhea, confusion, ↓ BP, ↓ weight, bronze-colored skin.
- ↑ adrenocorticotropic hormone (ACTH), ↓ serum cortisol, ↓ 17-ketosteroids, ↓ 17-hydroxysteroids, ↑ K, ↓ Na.
- *Addisonian crisis:* Pallor or cyanosis, anxiety, ↑ P, ↑ R, ↓ BP due to acute stress (surgery, emotions, cold exposure, infection).

Treatment

- Glucocorticoid replacement (hydrocortisone or cortisone acetate); mineralocorticoid replacement (fludrocortisone); ↑ dose under stress to ↓ risk of Addisonian crisis.
- F&E replacement.

Nursing Care

- Assess for S&S of Addisonian crisis.
- Encourage ↑ protein and ↑ CHO diet with added salt.
- Hydrocortisone: Administer prescribed larger dose in a.m. (mimics circadian rhythm, ↓ side effects); assess fluid balance, daily weight; protect from infection due to masking of S&S.
- Fludrocortisone: Assess fluid retention, electrolyte imbalances; ↓ BP may indicate inadequate dose.
- Teach need for lifelong therapy, avoidance of stress, balance of rest and exercise, and use of medical alert band.

Cushing Syndrome

- Adrenocortical disorder exhibited by ↑ secretion of adrenocortical hormones (glucocorticoids, mineralocorticoids, and androgens), which → ↓ immune response; ↑ Na; fluid retention; ↑ serum glucose.
- Causes: Adrenal tumor or ↑ ACTH from pituitary, steroid therapy.

Signs and Symptoms

- Truncal obesity, thin extremities due to muscle wasting, buffalo hump and moon face due to fluid retention, acne, hirsutism, purple abdominal striae, ↓ libido, S&S of hypervolemia.
- ↑ serum cortisol, ↑ 17-ketosteroids, ↑ 17-hydroxysteroids, ↓ K, ↑ Na, ↓ ACTH (↑ ACTH if due to a pituitary problem), ↑ glucose.
- ↑ risk of infection, osteoporosis, psychosis.

Treatment

- Adrenalectomy or removal of pituitary tumor **(hypophysectomy)**, depending on cause.
- Adrenal enzyme inhibitors: Mitotane, ketoconazole.
- If resulting from steroid therapy, reduce steroids slowly.
- Treat complications such as DM, osteoporosis.

Nursing Care

- Assess for S&S.
- Encourage ↓ Na and ↑ K in diet as prescribed.
- Protect from infection and injury because of ↑ risk for fractures due to osteoporosis.
- Assess for effects of excessive adrenal inhibitors: fatigue, orthostatic hypotension, ↓ weight, dehydration, GI distress, shock; mitotane—assess for ↓ hepatic function.
- Administer meds or their reduction as prescribed.
- Encourage use of medical alert band.
- Provide emotional support for altered body image and labile mood.

Diabetes Mellitus (DM)

- *Normal glucose metabolism:* Blood glucose regulated by the hormones insulin and glucagon; glucose is stored as glycogen in liver and muscles or as fat in adipose tissue.
- *Action of insulin:* Secreted by beta cells in islets of Langerhans in pancreas; insulin decreases blood glucose by promoting its entry into cells.
- *Action of glucagon:* Secreted by alpha cells in pancreas as blood glucose falls; promotes release of glycogen from liver.
- *DM:* Decreased amount of insulin or ↓ response to insulin leads to ↑ blood glucose **(hyperglycemia)**.

Type 1

- 10% of clients with DM; beta cell destruction → little or no insulin for cellular metabolism of glucose; requires exogenous insulin.
- Associated with specific human leukocyte antigens; autoantibodies; viruses; presents at <30 yr of age.

Type 2

- 90% of clients with DM; ↓ sensitivity to insulin **(insulin resistance)** and ↓ secretion of insulin; may be controlled by diet, exercise, and hypoglycemics; may need insulin when stressed.
- Associated with obesity, genetics, inactivity, gestational diabetes; usually presents at >45 yr of age; increasing incidence in children.

Signs and Symptoms

- *The 3 Ps:* Polyuria, Polydipsia, Polyphagia (excessive urination, thirst, hunger).
- Fasting blood glucose >126 mg/dL, random blood glucose >200 mg/dL.
- >7% glycated Hb (Hb A_{1C}) indicates lack of glucose control over prior 3 mo; glycosuria.
- Risk for infection; ↓ healing; type 1—↓ weight; type 2—↑ weight.
- Long-term complications
  - *Microvascular changes:* Retinopathy, neuropathy, nephropathy.
  - *Macrovascular changes:* Peripheral vascular disease, ischemic heart disease, cerebral vascular disease.

Alterations in Blood Glucose Associated With DM

Hyperglycemia	Hypoglycemia
• Blood glucose >110 mg/dL. • **Causes**: Stress, omission of hypoglycemic med or insulin, excess food intake; develops over days. • **S&S**: Polyuria; thirst; dry, hot, red skin; blurred vision; confusion; ↑ P; ↓ BP; dehydration.	• Blood glucose <60 mg/dL. • **Causes**: Excess insulin or oral diabetic meds; ↑ exercise or ↓ food while taking antidiabetic meds; develops rapidly. • **S&S**: Nervousness; pallor; cool, clammy skin; ↑ P; tremors; slurred speech; seizure.

Alterations in Blood Glucose Associated With DM—cont'd

Hyperglycemic Hyperosmolar Nonketotic Syndrome (HHNS)	Diabetic Ketoacidosis (DKA)
• Serum glucose >600 mg/dL without ketonuria; associated with type 2 DM. • **Causes:** Stress (surgery, infection), ↓ hypoglycemic meds, ↑ food intake. • **S&S:** Hyperglycemia, no ketones in urine, no S&S of metabolic acidosis.	• Serum glucose >300–600 mg/dL; breakdown of fat to meet energy needs causes ketonuria; associated with type 1 DM. • **Causes:** Stress (surgery, infection); ↓ exogenous insulin; ↑ food intake; meds such as steroids. • **S&S:** Hyperglycemia, ketonuria, metabolic acidosis.
Somogyi Effect	**Dawn Phenomenon**
• Hypoglycemia ↑ release of epinephrine, corticosteroids, and growth hormone, causing rebound hyperglycemia; hyperglycemia at hours of sleep with hypoglycemia at 2 a.m. followed by rebound hyperglycemia later in a.m.	• Marked increase in insulin requirements between 6–9 a.m. compared to midnight–6 a.m.

Treatment

- Regular exercise to control weight and ↓ insulin resistance.
- Balance diet (50%–60% CHO, 20% protein, 20%–30% fat) based on glycemic food index; ↑ soluble fiber → slow glucose absorption.
- Insulin and/or oral hypoglycemics, pregabalin for neuropathy.
- Pancreatic or islets of Langerhans transplants.
- *DKA and HHNS:* IVF, rapid or short-acting insulin, eventual Na and K replacement.
- *Hypoglycemia:* 10–15 g of simple sugar followed by complex CHO and protein if conscious; glucagon injection or 50% dextrose IV if unconscious.
- *Somogyi effect:* Requires increased insulin adjustment.
- *Dawn phenomenon:* Requires decreased insulin adjustment.

Nursing Care

- *Assess for S&S of alterations in blood glucose:* Hyperglycemia, hypoglycemia, DKA, HHNS, Somogyi effect, and dawn phenomenon.
- Teach about foot care
  - Inspect daily for lesions.
  - Wash/dry between toes daily; wear seamless, square toe box, moisture-wicking socks; wear well-fitting shoes; avoid heat/cold.
- Encourage weight-control efforts and continued health-care supervision (certified diabetic educator, dietician, podiatrist, ophthalmologist).
- Provide emotional support.
- Teach self-monitoring of blood glucose.
- Teach S&S of alterations in blood glucose.
- Teach administration of meds (insulin injection, insulin pump).
- Explain need for medical alert ID.

Hypothyroidism

- *Primary hypothyroidism:* Autoimmune lymphocytic destruction **(Hashimoto thyroiditis)**, atrophy with aging, genetics, meds (iodides, lithium), toxic effect of hyperthyroidism therapy (thyroidectomy, ^{131}I).
- *Secondary hypothyroidism:* Hypothalamus and/or pituitary problems, causing ↓ thyrotropin-releasing hormone (TRH) or ↓ thyroid-stimulating hormone (TSH).

Signs and Symptoms

- ↓ VS; ↑ weight; dry, pale skin; brittle hair/nails; cold intolerance.
- Constipation, periorbital edema, anemia, enlarged tongue.
- Dull expression, apathy, lethargy.
- ↓ T_3, ↓ T_4, ↑ TSH, ↑ cholesterol, ↓ HDL, ↑ LDL.
- Severe hypothyroidism **(myxedema)** may cause coma.

Treatment

- Hormone replacement with levothyroxine.
- TSH levels are monitored as dose is ↑ to determine optimum dose.

Nursing Care

- Assess for S&S; explain that S&S ↓ with hormonal replacement.
- Teach to ↑ rest, measures to stay warm; ↑ fluids and fiber to ↓ constipation.
- Teach S&S of hyperthyroidism that may result from excessive hormonal replacement; hold med if P is ≥100 per min, report to primary health-care provider; see Nursing Care section in Hyperthyroidism, p. 189.
- Assess for toxic effects of meds especially CNS depressants due to ↓ metabolism.

Hyperthyroidism (Graves Disease, Thyrotoxicosis)

- Excessive production of thyroid hormones; T_3 (triiodothyronine) and T_4 (thyroxine); caused by stimulation of thyroid gland by circulating immunoglobulins; has an autoimmune component **(Graves disease)**; often precipitated by stress or infection, resulting in ↑ metabolic rate and sensitivity to catecholamines.
- Generally occurs between 20–40 yr of age; more common in females.
- Sudden, severe, life-threatening hyperthyroidism (**thyroid storm, thyrotoxic crisis**).
- Can precipitate osteoporosis, amenorrhea, heart failure.

Signs and Symptoms

- ↑ VS, ↑ BP, hunger, ↓ weight, diarrhea, enlargement of gland **(goiter)**.
- Fine hand tremors, nervousness, bulging eyes **(exophthalmos)**.
- ↑ sweating, flushed skin, heat intolerance.
- Increase in radioactive iodine uptake, T_3, and T_4; ↓ TSH; positive thyroid scan.
- *Thyroid storm/thyrotoxic crisis:* ↑ T, P >120 bpm, delirium, heart failure, coma.

Treatment

- Radioactive iodine (^{131}I) destroys thyroid cells.
- Propylthiouracil or methimazole to ↓ T_4; beta-blocker to ↓ heart rate.
- Subtotal thyroidectomy
- *Thyroid storm/thyrotoxic crisis:* O_2; antithyroid meds; hydrocortisone to ↓ conversion of T_4 to T_3; sedative to ↓ aggitation; cholestyramine to rapidly ↓ thyroid hormone levels.

Nursing Care

- Assess for S&S of thyroid storm/thyrotoxic crisis.
- Provide calm, cool environment; high-protein, high-calorie diet.
- Teach S&S of hypothyroidism that may result from treatment, see Nursing Care section in Hypothyroidism, p. 188.
- Administer eye care (drops, taping eyes shut when sleeping) for exophthalmos.
- *Radioactive iodine:* Use precautions for 6–8 hr to 3–7 days as prescribed (discard vomitus and excreta with multiple toilet flushes, avoid holding or hugging others, isolation from others).
- *Thyroid storm/thyrotoxic crisis:* Maintain prescribed hypothermia blanket; administer prescribed O_2 and meds.

Cardiovascular Disorders

Ischemic Heart Disease (IHD): Angina and Myocardial Infarction (MI)

Angina
- Fatty deposits in intima of coronary arteries precipitate inflammatory process → plaques **(atheromas)** → further obstruction of blood flow → chest pain due to myocardial ischemia.

Myocardial Infarction
- Rupture of atheroma → thrombus → severe ischemia and myocardial cell death.
- Other causes of MIs include ↓ myocardial O_2 supply (vasospasm, hemorrhage), ↑ O_2 demand (drug misuse such as cocaine; hyperthyroidism).

Risk Factors
- Aging, family history, race (African ancestry), gender (males more than premenopausal females).
- HTN, DM, metabolic syndrome (insulin resistance, abdominal obesity, abnormal lipid profile).
- Modifiable risk factors: Smoking, obesity, sedentary lifestyle.
- ↑ cholesterol, ↑ triglycerides, ↑ LDL, ↓ HDL, ↑ C-reactive protein.

Signs and Symptoms

Angina
- Chest pain/pressure may be substernal and/or radiate to neck, jaw, left arm.
- Precipitated by exertion (↑ O_2 demand); cold exposure (vasoconstriction); stress (SNS response); heavy meal (blood diverted to GI tract ↓ blood to heart).
- Pain subsides with rest and/or nitroglycerin.

Myocardial Infarction
- May have sudden chest pain (see Angina) unrelieved by rest/nitroglycerin.
- SOB; restlessness; cool, pale, clammy skin; diaphoresis; N&V.
- Pulse deficit if atrial fibrillation is present.
- *S&S in women:* Extreme fatigue, dizziness, indigestion, anxiety, insomnia.

Diagnostic Tests
- ECG: ↑ ST segment, inverted T wave, presence of Q wave.
- Echocardiogram: Identifies ↓ ventricular wall motion and ↓ ejection fraction.
- Coronary angiogram: Identifies extent of obstruction of coronary arteries.
- Myoglobin: ↑ in 1–3 hr, returns to baseline in 12 hr.

- Isoenzymes specific to heart muscle damage
  - Cardiac troponin T (cTnT): ↑ in 3–6 hr and remains ↑ 14–21 days.
  - Cardiac troponin I (cTnI): ↑ in 7–14 hr and remains ↑ 5–7 days.
  - CK–MB: ↑ in 4–6 hr, returns to baseline in 3 days.

Treatment

- ↓ cardiac demands and ↑ O_2 to cardiac muscle.

Angina

- ↓ modifiable risk factors; percutaneous coronary interventional (PCI) procedures (angioplasty, atherectomy, stent); coronary artery bypass graft (CABG).
- Meds: Nitroglycerin, beta-blockers, calcium channel blockers, antiplatelets, anticoagulants, antilipidemics, selective sinus node inhibitor.
- O_2 prn; cardiac rehab to ↑ exercise tolerance and quality of life.

Myocardial Infarction

- Provide O_2; morphine to ↓ pain.
- IV thrombolytics within 3 hr of start of MI to dissolve clot and ↓ damage.
- Meds: Opioid analgesics, beta-blockers, ACE inhibitors, stool softeners, anticoagulants.
- Emergency PCI; additional care (see Angina above).

Nursing Care

Angina

- Assess for S&S; balance activity/rest; give sublingual nitroglycerin and O_2 prn.
- Teach meds and to ↓ modifiable risk factors.

Myocardial Infarction

- Assess cardiac function (ECG, hemodynamic parameters, arterial blood gases); ↑ HOB; administer prescribed O_2 and opioid.
- Maintain IV access; avoid fluid overload; maintain BR until stable.
- Identify S&S of complications: HF, pulmonary edema, dysrhythmias, cardiogenic shock.
- **Percutaneous transluminal coronary angioplasty (PTCA)**
  - Assess for bleeding (restlessness, back pain due to retroperitoneal bleed, ↑ P, ↓ BP, ↓ Hb, ↓ Hct).
  - Apply pressure to insertion site; keep limb extended.
- Assess distal pulses of extremity.
- **Postoperative coronary artery bypass graft (CABG)**
  - Assess hemodynamic status, which may be ↑ due to HF or fluid overload or ↓ due to fluid deficit or bleeding.
  - Monitor ECG for dysrhythmias.
  - Assess pulses distal to vein harvest site if a lower extremity vein is used.
  - Assess urine output; notify primary health-care provider if <30 mL/hr because it may indicate ↓ renal perfusion.

- Monitor electrolytes and coagulation profile.
- Maintain chest tube drainage and ventilator as needed, then encourage incentive spirometer, splinting, coughing, and deep breathing.
- Provide for alternate communication while intubated.
- Provide pain control.
- Refer to cardiac rehab and Mended Hearts Club.

Hypertension (HTN)

- ↑ systolic blood pressure (SBP) and/or ↑ diastolic blood pressure (DBP).
- *Prehypertension:* SBP 120–139 mm Hg, DBP 80–89 mm Hg.
- *Stage 1:* SBP 140–159 mm Hg, DBP 90–99 mm Hg.
- *Stage 2:* SBP ≥160 mm Hg, DBP ≥100 mm Hg.
- *Hypertensive emergency:* ≥ SBP 180 mm Hg, DBP ≥110 mm Hg.
- *Contributing factors:* ↑ peripheral resistance; ↑ cardiac output, and/or ↑ blood volume due to ↑ renin, ↑ angiotensin, ↑ aldosterone, Na, and water retention, ↑ SNS activity, pregnancy, meds, renal disease.
- *Complications of HTN:* HTN → vascular changes → ventricular hypertrophy, heart failure, MI, kidney disease, retinopathy.
- *Preload:* Stretch of cardiac muscle fibers at end of diastole.
- *Afterload:* Resistance to ejection of blood from left ventricle.

Treatment

- Lifestyle modifications (see Nursing Care below).
- Meds such as diuretics, beta-blockers, alpha-blockers, ACE inhibitors, angiotensin II receptor blockers, calcium channel blockers, vasodilators, antilipidemics.

Nursing Care

- Assess BP and S&S of target organ damage (SOB, angina, ↓ vision, epistaxis, headache, edema).
- Teach health promotion: ↓ smoking, ↓ weight, ↓ alcohol intake, ↑ aerobic activity, ↓ stress.
- Teach balanced diet: Restrictions in Na, saturated fats, cholesterol; ↑ fruits, vegetables, whole grains, fish, poultry, nuts in diet.

Heart Failure (HF)

- Cardiac output insufficient due to ↓ ventricular filling or ↓ ventricular contraction.
- Decreased cardiac output stimulates SNS → ↑ cardiac workload and ventricular hypertrophy → ↓ renal perfusion.
- ↓ renal perfusion → renin/angiotensin response → vasoconstriction and ↑ aldosterone.
- ↑ aldosterone → Na and fluid retention → further ↑ cardiac workload.

- Pressure may ↑ in pulmonary circulation **(left-sided HF)** or in systemic circulation **(right-sided HF)**.
- Severe HF may → cardiomegaly, pulmonary edema, and/or cardiogenic shock.

Risk Factors

- Coronary artery disease; inflammation/infection of cardiac structures; damage to heart muscle from disease such as DM; alcohol/drug misuse; some chemotherapy meds.
- Structural disorders of valves (mitral regurgitation, aortic stenosis).
- Dysrhythmias such as rapid atrial fibrillation.
- ↑ cardiac demands related to HTN, anemia, thyrotoxicosis, fever, obesity.

Signs and Symptoms

- ↑ P, ↑ R, fatigue, dyspnea, restlessness, confusion, 3rd heart sound **(ventricular gallop)**, cardiomegaly, ↓ urine output.
- *S&S of systemic circulation congestion:* Ankle edema, anorexia, nausea, hepatomegaly, ascites, jugular vein distention.
- *S&S of pulmonary circulation congestion:* Crackles, cyanosis, frothy sputum.

Diagnostic Tests

- ↑ brain natriuretic peptide; ↑ *N*-terminal prohormone; these neurohormones are released in response to hemodynamic stress.
- Echocardiogram, chest x-ray to identify cardiomegaly.

Treatment

- Treat cause, O_2, ventricular pacing.
- ACE inhibitors to ↓ preload and ↓ afterload.
- Beta-blockers to counteract SNS overstimulation; ivabradine slows heart and ↑ cardiac perfusion.
- Diuretics to ↓ fluid overload, digoxin to ↑ cardiac output.
- Ventricular assist device or heart transplant in advanced stage.
- *Acute heart failure:* Intubation, mechanical ventilation, and positive end-expiratory pressure (PEEP) to ↓ hypoxia; diuretics; opioid; cardiac stimulant to ↑ cardiac output.

Nursing Care

- Assess apical pulse for galloping rhythm; radial pulse for rate, rhythm, volume; compare apical and radial pulses for pulse deficit; daily weight; breath sounds (crackles).
- Teach to ↓ smoking, ↓ weight, gradually ↑ exercise, ↓ Na in diet, ↑ potassium in diet (dried fruit, bananas, oranges, melon).
- ↑ HOB to ↓ venous return; give O_2; teach about meds.
- *Ivabradine:* Teach that med may cause fetal toxicity; use of effective contraceptives.

Anemia

- Features common to all types of anemia (see Anemia in Pediatrics Tab, p. 117, for iron deficiency, sickle cell, and β-thalassemia anemias).
- ↓ RBC due to blood loss, ↓ production or ↑ destruction of RBC: causes ↓ O_2- carrying capacity of blood, ↑ cardiac workload, HF.
- *S&S:* ↑ P, ↑ R, fatigue, weakness, pallor, confusion, ↓ Hb, ↓ Hct.

Treatment

Correction of cause; O_2; blood transfusions; meds depending on type of anemia.

Nursing Care

Assess for S&S; balance rest/activity; ↑ protein, fiber, and fluids; teach iron supplements cause black stools and constipation; give prescribed blood transfusions.

Microcytic Anemia

- ↓ iron due to ↓ dietary intake (vegetarians, teens); blood loss from GI bleeding (ulcers, cancer, inflammation) or menorrhagia; ↓ iron absorption after gastric surgery.
- *S&S:* Mean corpuscular volume (MCV) <80 fL; ↓ ferritin; ↓ serum iron; ↓ transferrin; inflammation of tongue **(glossitis)** and lips **(cheilitis)**; craving for ice, clay, starch, etc. **(pica)**.

Treatment and Nursing Care

Give prescribed oral iron with orange juice between meals (vitamin C and empty stomach ↑ absorption); dilute liquid iron, use straw, rinse mouth after (stains teeth); ↑ dietary sources of iron, such as raisins, eggs, meat (liver), green vegetables.

Macrocytic Anemia

- ↓ folate due to ↓ dietary intake, alcohol consumption; B_{12} deficiency due to lack of intrinsic factor **(pernicious anemia)**; ↓ folate absorption after gastric surgery or Crohn disease.
- *S&S:* MCV >100 fL; ↓ folate; ↓ B_{12} (Schilling test for pernicious anemia); sore, smooth, red tongue; diarrhea; neurological changes due to ↓ myelin (paresthesias, ataxia); screen for stomach Ca.

Treatment and Nursing Care

Give prescribed oral folic acid; IM B_{12}; teach to avoid alcohol; ↑ dietary sources of folic acid (green vegetables, liver, mushrooms).

Normocytic Anemia

- *Hemolytic anemia (HA):* RBC break down rapidly → ↑ bone marrow release of reticulocytes; examples include toxins that precipitate HA, sickle cell anemia, β-thalassemia.
- *Anemia in renal disease:* ↓ erythropoietin → ↓ RBC synthesis.
- *S&S:* MCV 80–100 fL; ↑ reticulocytes; jaundice due to Hb breakdown; hepatomegaly; S&S of acute hemolysis (↑ T, chills, abdominal and back pain, hemoglobinuria).

Treatment and Nursing Care

- *HA:* Depends on etiology.
- *Renal disease:* Administer prescribed iron, folate, recombinant erythropoietin.

Peripheral Artery Disease (Arterial Insufficiency)

Atherosclerosis → ischemia of extremities (↑ incidence in distal legs); ↓ sensation → ↑ risk of injury.

Risk Factors

- ↑ age, males, heredity, smoking, obesity, inactivity, HTN, hyperlipidemia, diabetes.

Signs and Symptoms

- Leg pain when walking relieved by rest **(intermittent claudication)**.
- Cool, pale, shiny leg with faint/absent pulse.
- ↓ hair on legs; thick, yellow toenails; ulcers on toes that may extend to dry gangrene.

Treatment

- ↓ risk factors.
- Anticoagulants to ↓ platelet aggregation; pentoxifylline to ↓ blood viscosity; vasodilators.
- Bypass grafts to ↑ blood flow.

Nursing Care

- Assess for S&S; administer prescribed meds.
- Position legs ↓ than heart; keep legs/feet warm (socks, blankets).
- Teach to ↓ smoking and exposure to cold; avoid constrictive clothing.
- Teach foot care: Inspect feet daily; wear shoes and socks and dry feet well to protect feet; apply prescribed dressings to ulcers.

Aortic Aneurysm

Weakness in vessel → protrusion and possible rupture.

Risk Factors
- Atherosclerosis, trauma, congenital weakness, infection, inflammation, HTN, smoking, family history.

Signs and Symptoms
- May be symptom-free; may be able to palpate a pulsating mass.
- Diagnosis confirmed with CT, MRI, sonogram.
- *Dissecting aneurysm:* Sudden severe chest pain extending to back, shoulder, epigastrium, abdomen; diaphoresis; ↑ P.

Treatment
- Surgical replacement with synthetic graft; fabric-covered stent **(endograft)**.
- Antihypertensives to ↓ BP and risk of extension or rupture.
- Smoking cessation, maintenance of healthy weight and diet, ↓ cholesterol level.

Nursing Care
- Assess BP; monitor Hb and Hct.
- Assess for sudden ↑ pain that may signal impending rupture.
- Teach to avoid activities that ↑ intra-abdominal pressure (sneezing, coughing, vomiting, straining at stool).
- Encourage smoking cessation, healthy diet, exercise program.

Deep Vein Thrombosis (DVT)

Virchow triad: Venous stasis, damage to vein, ↑ blood coagulation.

Risk Factors
- ↑ age, obesity, immobility, oral contraceptives, varicose veins, popliteal pressure, fractures.

Signs and Symptoms
- Lower extremity edema; ache in calf, calf pain on foot dorsiflexion **(Homan sign)**; Homan sign should not be elicited deliberately because it may cause a thrombus to become an embolus.
- ↑ P, dyspnea, chest pain if thrombus dislodges, causing a PE.

Treatment
- Thrombolytics, anticoagulants.
- Thrombectomy; insertion of vena cava filter to prevent PE.

Nursing Care
- *Prevention:* Provide prescribed antiembolism stockings or sequential compression device, encourage exercise, ↑ fluids, give prescribed prophylactic anticoagulant; teach ankle-pumping exercises and need to walk every 2 hr when traveling in car, train, or airplane.
- *Acute phase:* Maintain bedrest, elevate extremity, apply prescribed warm soaks, give prescribed anticoagulant.

Peripheral Venous Disease (Venous Insufficiency)

Incompetent valves and ↑ venous pressure → vein dilation; ↓ sensation →; ulcers around ankles and lower legs.

Risk Factors

- Varicose veins, thrombophlebitis, aging, smoking, inactivity (lack of muscle contraction).

Signs and Symptoms

- Leg edema, pain, fatigue, and heaviness that ↑ over day, varicose veins.
- Brownish pigmentation of legs **(hemosiderin deposition)**.
- Stasis ulcers with exudate around ankles and lower legs.

Treatment

- Positioning, compression therapy (Unna boot, Velcro wrap) to ↓ venous pressure; antibiotics for infection.
- Sclerotherapy; in 10% of clients—surgical ligation, repair, vein transplant.
- Surgical and nonsurgical debridement of necrotic tissue.

Nursing Care

- Elevate legs; apply elastic stockings before legs are dependent; teach to avoid constrictive clothing and crossing legs when sitting.
- Teach foot care: Inspect feet daily, wear shoes and socks, dry feet well (particularly between toes).
- Administer prescribed antibiotics; wound care for ulcers.

Respiratory Disorders

Features common to most respiratory disorders:

- ↓ ventilation due to obstruction or ↓ surface area for gas exchange.
- Results in ↓ O_2 to below physiological level **(hypoxia)** and ↑ CO_2 to an excessive level **(hypercapnia)** → ↑ $Paco_2$, ↓ arterial pH **(respiratory acidosis)**.

Signs and Symptoms

- ↑ P, ↑ R, fatigue, weakness, restlessness, confusion.
- Adventitious breath sounds, dyspnea, orthopnea, use of accessory muscles of respiration, ↓ pulse oximetry.

Treatment

- Based on cause; see various respiratory diseases.
- O_2, prophylactic influenza/pneumonia vaccines for those at ↑ risk.

Nursing Care

- Assess for S&S; ↑ HOB, administer O_2, prescribed meds.
- Teach to balance activity/rest; stop smoking.

Pneumonia

- Microorganisms from upper airway/blood, aspiration of food/gastric contents → inflammation.
- Alveoli fill with exudate and WBC **(consolidation)** → ↓ ventilation and ↓ diffusion of gases; aerosolized or droplet transmission.

Risk Factors

- ↑↓ age, smoking, immunosuppression.
- Winter (Streptococcal pneumonia); summer and fall (*Legionella*).

Signs and Symptoms

- ↑T and WBC, adventitious breath sounds, cough, sputum (character depends on organism).
- Chest x-ray indicates patchy or lobe consolidation or infiltrates.

Treatment

- Antibiotic regimen based on C&S results, O_2, bronchodilator, mechanical ventilation.
- Replacement of fluid losses due to ↑ T and ↑ R.

Nursing Care

- Assess for signs of respiratory distress: ↑ R, use of accessory muscles of respiration, dyspnea, ↓ LOC.
- Administer prescribed chest PT, ↑ fluids, O_2, meds.
- Teach how to prevent recurrence and ↓ transmission (hand hygiene, correct tissue disposal).
- Teach need to finish antibiotic regimen to ↓ recurrence and/or resistance.

Tuberculosis (TB)

- Infection of lungs caused by *Mycobacterium tuberculosis*; granulomas of bacilli become fibrous tissue mass **(Ghon tubercle)** that can calcify and become dormant or ulcerate and activate the bacilli; transmitted via inhalation of infected respiratory droplets.
- *Miliary TB:* Bacilli may travel to bone, kidneys, or brain.

Risk Factors

- ↓ immune response (HIV, steroids), crowded living conditions (prisons, long-term care facilities), debilitating physical conditions.

Signs and Symptoms

- Night sweats, ↓ weight, cough, hemoptysis.
- Positive PPD/Mantoux: 10 mm induration indicates immune response (exposure to but not necessarily the disease).
- Chest x-ray reveals active/calcified lesions; acid fast bacteria in sputum.

Treatment

- Combination of antituberculars for 6–12 mo.
- Prophylactic isoniazid for exposure.

Nursing Care

- Use airborne precautions during active disease.
- Teach need for long-term adherence to med regimen.
- Teach prevention of transmission: Frequent hand hygiene, use of disposable tissues, covering cough, use of separate eating utensils.

Chronic Obstructive Pulmonary Disease

- **Emphysema:** Alveolar wall becomes distended, inelastic, or destroyed → ↓ effective surface area for gas exchange, air trapping, ↑ residual volume.
- **Chronic bronchitis:** Bronchial tubes become inflamed causing reduced air flow.
- Both result in ↑ work to exhale; chronic hypercapnia (↑ $Paco_2$); may cause right-sided HF **(cor pulmonale)**.

Risk Factors

- ↑ age, smoking, secondhand smoke, inhaled pollutants, alpha-antitrypsin deficiency.

Signs and Symptoms

- *Emphysema:* Barrel chest, clubbing of fingers, cyanosis, pursed-lip breathing, use of accessory muscles of respiration; ↓ forced expiratory volume; ↑ residual lung capacity.
- *Chronic bronchitis:* ↑ mucus, SOB.

Treatment

- Smoking cessation, ↑ fluid intake to liquefy secretions.
- Steroids and bronchodilators.
- *Emphysema:* O_2 at less than 2 L/min because excessive exogenous O_2 ↓ the respiratory drive and results in ↓ breathing and ↑ CO_2 retention. Normally ↑ CO_2 stimulates breathing. With emphysema, there is chronic ↑ CO_2 and as a result, low O_2 stimulates breathing. In addition, the Haldane effect suggests that the adverse effects of ↑ O_2 are caused by the inability of oxygen-saturated hemoglobin molecules to transport CO_2. Both issues relate to CO_2 narcosis; lung volume reduction or lung transplant may be done for severe cases.
- *Chronic bronchitis:* Chest PT, postural drainage.

Nursing Care
- Maintain O_2 at ≤2 L; balance activity and rest.
- *Emphysema:* Teach diaphragmatic and pursed-lip breathing to extend exhalation and keep alveoli open.
- *Chronic bronchitis:* Assist with postural drainage; arrange chest PT by respiratory therapist.

Lung Cancer

- Altered DNA → altered cellular replication; may be primary or metastatic; primary lung cancer often metastasizes to lymph nodes, bone, brain.
- Types: Adenocarcinoma, small cell (oat cell), large cell (undifferentiated), squamous cell carcinoma.

Risk Factors
- Inhalation of carcinogens (tobacco smoke, asbestos, exposure to radon).
- Heredity, primary cancer at another site.

Signs and Symptoms
- Dry, chronic cough; hoarseness; ↓ weight; lymphadenopathy.
- Sputum positive for cytology.
- Chest x-ray and scans indicate lesion and possible effusion.
- Biopsy indicates source (primary or secondary).

Treatment
- Thoracentesis with chest x-ray before/after, lobectomy, pneumonectomy.
- Chemotherapy, radiation, palliative care to ↓ pain.

Nursing Care
- Lobectomy: Manage chest tubes.
- Pneumonectomy: Place on operative side to allow remaining lung to aerate.
- Chemotherapy: Manage side effects (see Nursing Care for Clients With Cancer or Experiencing Nontherapeutic Effects of Antineoplastic Therapies, p. 172).
- Thoracentesis: Assess respiratory status before/after (pneumothorax and subcutaneous emphysema are complications); support client in orthopneic position during procedure; tell client to hold breath during needle insertion; position on opposite side of insertion for 1 hr after.
- Support decision for hospice or palliative care.

Acute Respiratory Distress Syndrome (ARDS)

- Direct or indirect lung damage/disruption → inflammation → fluid movement into alveolar spaces and ↓ surfactant → atelectasis → hypoxia and ↑ dead space.
- Due to trauma, aspiration, shock, infection.

Signs and Symptoms

- Early: Dyspnea, anxiety, ↓ O_2 sat, ↓ Pao_2.
- Late: ↑ CO_2, cyanosis, lung infiltrate on x-ray.

Treatment

- Treat cause; mechanical ventilation and positive end—expiratory pressure (PEEP) keeps alveoli open.
- Steroids, interleukin-1 receptor antagonists, surfactant therapy.
- Sedatives or neuromuscular blocks to ↓ fighting the ventilator.

Nursing Care

- Assess for S&S, arterial blood gases, O_2 sat; suction airway.
- Client on a mechanical ventilator
  - Assess breath sounds: Absence indicates pneumothorax due to PEEP; unilateral aeration indicates endotracheal tube (ET) may be in 1 bronchi (usually right).
  - Maintain trach or ET cuff pressure seal to ensure full volume delivery.
  - Check ventilator settings and alarms; high-pressure alarm responds to obstruction due to mucus or tubing kinks; low-pressure alarm responds to ↓ cuff pressure or separation of tubing.
  - Provide alternate mode of communication.

Pneumothorax

- Disruption of lining of lung **(visceral pleura)** or lining of thoracic cavity **(parietal pleura)** permitting air **(pneumothorax)** and/or blood **(hemothorax)** into pleural space → lung collapse.
- Due to rib fracture, stab or gunshot wound, thoracentesis, emphysema.

Signs and Symptoms

- Sudden unilateral chest pain; air/blood in pleural space on x-ray.
- ↑ P, ↑ R, dyspnea, ↓ breath sounds on affected side, ↓ Pao_2.

Treatment

- O_2, chest tube/water seal drainage to reestablish negative pressure (pneumothorax—2nd anterior intercostal space, hemothorax—lower and more posterior space).

Nursing Care

- Assess for S&S; relieve pain.
- Assess water seal chamber fluid level (↑ on inspiration and ↓ with exhalation) and for bubbling in water seal chamber (continuous bubbling suggests air leak and absence suggests full lung expansion or blocked tube).
- Instruct client to exhale and bear down when removing chest tube, then apply occlusive dressing.

- *Subcutaneous emphysema:* Palpate around insertion site for crackles, which indicates air in subcutaneous tissue **(crepitus)**.

Asthma

See Asthma in Pediatrics Tab, pp. 112–113.

Musculoskeletal Disorders

Fractures

- Break in bone continuity from excessive force; traumatizes muscles, blood vessels, and nerves leading to inflammation and possible hemorrhage.
- Types of fractures
  - *Simple (closed):* Skin remains intact.
  - *Compound (open):* Fragments penetrate skin.
  - *Transverse:* Straight across.
  - *Oblique:* Angled across.
  - *Spiral:* Twists around shaft.
  - *Comminuted:* Multiple bone fragments.
  - *Compression:* Compressed bone mass.
  - *Depressed:* Bone fragments forced inward.
  - *Greenstick:* Break partially extends across and then along length; common in children.
  - *Pathological:* Less force than usual needed to break bone due to ↑ age; porous, brittle bones **(osteoporosis)**; metastatic or primary tumors.

Signs and Symptoms

- Pain, spasms, shortening of extremity, ecchymosis, swelling.
- Grating sound when moved **(crepitus)**; x-ray reveals fracture.
- ↓ mobility, deformity, paresthesias due to nerve damage.
- Bleeding; shock due to hemorrhage.
- *Fat emboli:* Dyspnea; ↑ VS; copious white sputum; crackles; ↓ mentation; buccal, conjunctival, and chest petechiae.
- *Compartment syndrome:* ↑ pressure within closed fascial compartment due to edema/bleeding → ↓ circulation → tissue hypoxia and tissue damage; peripheral neurovascular assessment reveals ↓ peripheral pulses, skin pallor and cool to touch, capillary refill more than 2–3 sec, ↓ motor/sensory function.

Treatment

- Closed reduction: Bone fragments aligned and stabilized with cast, splint, traction.
- Open reduction internal fixation (ORIF): Bone fragments stabilized with devices such as wires, pins, nails, rods, plates.
- Ultrasound device (Exogen) applied 20 min daily speeds bone healing.
- Total hip replacement: Surgical insertion of a prosthetic system with hardware for each surface of the joint.
- Vertebrae fracture: ↓ activity; back brace; bone reabsorption inhibitors, analgesics, antispasmodics; acrylic cement into collapsed vertebra **(vertebroplasty)**; spinal fusion.

Nursing Care

- Immobilize to ↓ trauma and pain; pain management.
- Elevate limb and notify health-care provider if neurovascular status is impaired.
- *Client with a cast:* ↑ limb on pillow; uncover to ↑ drying; handle with palms not fingertips until dry; encourage isometric exercise to ↓ atrophy; odor may indicate infection; use cast cover or plastic bag/wrap to keep it dry when bathing.
- *Client with traction:* Hang weights freely; maintain functional alignment; provide prescribed pin care for skeletal traction.
- *Client with external fixation device:* Observe for S&S of infection at pin sites; provide prescribed pin care; support limb when moving client; encourage use of nonrestrictive clothing.
- *Postoperative care for client after total hip replacement*
  - Manage pain: Prescribed patient-controlled analgesia and/or IM, Sub-Q, oral opioids.
  - Avoid displacement of prosthesis: Abduction pillow and high toilet seat/chair; avoid internal rotation or hip flexion >90°.
  - Prevent DVT: Prescribed anticoagulants, compression devices; avoidance of dorsiflexion, popliteal pressure.
  - Prevent atelectasis/pneumonia: Incentive spirometry; coughing and deep breathing.
- Postoperative care for client after spinal surgery: Log roll side to side every 2 hr; progress activity as prescribed.
- See Postoperative Nursing Care, p. 235.

Arthritis

Rheumatoid Arthritis (RA)	Osteoarthritis (OA)	Gouty Arthritis
• Immune response → inflammation, breakdown of collagen, synovial edema, pannus formation, narrowed joint space, bone spurs.	• Involves chondrocyte response → cartilage breakdown.	• Purine metabolism defect → ↑ serum uric acid → urate deposits that become porous stone **(tophi)**.
Risk Factors		
• ↑ in female.	• ↑ age, obesity, joint injury, repetitive use, congenital hip subluxation.	• Starvation, organ meat and shellfish intake, ↑ cell proliferation (leukemia, psoriasis), ↑ in males.
S&S		
• Acute bilateral inflammation of joints (hands, wrists, feet, and later other joints). • Pain unrelieved by rest; a.m. stiffness longer than 1 hr. • Deformities (ulnar drift, swan neck, Boutonniere deformity). • ↑ erythrocyte sedimentation rate (ESR), ↑ C-reactive protein, ↑ rheumatoid factor, ↑ antinuclear antibody (ANA); synovial fluid has complements and WBC. • Fatigue, anemia, ↑T, ↑ node size.	• Morning stiffness of hips, knees, cervical/lumbar spine, small joints of hands and feet for less than 1 hr; improves with activity. • Bony hypertrophy occurring in fingers **(Heberden, Bouchard nodes)**; if inflamed, they enlarge and are tender, joint spaces narrow, crepitus occurs with joint movement.	• Acute asymmetrical joint pain and inflammation. • Located most often in big toe but may affect ankle, knee, elbow, wrist, or fingers. • Tophi in periphery (outer ear, feet, hands, elbows, knees). • ↑ serum uric acid, uric acid crystals in synovial fluid, urate renal calculi and nephropathy.

Rheumatoid Arthritis (RA)	Osteoarthritis (OA)	Gouty Arthritis
Treatment		
• Meds: Steroids; NSAIDs; analgesics; disease-modifying antirheumatic drugs (DMARDs) such as hydroxychloroquine, leflunomide, sulfasalazine, methotrexate; biologic response modifiers that are genetically engineered to target a specific protein or cell related to inflammatory types of arthritis such as adalimumab, abatacept, tofacitinib. • Synovectomy; joint fusion or replacement.	• Meds: Glucosamine, chondroitin; NSAIDs such as celecoxib, piroxicam; tramadol for pain; topical capsaicin; knee-joint injections of hyaluronic acid; cortisone injections in joints. • Heat and cold therapy; PT. • Arthroplasty.	• Meds: Allopurinol and febuxostat to ↓ uric acid level; NSAIDs and colchicine for pain; corticosteroids. • ↓ intake of purines (organ meats) and alcohol. • ↑ fluid intake to ↓ renal calculi.
Nursing Care		
• Assess for S&S; balance rest/activity; provide or teach ROM; keep joints in functional alignment; apply prescribed heat or cold; • Give prescribed meds; implement nondrug pain relief measures; • Encourage ↓ weight; teach use of adaptive devices to ↑ independence; • Refer to Arthritis Foundation. • *Gouty arthritis:* Teach to avoid organ meats and alcohol.		

Neurological Disorders

Multiple Sclerosis

- Autoimmune response → formation of scattered sclerotic plaques on demyelinated axons → ↓ impulse conduction.
- Remissions and exacerbations with downward plateaus.
- Frequently affected areas: Optic nerves, cerebrum, brain stem, cerebellum, spinal cord.

Risk Factors

- Caucasian race 20–40 yr of age; female gender.

Signs and Symptoms

- Vary depending on nerves involved.
- *Charcot triad:* Intention tremor, nystagmus, scanning speech.
- Visual disturbances: Diplopia, visual field deficits.
- Fatigue, paresthesias, dysphagia, incoordination, slurred speech, spasticity, bladder dysfunction, emotional lability.

Treatment

- Disease-modifying therapy: Interferon beta-1a and -1b; glatiramer acetate; teriflunomide; alemtuzumab and daclizumab are monoclonal antibodies.
- Corticosteroids, antispasmodics.
- Palliative care: PT, OT.

Nursing Care

- Assess for S&S, balance activity/rest, provide cool environment.
- Ensure safe mobility: Wide base of support, assistive devices.
- Prevent pressure ulcers: Change position every 1–2 hr, skin care, pull sheet to ↓ shearing, pressure-relieving devices.
- Improve elimination pattern: Respond to urge, follow bowel and bladder toileting schedule, ↑ fiber and fluids, give prescribed ascorbic acid to acidify urine.
- Encourage PT, ↓ fat in diet; administer prescribed meds.
- Encourage expression of feelings, refer to National Multiple Sclerosis Society.

Seizures

- Sudden, abnormal electrical discharge from cerebral neurons → generalized seizures (affect both hemispheres) or partial seizure (start in one area of the brain).
- Secondary to cerebrovascular disease, head trauma, brain tumor, drug or alcohol withdrawal, hypoglycemia, high T in children.

Signs and Symptoms

Focal Seizures (Formerly Partial Seizures)

- **Simple:** Motor, sensory, or emotional disturbances; retains awareness.
- **Complex:** Lip smacking, chewing, fidgeting, other repetitive movements; impaired awareness.

Generalized Seizures

- **Tonic–clonic (formerly grand mal seizure)**
  - Intense muscle contractions (tonic phase); alternating with relaxation (clonic phase).
  - Often preceded by flash of light or specific noise **(aura)**.
  - Unconsciousness, shallow/absent breathing, bladder/bowel incontinence.
  - Confusion, drowsiness, and/or sleep following seizure.
- **Absence (formerly petit mal seizure)**
  - Abrupt, brief (3–5 sec) event; vacant, blank stare; unresponsive.
- **Myoclonic**
  - Short (few min) sporadic periods of muscle contractions.
- **Tonic**
  - Increase in muscle tone; loss of consciousness.
  - Autonomic changes for 30 sec to several min.
- **Atonic**
  - Sudden loss of muscle tone for several sec resulting in a fall.
- **Clonic**
  - Muscle contraction and relaxation lasting several min.
- **Status epilepticus**
  - Continuous tonic–clonic seizure activity for >30 min; life threatening.
- **Febrile**
  - Tonic–clonic seizure with T >101.8°F; most common in children; self-limiting.

Treatment

- Antiseizure agents, treatment of underlying cause (brain tumor, fever).

Nursing Care

- Assess seizure activity: Precipitating event, presence of aura, specific origin and progression of motor activity, length, client response.
- Identify presence of status epilepticus.
- Protect client: Ease to floor if out of bed, protect head, loosen clothes, do not insert airway or restrain client, position laterally if possible.
- Teach need to adhere to antiseizure therapy to maintain therapeutic levels; continue health-care supervision; wear medical alert band.

- Teach to avoid factors that may precipitate a seizure (flickering lights, alcohol, sleep deprivation, excessive exercise, emotional stress).
- Provide emotional support related to client's concerns (fear of seizure, stigmatization, incontinence during a seizure, inability to drive until condition is controlled); refer to Epilepsy Foundation of America.

Parkinson Disease

- Neuronal destruction of substantia nigra in basal ganglia → ↓ dopamine → neurotransmitter imbalance.
- Progressive degeneration; may lead to complete dependence.

Risk Factors

- Genetics, male gender, 50–60 yr of age, atherosclerosis.

Signs and Symptoms

- Pill-rolling motion of thumb against fingers **(resting, nonintention tremor)**.
- Propulsive, shuffling gait **(cogwheel gait)**; no arm swing; slow voluntary movement **(bradykinesia)**.
- Stooped posture, masklike facies, rigidity, monotone voice, dysphagia, constipation, incontinence, ↓ cognition.

Treatment

- *Antiparkinson agents:* Dopaminergics, anticholinergics, antivirals, dopamine agonist, MAO inhibitors.
- Deep brain stimulation; destruction of thalamus for tremor and globus pallidus for bradykinesia.
- Palliative care: PT, OT.

Nursing Care

- Maintain airway, suction as needed; give prescribed meds.
- Provide safe mobility: Wide base of support, assistive devices, encourage to walk erect and take longer steps, ride stationary bicycle, balance activity and rest.
- Provide warm baths and active ROM to ↓ rigidity; splints to ↓ contractures.
- Promote bowel elimination: ↑ fluids, ↑ roughage, raised toilet seat.
- Promote nutrition: Assistive devices, bite-size pieces, thicken liquids.
- Provide emotional support: ↑ expression of feelings; refer to National Parkinson Foundation.

Neurological Disorders With Respiratory Insufficiency

Myasthenia Gravis	Guillain-Barré Syndrome	Amyotrophic Lateral Sclerosis (ALS; Lou Gehrig Disease)
• Autoimmune response → antibody attachment to acetylcholine receptor sites causing destruction of acetylcholine → ↓ impulse transmission → muscle weakness that worsens with activity and improves with rest; remissions and exacerbations.	• Autoimmune response → ascending peripheral nerve myelin destruction → ↓ ability to transmit impulses. • Schwann cells eventually produce myelin → recovery, but may take 2 yr and leave residual deficits.	• Cause unknown; possible autoimmune response or excess nerve stimulation by glutamate → progressive loss of upper and lower motor neurons → lack of muscle stimulation → progressive atrophy. • Life expectancy about 3–5 yr.
Risk Factors		
• Females, 20–40 yr of age; males, 60–70 yr of age. • Evidence of familial inheritance.	• Vaccination, recent infection, recent surgery.	• Males, 50–60 yr of age. • Evidence of familial inheritance.

Continued

Myasthenia Gravis	Guillain-Barré Syndrome	Amyotrophic Lateral Sclerosis (ALS; Lou Gehrig Disease)
S&S		
• Double vision **(diplopia)**, eyelid droop **(ptosis)**, snarl **(myasthenic smile)**, voice change **(dysphonia)**, difficulty swallowing **(dysphagia)**, temporary ↑ in muscle strength after IV Tensilon **(Tensilon test)**. • **Myasthenic crisis:** Weakness, aphagia, respiratory failure.	• Ascending symmetrical weakness/paralysis, areflexia, paresthesias; respiratory paralysis; aphagia; autonomic nerve dysfunction → labile P and BP rates.	• Fatigue, weakness, impaired coordination, muscle twitching **(fasciculations)**, nasal-sounding voice, ↑ deep tendon reflexes, dysarthria, dysphagia, dyspnea.
Treatment		
• Anticholinesterase agents, steroids, plasmapheresis, immunoglobulin, thymectomy to ↓ antibodies.	• IgG IV, O_2, plasmapheresis, tracheostomy and mechanical ventilation.	• Riluzole, a glutamate antagonist, may prolong life; antispasmodics (baclofen); enteral feedings; mechanical ventilation.

Nursing Care

- Support respirations: Assess respiratory status and O_2 sat; Fowler position; suctioning; chest PT; incentive spirometer; maintain ET tube, tracheostomy, mechanical ventilator if present.
- Prevent DVT and PE: ROM; prevent popliteal pressure; provide sequential compression devices and anticoagulant as prescribed.
- Prevent pressure ulcers: Reposition every 1–2 hr, skin care, pull sheet to ↓ shearing, pressure-relieving devices.
- Support independence; OT; PT.
- Support nutrition: Assess weight; assist with oral intake and prevent aspiration (↑ HOB, feed slowly, use thickening product); provide prescribed parenteral or enteral feedings.
- Recognize LOC and mental status are not affected but may be unable to speak; devise alternate means of communication; speech therapy.
- Refer to MG Foundation, GB Foundation, or ALS Association.
- **Nursing care for clients with myasthenia gravis**
  - Distinguish between myasthenic and cholinergic crises; both cause respiratory muscle weakness, difficulty swallowing **(dysphagia)**, and difficulty speaking **(dysarthria)**.
  - Give prescribed rapid-acting anticholinesterase (improves symptoms of myasthenic crisis and intensifies symptoms of cholinergic crisis).
  - Give meds at precise times and schedule meals at peak action; provide rest periods.

Brain Attack (BA)/Cerebrovascular Accident (CVA)

- Irreversible neurological deficit caused by cerebral ischemia.
- Caused by embolus, thrombus, subarachnoid or intracerebral bleeding.

Risk Factors

- Transient ischemic attack (TIA) in which deficits last <24 hr; may precede BA.
- ↑ age, male gender, ↑ BP, DM, cardiac disease, hyperlipidemia.
- African heritage, obesity, smoking, oral contraceptives.

Signs and Symptoms

- Based on location/extent of damage; indicated by CT scan, MRI, cerebral angiogram.
- ↑ *intracranial pressure (ICP):* Headache, restlessness, ↓ LOC, ↑ systolic BP, widening pulse pressure, ↑ T, ↓ P, ↓ R, vomiting, vision problems, unilateral pupil changes, seizures.
- *Posturing:* Arms extended and turned in **(extension, decerebrate)**, due to disruption in midbrain and brain stem; arms flexed, legs internally rotated **(flexion, decorticate)**, due to disruption in cerebral cortex.

- *Motor:* Unilateral weakness **(hemiparesis)** or unilateral paralysis **(hemiplegia)** on side of body opposite to affected side of brain; difficulty swallowing **(dysphagia)**.
- *Bowel/bladder:* Constipation; urinary frequency and urgency; incontinence.
- *Sensory:* Unilateral paresthesia, loss of 1/2 visual field **(hemianopsia)**; ↓ proprioception.
- *Communication:* ↓ articulation **(dysarthria)**; difficulty communicating thoughts in words **(expressive or Broca aphasia)**; difficulty understanding communication **(receptive or Wernicke aphasia)**.
- *Cognitive/emotional:* Lability of mood, ↓ memory, ↓ attention span, ↓ judgment.

Treatment

Prevention

- ↓ weight, ↓ fat in diet, smoking cessation.
- Antihypertensives for HTN, anticoagulant for atrial fibrillation (AF), glucose control for DM.
- Carotid endarterectomy.

Acute phase

- *Ischemic BA:* Thrombolytic therapy within 3 hr; anticoagulants; mechanical clot removal; angioplasty; stents.
- *Hemorrhagic BA:* Antidote if on anticoagulant; meds to ↓ ICP, ↓ BP, prevent vasospasm; surgery to remove blood, repair vessel.
- Steroids to ↓ ICP due to cerebral edema.
- PT, OT, speech therapy, NGT feedings if necessary.

Rehabilitation phase

- Multidisciplinary depending on needs.

Nursing Care

- **Teach public awareness of S&S (FAST): F**ace—ask to smile, does one side of face droop; **A**rms—ask to raise both arms, is one arm unable to raise up; **S**peech—slurred or strange; **T**ime—call 911 immediately with any of these signs.
- Assess for S&S, balance activity/rest, maintain low semi-Fowler position to ↓ ICP.
- Employ seizure precautions: Bed in ↓ position, quiet environment, pad side rails.
- Prevent aspiration: Suction to maintain patent airway; feed slowly; ensure mouth is empty between each mouthful and at end of meal; thicken liquids; ↑ HOB when giving prescribed enteral tube feedings.
- Maintain mobility/prevent contractures: ROM, position changes, splints.
- Prevent DVT: Give prescribed anticoagulants, ↓ popliteal pressure, ROM, sequential compression devices, leg exercises.

- Prevent pressure ulcers: Position change every 1–2 hr, skin care, pull sheet to ↓ shearing, pressure relief devices.
- Promote communication: Use picture board, simple sentences with visual clues for receptive aphasia, have patience and avoid completing client's message for expressive aphasia.
- Support elimination: Respond to urge; bowel and bladder training.
- Involve client with planning; accept emotional lability and grieving for losses.

Spinal Cord Injury

- Injury due to contusion, compression, laceration, transection.
- Edema and bleeding → ischemia → ↑ injury.
- Frequently affects C5–7, T12–L1.

Risk Factors

- <30 yr of age; >60 yr of age; risky behavior; male gender.
- Automobile or diving accident, violence, falls, contact sports, tumors, disk degeneration, metastasis to vertebrae.

Signs and Symptoms

- Varies on level of injury; CT scan, MRI, x-ray indicate level.
- *Spinal shock:* Flaccid paralysis; loss of sensation and reflexes below injury; loss of bowel and bladder function.
- *Neurogenic shock:* ↓ BP, ↓ P, inability to sweat due to ↓ autonomic nerve activity.
- *Paralysis:* Depends on level of injury; all four extremities **(quadriplegia)**; both legs **(paraplegia)**.
- *Bladder dysfunction*
    - *Spastic bladder:* Empties automatically when detrusor muscle is stretched; occurs with injury above conus medullaris.
    - *Flaccid bladder:* Atonic bladder distends and periodically overflows but does not empty; occurs with injury at or below conus medullaris (around L1 and L2 vertebra).
- *Autonomic hyperreflexia*
    - Exaggerated SNS response with cord injury ≥T6.
    - Mainly due to bladder or bowel distention.
    - Headache, ↑ BP, ↓ P, “goose bumps” **(piloerection)**, nasal congestion, diaphoresis, nausea.
- *Respiratory paralysis:* Lack of voluntary breathing with injury above C3–4.

Treatment

- Stabilize head, neck, and spine on backboard for transport.
- IV corticosteroids to ↓ cerebral edema, antispasmodics, pain meds.
- Respiratory support due to paralyzed or weak intercostal muscles.
- Surgery to ↓ compression, correct alignment, ↑ spine stability.
- Traction with skeletal tongs or halo device.
- NGT for gastric decompression due to paralytic ileus.
- Urinary retention catheter to ↓ bladder distention.
- Multidisciplinary rehabilitation (RT, PT, OT, vocational education).

Nursing Care

- Identify and treat autonomic hyperreflexia: ↑ HOB; loosen clothing; avoid cutaneous stimulation; ensure empty bladder; catheterize to ↓ urinary distention prn; remove fecal mass after application of anesthetic ointment prn.
- Use American Spinal Injury Association scale to determine extent of motor and sensory dysfunction.
- Assess R, P, O_2 sat, ABGs; encourage coughing and deep breathing; maintain hydration; arrange for chest PT.
- Prevent DVT and PE: Assess calf and thigh circumference; give prescribed anticoagulants; use sequential compression devices; avoid popliteal and calf pressure.
- ↓ spasticity and prevent contractures: Use ROM, splints to ↓ footdrop, trochanter rolls to ↓ external hip rotation; give prescribed antispasmodics.
- Maintain skin integrity: Change position frequently (teach to shift weight if able); provide hygiene and back rub; provide special bed, mattress, chair cushion; ↑ protein and vitamin C in diet.
- Provide pin site care with halo traction: Cleanse with prescribed solution; apply prescribed topical antibiotic.
- Promote fecal elimination: ↑ fluid and fiber intake; assist with bowel training; perform digital stimulation of rectum after meal.
- Promote urinary elimination: Use Credé maneuver; cutaneous stimulus to instigate urination (pull pubic hair, stroke inner thigh); intermittent catheterization if prescribed.
- Support independence: Modern wheelchair, voice-controlled electronic aids, devices to accomplish daily tasks, OT, PT.
- Involve client with planning; assist with coping with losses; discuss sexual concerns, residence, marriage, employment, education.

Morbid Obesity

- ≥100 lb more than ideal body weight, body mass index (BMI) ≥40.
- Causes: Inactivity, unhealthy diet, dysfunctional eating habits.
- ↑ risk for cardiovascular disease, arthritis, asthma, bronchitis, DM, impaired body image, ↓ self-esteem, depression.

Treatment

- Weight-reduction diet, behavior modification, exercise, counseling.
- Bariatric surgery if conservative treatment is unsuccessful (gastric bypass, gastric sleeve, vertical banded gastroplasty).
- After surgery ↑ risk for peritonitis, obstruction, atelectasis, pneumonia, thromboembolism, nutritional deficiencies, metabolic disturbances due to N&V.
- Antisecretories; vagal nerve blockade with implantable device that blocks sense of hunger during waking hr.

Nursing Care

- Support weight loss, diet modification, exercise regimen; encourage participation in support group.
- **Provide postoperative care**
  - NPO; 6 small feedings daily as prescribed (600–800 calories total) when bowel sounds return; ↑ oral fluids to ↓ risk of dehydration.
  - Assess for bleeding, peritonitis, thromboembolism, F&E imbalances.
  - Teach to eat small amounts slowly and chew completely to prevent vomiting and painful esophageal distention.
  - Provide emotional support (body image, dietary restrictions, need for body contouring surgery if desired).

Gastroesophageal Reflux Disease (GERD) and Hiatal Hernia

	Pathophysiology and Etiology	Signs and Symptoms	Treatment
GERD	• Gastric contents enter esophagus, causing inflammation. • May cause a precancerous condition **(Barrett esophagus)**; esophageal stricture. • Related to ↓ tone of lower esophageal sphincter (LES), obesity, hiatal hernia, pregnancy.	• Heartburn **(pyrosis)**, chest pain, sore throat, hoarseness, wheezing, dysphagia. • Acidic esophageal pH. • Endoscopy reveals tissue damage; barium swallow shows impaired silhouette of esophagus and stomach.	• Meds: Proton pump inhibitors, H_2 receptor blockers, antacids, cholinergics. • Surgery to tighten esophageal fundus.
Hiatal Hernia	• Part of stomach slides upward into thoracic cavity; may cause reflux, obstruction, hemorrhage. • Related to obesity, congenital weakness, pregnancy, female gender.	• May be asymptomatic. • Sense of fullness, regurgitation, pyrosis, dysphagia, nocturnal dyspnea. • Evident in barium swallow.	• Paraesophageal hernias may require emergency surgery to ↓ restricted blood flow. • Meds: See Treatment under GERD.

Nursing Care

- Assess for S&S; support weight control.
- Teach to have small, frequent, low-fat meals; drink fluids between meals; remain upright 1 hr after meals.
- Teach to ↑ HOB to prevent nighttime distress.
- Advise to avoid tight belts and waistbands and to avoid chocolate, caffeine, alcohol, and peppermint, which ↓ LES tone and to continue prescribed meds.

Peptic Ulcer Disease and Gastric Carcinoma

Peptic Ulcer Disease (PUD)

Etiology and Pathophysiology	Risk Factors	S&S	Treatment
• ↑ pepsin, ↑ HCl acid or ↓ tissue resistance to acid → gastric or duodenal ulcers. • May → hemorrhage, perforation, or peritonitis.	• *H. pylori*, NSAIDs, alcohol, stress, smoking, Zollinger-Ellison syndrome (↑ HCl).	• Gnawing epigastric pain. • Duodenal ulcer pain occurs 2–3 hr after meals and is relieved by food. • Gastric ulcer pain occurs <1 hr after meals and is relieved by vomiting.	• Proton pump inhibitors, H_2 receptor blockers, antacids, sucralfate or misoprostol to protect tissue that lines stomach and small intestine, antibiotics for *H. pylori*. • Surgery: Partial gastrectomy, vagotomy, pyloroplasty for perforated or bleeding ulcer.

Gastric Carcinoma

Etiology and Pathophysiology	Risk Factors	S&S	Treatment
• Generally caused by adenocarcinoma, which can metastasize to liver, bone, pancreas, or esophagus before diagnosis.	• Smoked food, pernicious anemia, gastric ulcers, *H. pylori*, smoking. • Japanese descent. • Male.	• May be asymptomatic. • Full after small meal, ↓ weight, stomach pain, N&V, heartburn. • Biopsy identifies cancer cells. • Bone and liver scans identify metastasis.	• Gastrectomy, radiation, monoclonal antibodies, chemotherapy. • Tumor markers used to check progress (carcinoembryonic antigen, CA19-9).

Nursing Care

- Assess VS; note amount of coffee ground–like or frank bloody emesis or melena; assess for S&S of shock.
- Manage NG tube and normal saline lavage for bleeding.
- Assess for GI perforation: ↑ P, ↓ BP, abdominal pain, rigid boardlike abdomen, diaphoresis.
- **Dumping syndrome may occur after gastrectomy**
  - Hypertonic gastric contents move rapidly into intestine → shift of intravascular fluid into intestine causing ↓ peripheral vascular resistance, visceral pooling of blood, and reactive hypoglycemia.
  - Results in ↑ P, ↓ BP, diaphoresis, fainting.
  - Teach to not drink fluid with meals; eat small, frequent meals; avoid simple CHO; recline 1 hr after meals.

Lower GI Disorders

Inflammatory Bowel Disease (IBD)

Regional Enteritis	Ulcerative Colitis	Diverticulosis and Diverticulitis	Colorectal Cancer
• Crohn disease affects distal ileum and colon. • Mucosal thickening with discrete ulcers. • May → fissures and abscesses that → thick walls and narrow lumen.	• Affects colon and rectum. • Superficial ulcerations cause edema, bleeding; abscesses → thick walls and narrow lumen; ↑ risk of colon cancer.	• Pouchlike herniations in muscle layer of colon **(diverticulosis)**. • Trapped food or feces cause inflammation **(diverticulitis)** that may lead to bleeding, obstruction, perforation, and/or peritonitis.	• Adenocarcinoma of epithelial lining invades surrounding tissue by direct extension into lumen → colon narrowing and ulcerations, or metastasis via blood or lymph to other sites.
Risk factors Genetics (Caucasian, Eastern European Jewish heritage), young adults, smoking.	**Risk factors** Genetics (Caucasian, Eastern European Jewish heritage), 30–50 yr of age.	**Risk factors** ↑ age, genetics, lack of fiber, constipation, obesity, smoking, meds (steroids, opioids, NSAIDs).	**Risk factors** Polyps, IBD, ↑ age, genetics (African American); ↑ fat, ↑ protein, ↓ fiber in diet.

<table>
<tr><th>Regional Enteritis</th><th>Ulcerative Colitis</th><th>Diverticulosis and Diverticulitis</th><th>Colorectal Cancer</th></tr>
<tr>
<td>S&S
Right lower quadrant (RLQ) cramping pain after meals, ↑ T, ↓ weight, malnutrition, severe diarrhea, rectal bleeding.</td>
<td>S&S
Left lower quadrant (LLQ) abdominal cramps, ↓ weight, rectal bleeding, diarrhea.</td>
<td>S&S
LLQ abdominal pain, ↑ T, ↑ WBC, fatigue, N&V, constipation, CT scan confirms diagnosis.</td>
<td>S&S
Change in bowel habits, ribbon or pencil-shaped stool, ↓ weight, rectal bleeding, cramps, gas, abdominal pain, fatigue.</td>
</tr>
<tr>
<td colspan="2">Treatment
• Meds: Antidiarrheals; antispasmodics; anti-inflammatories; immune system suppressors; antibiotics; pain relievers; iron, calcium, vitamin D and B_{12} supplements.
• Exacerbation: NPO, TPN, IVF; then rest bowel with ↓ residue, ↑ protein, ↑ calorie diet.
• Colectomy with ileoanal anastomosis, ileostomy, continent ileostomy (Kock pouch) if needed.
• Remission: Maintain balanced diet avoiding foods that aggravate GI mucosa; bulk laxatives to ↓ diarrhea with Crohn disease.</td>
<td>Treatment
• Meds: Antibiotics, antispasmodics, acetaminophen for pain.
• Exacerbation: NPO to liquid then to ↓ residue diet until inflammation subsides.
• Temporary colostomy or colon resection if needed.
• Remission: Fluids, dietary fiber and bulk laxative to prevent constipation and ↓ intraluminal intestinal pressure.</td>
<td>Treatment
• Chemotherapy: 5-Fluorouracil, capecitabine, irinotecan, oxaliplatin.
• Hemicolectomy or abdominal perineal resection with colostomy.
• Radiation.
• Targeted therapy: Antiangiogenic agent; monoclonal antibodies.
• Monitor carcinoembryonic antigen and CA 19-9 to mark tumor and response to treatment.</td>
</tr>
</table>

Nursing Care for Clients With Lower GI Disorders

- Assess for S&S, bowel sounds.
- Assess for S&S of perforation/peritonitis: Rigid boardlike abdomen, diaphoresis, ↑ T, ↑ P, ↓ BP.
- Assess stool shape and consistency; blood in stool **(frank blood, melena)**.
- Support coping with disease chronicity; teach diet.

Provide Preoperative Care

- Provide prescribed liquid diet for 48 hr; prescribed antibiotics to ↓ intestinal flora, laxatives and enemas before surgery to empty bowel.

Provide Postoperative Care

- Assess VS, breath and bowel sounds; maintain nasogastric decompression until peristalsis resumes, then advance diet as prescribed; teach to avoid gas-forming foods; provide prescribed IVs for F&E balance and meds; perform wound care (irrigations or sitz baths for hygiene, comfort, packing removal).
- Prevent pneumonia: Teach coughing, deep breathing, use of incentive spirometry.
- Prevent DVT: Teach ankle pumping, early ambulation, apply prescribed sequential compression devices, avoid pressure behind the popliteal space.

Provide Care for the Client With a Colostomy

- Assess stoma: Pink/brick red is normal; pale, purple, or black indicates ischemia; notify primary health-care provider if stoma is ischemic.
- Assess bowel sounds, distention, character/amount of stool that usually begins in 3–6 days.
- Determine consistency of stool; intestinal site determines nature of stool (ileostomy constantly drains liquid stool; sigmoid colostomy stool usually is formed).
- Apply appliance with 1/8–1/4 inch clearance around stoma to avoid stoma constriction or excess skin exposure to stool.
- Clean area with soap and water; use prescribed protective barrier and antifungal agent on skin under appliance.
- Empty appliance when 1/2 full to ↓ leakage.
- Irrigate distal colostomy with 105°F water at same time daily to regulate elimination.
- Refer to United Ostomy Association or enterostomal therapist.

Disorders of Accessory Organs of Digestion

Cholecystitis

- Impaired bile flow → gallbladder inflammation **(cholelithiasis)**, distention, and autolysis leads to gangrene or perforation; blocked bile flow may → obstructive jaundice.
- Usually due to gallstones; bile duct blockage; tumor.

Risk Factors

- 4 Fs: Fair, Fat, ≥ Forty yr of age, Female.
- Rapid weight loss, estrogen therapy, multiple pregnancies, cirrhosis, DM.

Signs and Symptoms

- RUQ abdominal pain usually radiating to back subscapular area especially after high-fat meal.
- N&V, ↑ T, rebound tenderness, obstructive jaundice, yellow skin and sclera, dark urine, clay-colored stools.
- Signs of bleeding due to decreased fat digestion causing ↓ absorption of the fat-soluble vitamin K.
- ↑ WBC, ↑ serum bilirubin, ↑ alkaline phosphatase, ultrasound identifies gall stones, CT scan identifies presence and location of pathology.

Treatment

- NPO, IV fluids, antibiotics, pain meds.
- Laparoscopic or abdominal removal of gallbladder **(cholecystectomy)**.

Nursing Care

- Assess for S&S.
- Administer prescribed preoperative vitamin K, analgesics.
- Postoperative: Teach low-fat diet, use of incentive spirometer, coughing and deep breathing (client may be reluctant to deep breathe because surgical trauma is near diaphragm), provide prescribed antibiotic and analgesic, encourage maintenance of a healthy weight.
- Maintain T-tube drainage if bile duct explored; T tube is removed when ductal edema subsides indicated by stool regaining brown color.

Hepatitis

- Inflammation of liver due to infection, parasitic infestation, alcohol, toxins, meds.
- *Hepatitis A (HAV)* and *E (HEV):* Spread via fecal-oral route; due to ↓ sanitation and eating shellfish from contaminated water.
- *Hepatitis B (HBV), C (HCV),* and *D (HDV):* Spread via contaminated blood and body fluids; sexual contact; shared contaminated sharps (needles, razors).

Risk Factors

- Health-care professionals, multiple sexual partners, intravenous drug users.
- Hemophiliacs due to frequent transfusions of clotting factors.
- 30% have unidentifiable sources.

Signs and Symptoms

- May be asymptomatic.
- *Preicteric stage*: Flulike symptoms, RUQ discomfort.
- *Icteric stage:* N&V, anorexia, malaise, jaundice, presence of specific hepatitis antigens and antibodies, ↑ aspartate aminotransferase (AST), ↑ alanine aminotransferase (ALT), gamma-glutamyl transpeptidase (GGT).

Treatment

- Vaccines against HAV and HBV before exposure provide active immunity.
- Antivirals (interferon); immune globulins provide passive immunity post-exposure.
- Antiretrovirals: Hepatitis B: Lamivudine; hepatitis C: Sofosbuvir; protease inhibitors; combination drugs Sepatier, Dakinza, Viekira Pak, Harvoni.

Nursing Care

- Assess for S&S; contact precautions for HAV and HEV.
- ↑ calories, ↑ protein, ↓ fat in diet as prescribed; encourage rest.
- Teach to avoid toxins (acetaminophen, alcohol, carbon tetrachloride).

Cirrhosis

- Fibrous scar tissue and fat accumulate in liver → hepatomegaly and portal hypertension; results in esophageal varices, hemorrhoids, obstructive jaundice, and ascites.
- ↓ liver function → ↓ metabolism → ↑ ammonia (a metabolized protein by-product) → encephalopathy.

Risk Factors

- Alcoholism (most common), hepatitis or biliary disease.
- Industrial chemicals, male gender, 40–60 yr of age.
- Acetaminophen more than 4,000 mg daily; ↑ risk with lower doses if ingesting alcohol.

Signs and Symptoms

- ↑ liver enzymes (AST, ALT, LDH, GGT), jaundice, hepatomegaly.
- ↓ albumin, ↑ bilirubin, ↓ globulins, ↑ ammonia, ↑ prothrombin time.
- Distended abdomen caused by fluid in abdominal cavity **(ascites);** GI varices; edema due to ↓ albumin and ↑ aldosterone, which causes retention of Na and water.
- Confusion, agitation, flapping hand tremors **(asterixis)**.
- Liver biopsy to confirm diagnosis.

Treatment

- Treat underlying cause.
- Vitamins (A, D, E, K, B), zinc, K-sparing diuretics, antibiotics.
- Lactulose to ↓ ammonia, albumin.
- Portal caval shunt; sclerotherapy or balloon tamponade for varices.
- Paracentesis for ascites with dyspnea; liver transplant.

Nursing Care

- Assess for S&S, I&O, abdominal girth.
- Teach to avoid alcohol if appropriate, about products with acetaminophen and to ↓ its intake to less than 4,000 mg daily.

- *Liver biopsy:* Have client hold breath during needle insertion; keep on right side with pillow against insertion site; assess for bleeding.
- *Paracentesis*: Have client void before and maintain an upright position during procedure; assess respiratory status, S&S of shock, persistent leakage after procedure.
- *Balloon tamponade*: Provide oral suction; maintain traction on gastric balloon; monitor pressure of esophageal balloon.

Pancreatitis

- Obstruction of pancreatic duct causes reflux of trypsin, resulting in autodigestion of pancreas that leads to inflammation.
- Possible necrosis with calcification, perforation, hemorrhage.
- Pancreatic pseudocysts or abscesses may develop.
- May be idiopathic, acute, or chronic and result in DM.

Risk Factors

- Alcoholism in middle-age men; biliary disease in older females.
- Extremely high triglycerides >1,000 mg/dL, family history, smoking, multiple causes.

Signs and Symptoms

- Epigastric pain that ↑ with eating and may radiate to thorax/back.
- N&V, ↑ T, ↓ weight, abdominal distention and tenderness, jaundice.
- Steatorrhea and glucose intolerance with chronic pancreatitis.
- ↑ amylase, ↑ lipase, ↓ serum calcium, ↑ Ca 19-9; CT and MRI scans identify location and size of tumor; ultrasound identifies presence of pseudocyst.
- S&S of perforation: Rebound tenderness, rigid abdomen, shock.
- Complications: Pseudocyst, infection, DM, kidney failure, malnutrition, pancreatic cancer.

Treatment

- NPO; IVF and electrolyte replacement.
- NGT to remove secretions and ↓ GI motility.
- Antibiotics, analgesics, anticholinergics, pancreatic enzymes (lipase, trypsin, amylase) with meals for chronic pancreatitis.
- Surgery if due to biliary disease.

Nursing Care

- Give prescribed analgesics, antibiotics, anticholinergics, pancreatic enzymes, vitamins A and E.
- Provide diet as prescribed (usually low fat); provide small frequent meals.
- Assess I&O; S&S of hypocalcemia, and hyperglycemia.
- Support abstinence from alcohol; refer to Alcoholics Anonymous if appropriate.

Nursing Care for Clients Receiving Nutritional Support

Parenteral Nutrition (PN)

Introduction

- Nutrients given directly into bloodstream, bypassing GI tract.
- For clients who are unable to absorb nutrients or have high nutritive demands (severe burns, cancer, multiple trauma, stomach or intestinal problems, cancer); rests GI tract.
- PN solutions are hypertonic and formulated to meet individual needs; include amino acids, glucose, vitamins, minerals, trace elements, heparin, insulin; lipid emulsions containing essential fatty acids, triglycerides, and supplemental kilocalories may be given weekly.
- Catheter is advanced to superior vena cava to promote dilution of formula and prevent intima inflammation.
- **Total parenteral nutrition (TPN):** Catheter inserted into subclavian or jugular vein and advanced to superior vena cava; used when PN is required for a long period of time.
- **Partial parenteral nutrition (PPN):** Peripherally inserted central catheter (PICC); inserted into vein of arm and advanced to superior vena cava; used when PN is required for a short period of time or to supplement oral nutrition.

Nursing Care for Clients Receiving Parenteral Nutrition

- Ensure central catheter placement is confirmed by x-ray before use.
- Verify prescription for formula, amount, and rate of infusion; verify expiration date on formula; label solution bag with date, time, and formula type.
- Use an infusion pump; dedicate a port to prevent interactions with IVF or IV meds; assess insertion site for S&S of complications.
- Keep PN solution refrigerated; return to room temperature naturally because cold solution can cause pain, venous spasm, and hypothermia.
- Infuse slowly initially; ↑ rate in increments of 25 mL/hr until prescribed rate is reached; maintain consistent rate.
- Monitor for metabolic and F&E imbalances because they may indicate intolerance; may need to ↓ rate or halt flow until problem is corrected.
- Monitor blood glucose every 6 hr because PN solutions are high in glucose; administer insulin coverage as prescribed.
- Wean off PN to ↓ risk of metabolic problems (over 48 hr); if abrupt stopping is necessary give a 5% or 10% dextrose solution to prevent rebound hypoglycemia until primary health-care provider is notified.

Prevent Infection

- Use meticulous sterile technique when changing transparent occlusive dressing over insertion site every 72 hr; cleanse port before/after use with 70% alcohol or chlorhexidine gluconate-based pads.
- Change tubing every 24 hr; ensure tubing has in-line filter for PN; use set specific for lipids and use port below PN filter if given concurrently.
- Discard unused solution after 24 hr; avoid using if a leak, cloudiness, or floating particles are identified.

Monitor for Complications and Notify Health-Care Provider If One Occurs

- **Pneumothorax:** Puncture of lung during catheter insertion allows air in pleural cavity. *S&S:* Severe sudden chest pain, marked dyspnea, absent breath sounds on affected side. *Nursing care:* Elevate HOB, give O_2, monitor VS and O_2 sat, assist with chest tube insertion.
- **Catheter occlusion:** Debris or blood clot at tip of catheter. *S&S:* Sluggish or absent catheter flow rate. *Nursing care:* Stop infusion; flush with heparin or saline, aspirate clot, use thrombolytic agent as per protocol.
- **Infection:** Pathogens enter blood via catheter or insertion site. *S&S:* ↑ VS, chills, positive blood culture. *Nursing care:* Administer prescribed local and/or systemic antibiotics and antipyretics.
- **Hyperglycemia:** SNS stimulation of stress hormones and high glucose load of solution ↑ serum glucose level. *S&S:* Polyuria, polydipsia, headache, lethargy, increased serum glucose level. *Nursing care:* Administer insulin coverage as prescribed.
- Document client response, I&O, weekly weight (should gain about 3 lb).

Enteral Nutrition (Tube Feeding)

Introduction

- Liquid formula administered via tube into stomach or jejunum.
- For clients with intact GI systems but who have impaired swallowing, high nutritive demands, or are unable to meet nutritional needs orally.
- Tube advanced through nose into stomach (nasogastric [NG] tube), abdominal wall into stomach (percutaneous endoscopic gastrostomy [PEG] tube), or abdominal wall into jejunum (jejunostomy tube [J-tube]).
- Standard formulas balanced with 12%–20% protein, 45%–60% CHO, 30%–40% fats, vitamins and minerals; specialty formulas such as high-protein, high-fiber, renal, pulmonary, and hydrolyzed formulas are used for specific health problems.
- Feedings may be continuous, intermittent (bolus), or cyclical (continuous feeding administered for less than 24 hr a day).

Nursing Care for Clients Receiving a Tube Feeding

- Confirm tube placement: Radiographically before 1st use; before each use or every 4 hr for continuous/cyclical feedings via NG or PEG tube; use several methods.
  - Aspirate stomach contents: pH is normally acidic (1.5–3.5) greenish/yellow color; residual gastric volume should not exceed parameter such as >½ previous feeding; if excessive, hold feeding 1 hr and reassess; reinstill aspirate to prevent electrolyte and acid–base imbalances.
  - Instill 10–30 mL of air in tube while auscultating epigastric area; "whoosh" sound with gurgling is heard as air enters stomach.
- Secure NG tube to naris or cheek and assess skin every 4 hr; change sterile dressing to PEG or J-tube site every 8 hr until healed and then provide meticulous skin care.
- Verify prescription for formula, amount, and rate of infusion; verify expiration date on formula; label solution bag with date, time, and formula type.
- Wash hands; don clean gloves; raise HOB throughout feeding and 1 hr after bolus feeding; assess placement; measure and assess aspirate; flush tube with 30 mL water; instill bolus feeding or begin continuous/cyclical feeding; flush tube with 30 mL of water after bolus feeding or routinely with continuous/cyclical feeding; instill additional water as prescribed.

Monitor for Complications; Notify Primary Health-Care Provider If One Occurs.

- **Aspiration**: Gastric contents enter respiratory tract due to gastric reflux or vomiting. *S&S:* Coughing, SOB, dyspnea, restlessness, ↑ P, ↑ R, ↓ O_2 sat. *Nursing care:* ↑ HOB, O_2, suction airway, avoid oversedation.
- **Diarrhea**: Liquid stool due to hyperosmolar formula, rapid administration, malabsorption, cold formula, tube migration from stomach into small intestine, bacterial contamination. *S&S:* Frequent unformed stools, abdominal cramping. *Nursing care:* Assess bowel sounds and amount and character of stool, give prescribed antidiarrheal or probiotic such as *L. acidophilus*.
- **Dumping syndrome**: Hypertonic solution rapidly enters intestine pulling fluid from intestinal wall into lumen. *S&S:* ↑ peristalsis, ↑ bowel sounds, abdominal pain, vomiting, and release of insulin in relation to hyperglycemia ultimately causing weakness, shakiness, anxiety, sweating, ↑ P, confusion. *Nursing care:* Halt infusion, obtain prescription for slower rate or different formula, encourage rest/reclining position after a feeding.
- **Tube obstruction**: Occurs when tube is inadequately flushed, meds are inadequately crushed, feeding is on hold to provide nursing care, feeding runs out. *S&S:* Slow or absent flow rate; *Nursing care:* Ensure tube is not compressed or has dependent loops, reposition client with instructions to cough, flush tube with water or cranberry juice.
- Document client response, I&O, weekly weight (should gain about 3 lb).

Female Reproductive Cancers

Breast Cancer

- Development of malignant cells due to hormonal, genetic, and/or environmental factors.
- Localized or invasive; may affect lobules or ducts.
- Stage 0 (in situ), Stage 1 (tumor <2 cm), Stage 2 (tumor 2–5 cm), Stage 3 (tumor >5 cm), Stage 4 (metastasis).

Risk Factors

- ↑ age, female gender, family history, *BRCA-1* and *BRCA-2* genes.
- Nulliparity or late 1st pregnancy, estrogen replacement, early menarche, late menopause, postmenopausal hormone therapy.
- Alcohol, obesity, cancer in other breast, radiation exposure.

Signs and Symptoms

- Hard, nontender mass; often superior lateral breast; may attach to underlying tissue (fixed).
- Recent inversion or flattening of nipple; itchy, scaly nipple lesion.
- Unilateral venous prominence; enlarged axillary nodes.
- Orange peel appearance of breast tissue **(peau d'orange)**.
- Diagnostic tests: Mammogram; sonogram; MRI; estrogen receptor and progesterone receptor assays to determine tumor's sensitivity to hormones; scans and tumor markers (Ca 15–3, Ca-125).
- Sentinel node biopsy identifies primary axillary node for breast drainage and need for standard vs. invasive axillary node dissection.

Treatment

- Based on stage and type: Lumpectomy, mastectomy, nodal dissection, radiation, chemotherapy, hormonal therapy, bone marrow transplantation.
- Meds: Antiestrogens, aromatase inhibitors, monoclonal antibodies, antiangiogenic agents, combination chemotherapy.
- Reconstruction surgery may involve progressive addition of saline into temporary implants to expand tissue before insertion of final implants; client's own muscle flaps from abdomen or back are used to simulate breast tissue; tissue from inner thigh or labia is used to create nipple; tattoo to simulate areola.

Nursing Care

- Assess for S&S.
- Provide support of client and partner; refer to Reach to Recovery.
- Provide care for client receiving antineoplastic medications.

Teach Monthly Breast Self-Examination (BSE)

- Systematic light, medium, and deep palpation with finger pads over breasts and axilla once a mo; American Cancer Society does not recommend regular physical breast exams by clinicians or self because evidence does not show a benefit.
- 5–7 days after start of menses in premenopausal women and same day every mo in postmenopausal women.
- Inspect for symmetry, dimpling, or nipple inversion.

Provide Care for Client Receiving Radiation

- Balance rest/activity to manage fatigue.
- Prevent irritating site: Avoid sun, wearing bras, using ointments, lotions, or powders; wear soft cotton clothing.

Provide Care During Postoperative Period

- Provide for pain management.
- Maintain portable wound drainage device to ↓ edema.
- Teach postmastectomy exercises (wall climbing) to ↑ muscle strength, ↓ contractures, ↓ risk of lymphedema; encourage wearing of compression sleeve if prescribed.
- Protect upper extremity on side of surgery: No BPs, IVs, injections, or withdrawal of blood specimens; teach to avoid lifting or carrying heavy items, use electric razor for axillary hair, wear gloves for gardening.

Uterine (Endometrial) and Cervical Cancer

- **Cervical cancer**: Progresses through stages from dysplasia to invasive metastasis; 90% from squamous cells; 10% adenocarcinoma; high cure rate if diagnosed in situ.
- **Uterine cancer**: Arises from the endometrium of the uterus; can invade cervix, myometrium, regional lymph nodes, omentum, bowel.

Risk Factors

- *Cervical cancer:* 30–45 yr of age, human papillomavirus (HPV), repeated injury to cervix, sexual activity at young age, multiple sex partners, HIV, STI, weak immune system, smoking.
- *Uterine cancer:* Estrogen, ↑ age, nulliparity, late menopause, obesity, smoking, family history.

Signs and Symptoms

- *Cervical cancer*
  - Early: Watery vaginal secretion progressing to foul-smelling discharge, bleeding between menses **(metrorrhagia)** or after intercourse, pelvic pain or pain during intercourse **(dyspareunia)**, positive Pap smear.
  - Late: Back and leg pain, leg edema, dysuria, rectal bleeding, anemia, ↓ weight.

- *Uterine cancer*
  - Abnormal uterine bleeding usually after menopause, pain late in the disease, other signs relate to metastasis.
- Diagnostic tests: CT, MRI, and PET scans, to identify site of tumor; uterine cancer—endometrial biopsy; cervical cancer—Pap test, colposcopy, punch or cone biopsy.

Treatment

- *Cervical cancer:* Based on stage, cryotherapy or laser therapy, removal of part of cervix that maintains reproductive function **(conization)**, hysterectomy (simple, radical), loop electrocautery excision procedure; external radiation; intracavity radiation **(brachytherapy)**.
- *Uterine cancer:* Hysterectomy (simple, radical); antineoplastic therapy.

Nursing Care

- Provide emotional support.

Provide Care for Client Receiving External Radiation

- Assess for skin lesion, nausea, diarrhea, cystitis, fistulas.
- Encourage client to wear soft cotton underwear, avoid nylon underwear and pantyhose.
- Teach perineal care.

Provide Care for Client Receiving Internal Radiation

- Pregnant nurses must not care for clients receiving internal radiation.
- Provide private room; consider time/distance/shielding; organize care to ↓ time in room.
- Prevent dislodgment of intracavity device: Maintain supine position (usually 1–3 days); indwelling urinary catheter; low-residue diet and antidiarrheals.

Provide Postoperative Care

- Assess for bleeding and infection; provide pain management; encourage use of incentive spirometer.
- Teach DVT prevention such as ankle-pumping exercises, compression device.

Administer Prescribed Meds

- See Nursing Care for Clients With Cancer or Experiencing Nontherapeutic Effects of Antineoplastic Therapies, p. 172.

Ovarian Cancer

- 90% epithelial in origin.
- Lower incidence than other GYN cancers but ↑ mortality since most metastasize before diagnosis.

Risk Factors

- Breast cancer; *BRCA-1* and *BRCA-2* genes.
- High-fat diet, oral and intrauterine contraceptives, nulliparity, multipara, early menarche, late menopause, fertility treatment, smoking, obesity, endometriosis.

Signs and Symptoms

- May be asymptomatic until advanced.
- Enlarged ovary on palpation; ↑ abdominal girth due to tumor or ascites.
- Anemia; ↓ weight; change in bowel habits; flatulence; urinary frequency; leg or pelvic pain.
- ↑ Ca-125; tumor seen on transvaginal ultrasound, CT scan.

Treatment

- Total abdominal hysterectomy: Uterus, ovaries, fallopian tubes, omentum.
- Meds: Commonly carboplatin, paclitaxel, melphalan, cyclophosphamide, doxorubicin, cisplatin.
- Ca-125 levels to assess progress.
- Paracentesis for palliation.

Nursing Care

- Provide emotional support because usually diagnosed late with a poor prognosis.
- See Provide Postoperative Care under Uterine and Cervical Cancer, p. 229.

Infectious Diseases

Lyme Disease, Tetanus, and Zika Virus

	Lyme Disease	Tetanus (Lockjaw)	Zika Virus
Etiology and Pathophysiology	• *Borrelia burgdorferi:* Spirochete; infected deer or mouse → tick → human through tick's bite. • 3–30-day incubation.	• *Clostridium tetani:* Anaerobic bacillus; enters puncture wound, resulting in bacterial toxins affecting nervous system → muscle spasms.	• *Zika virus from genus flavivirus:* Spread through bite of infected *Aedes aegypti* mosquito. • Virus found in urine, semen, spinal, and amniotic fluid; present in semen longer than in blood.

	Lyme Disease	Tetanus (Lockjaw)	Zika Virus
		• 3–21-day incubation.	• Associated with neurological conditions (Guillain-Barré syndrome); miscarriage; stillbirth; microcephaly and other anomalies in newborns. • 3–12-day incubation.
Risk Factors	• Northeastern United States, wooded areas.	• No tetanus toxoid to produce active immunity.	• Perinatal transmission; transplacental. • Sexual contact with infected person; infected blood and body fluids. • Exposure in regions where Zika is found (Florida, French Polynesia, Caribbean, Latin America).
S&S	• Early: Bull's-eye rash. • Later: Arthritis, Bell palsy, meningitis, carditis, dementia, paralysis.	• Voluntary muscle spasms → pain; jaw clamping, ↑ BP, ↑ P, spasms where head and heels are bent backward and the body is bowed forward **(opisthotonic)** posturing. • Respiratory spasm.	• 80% asymptomatic. • Fever, malaise, rash, joint pain, headache, conjunctivitis.

Continued

	Lyme Disease	Tetanus (Lockjaw)	Zika Virus
Treatment	• Amoxicillin, doxycycline, ceftriaxone.	• Tetanus immune globulin, supportive care.	• Rest; fluids; acetaminophen when dengue has been ruled out to ↓ risk of bleeding.
Nursing Care	• Provide supportive care. • Teach to complete antibiotic therapy; wear long, light-colored clothes to see ticks; avoid tall grass; use bug repellent; inspect skin; use tweezers to remove tick.	• Maintain airway. • Administer immune globulin for brief passive immunity. • Provide wound care. • Teach need for tetanus toxoid booster every 10 yr for active immunity.	**Teach:** • Travel alert to high-risk regions; consult with primary health-care provider before traveling if pregnant, considering pregnancy, males or females of childbearing age. • Teach people to avoid vaginal, anal, or oral sex without a condom with a partner who has traveled to a high-risk area for 6 mo and throughout pregnancy; postpone pregnancy until risk factors are reduced. • Wear clothing to cover exposed skin, mosquito repellent; employ window screens and air conditioning. • ↓ standing water indoors/outdoors to minimize breeding areas for mosquitos.

HIV and AIDS

- Acquired immunodeficiency syndrome (AIDS) caused by human immunodeficiency virus (HIV).
- HIV infects helper T lymphocytes (T4/CD4 cells), B lymphocytes, macrophages, promyelocytes, fibroblasts.
- Opportunistic infections occur when T4/CD4 cell count <200/mcL (*Pneumocystis jiroveci* pneumonia, histoplasmosis, *Mycobacterium tuberculosis*, cytomegalovirus).
- Transmission: Contact with infected body fluids (blood, semen, vaginal secretions, blood tinged body fluids, breast milk, cerebrospinal fluid).
- Incubation period is 6 mo–10 yr or longer.

Signs and symptoms

- Anorexia, fatigue, chills, sore throat, dyspnea, night sweats, lymphadenopathy.
- Weight loss of 10% or more, constant fever, chronic diarrhea and weakness **(wasting syndrome)**.
- Memory loss, ↓ cognition, ↓ coordination, partial paralysis **(HIV encephalopathy)**.
- Opportunistic infections and malignancies such as Kaposi sarcoma.
- Diagnostic tests: HIV antigen can be detected within 2–4 wk after infection and HIV antibodies within 2–8 wk or longer.

Treatment

- Highly active antiretroviral therapy; 3 or more drugs from at least 2 classes that ↓ HIV replication; fusion inhibitor; integrase inhibitors; protease inhibitors; nonnucleoside reverse transcriptase inhibitors; nucleoside reverse transcriptase inhibitors; antivirals.
- Meds to treat opportunistic infections such as TB.
- Nucleoside reverse transcriptase inhibitors for postexposure prophylaxis such as after accidental needle sticks.
- Viral load and CD4 counts every 3–4 mo monitors response to treatment.
- Prevention: Noninfected high-risk people may take emtricitabine-tenofovir, consistent condom use if sex partner has HIV or HIV status is unknown.

Nursing Care

- Assess for S&S; VS, weight loss; progression of clinical manifestations; S&S of opportunistic infections.
- Maintain standard precautions; institute transmission-based precautions for client with opportunistic infections.
- Encourage expression of feelings; explain chronicity of condition.
- Encourage adherence to med regimen because nonadherence leads to resistant strains; assess for and teach common side effects.

- Teach to inform sexual contacts of diagnosis; use safer sex (condom with water-soluble jelly); avoid breastfeeding and sharing needles.
- Teach to protect self from infection: Avoid crowds, undercooked meats, small animals; perform hand hygiene often.
- Encourage ↑ calorie, ↑ protein diet with foods high in immune-stimulating nutrients such as vitamins A, C, and E, and selenium.

Perioperative Nursing Care

Preoperative Nursing Care

Identify Physical and Emotional Risk Factors

- *Cardiopulmonary status:* RBC, WBC, Hb, Hct, chest x-ray, ECG (over 40 yr of age or preexisting condition).
- *Bleeding/clotting risk:* Platelets, PT, PTT, INR, type and cross for blood transfusion.
- *Identification of preexisting conditions:* BUN and creatinine (kidney function); liver enzymes (liver function); fasting blood glucose (DM); hCG (pregnancy).
- *Emotional status:* Assess for positive or negative attitude regarding surgery and expected outcome; inform surgeon if client has an attitude of impending doom.

Provide Teaching

- *Expectations:* Such as pain management plan.
- *Skills:* Leg exercises, diaphragmatic breathing, coughing, use of incentive spirometer.
- *Care related to specific surgeries:* See specific diseases.

Preparation of Client on Day of Surgery

- *Secure informed consent:* Surgeon explains surgery/risks; nurse witnesses client's signature.
- *Prevent aspiration:* Restriction of oral intake; give prescribed anticholinergic to ↓ respiratory secretions and H_2 receptor antagonist to ↓ gastric acid.
- *Prevent surgical site infection:* Cleanse skin with prescribed antimicrobial agent such as chlorhexidine.
- *Limit anxiety and maximize anesthetic agent:* Give prescribed CNS depressant such as a sedative or opioid.
- *Implement "time-out" procedure:* Verify client name, type of surgery, site; ensure operative checklist is complete.

Postoperative Nursing Care

Maintain Airway

- Assess VS, O_2 sat, sputum characteristics, breath sounds for atelectasis or pneumonia.
- Administer O_2, remove artificial airway when gag reflex returns, suction airway if necessary, position on side if vomiting.
- Encourage coughing and deep breathing (splint incision), use of incentive spirometer.

Maintain Portable Wound Drainage Devices

- Empty and recompress self-contained suction devices (Hemovac, Jackson Pratt) when half full of drainage to reestablish negative pressure; as drainage increases negative pressure decreases, reducing effectiveness of suction device.
- Ensure patency, avoid dependent loops, assess amount and characteristics of drainage.

Manage Pain

- Assess location, characteristics, and extent of pain (use pain rating scale).
- Give prescribed analgesic (usually patient-controlled analgesia).
- Use nonpharmacological interventions (imagery, relaxation exercises).

Assess for S&S of Hypovolemic Shock Due to Hemorrhage

- Bloody drainage; weak, rapid pulse; ↑ R; ↓ BP; ↓ urine output (<30 mL/hr); ↓ Hb; ↓ Hct.
- Pallor; cold, clammy skin; maintain intravascular volume (administer prescribed transfusions, IVFs).

Assess for and Prevent Neurovascular Complications

- Assess for unilateral leg edema, inflammation, calf pain caused by dorsiflexion of foot (Homan sign) that may indicate thrombophlebitis; do not elicit Homan sign because it may cause a thrombus to become an embolus.
- Assess for sudden chest pain, SOB, ↓ Sao_2 that may indicate PE.
- Encourage early ambulation, leg exercises, use of sequential compression devices, ↑ fluids if permitted.
- Avoid popliteal pressure; give prescribed prophylactic anticoagulants.
- Assess peripheral neurovascular status after spinal anesthesia or extremity surgery such as peripheral pulse, capillary refill, color and temperature of skin, sensation, and mobility of distal extremity.

Prevent Urinary Retention

- Assess for inability to void, voiding small amounts often, suprapubic distention.
- Encourage frequent position change; ↑ fluids if permitted; may need to secure prescription to catheterize.

Prevent Paralytic (Postoperative) Ileus

- Assess for absence of bowel sounds, abdominal distention, vomiting.
- Maintain nasogastric tube to suction for decompression; assess amount and characteristics of drainage.
- Encourage early ambulation, fluids, dietary fiber as prescribed.

Identify Wound Complications

- Provide food high in vitamin C and protein within dietary prescription to facilitate wound healing.
- Assess approximation of wound edges especially between the 5th to 10th postoperative days; separation of wound edges **(dehiscence)**; protrusion of internal organs through incision **(evisceration)**; associated with obesity, coughing and straining; evisceration requires emergency care such as low-Fowler position, application of sterile moist saline dressing, notification of surgeon.
- Assess for S&S of infection such as inflammation, purulent exudate, ↑ T; use surgical asepsis for wound care; implement contact precautions.

Common Therapeutic Drug Classifications

Antacids: Decrease Gastric Acidity and Epigastric Pain and Protect Stomach Mucosa

Mechanism of Action	Examples	Nontherapeutic Effects
Bind with excess acid.	aluminum hydroxide (Amphojel) magnesium/aluminum hydroxide (Maalox, Mylanta)	• Aluminum salts ↓ stool transit causing constipation, hypophosphatemia. • Magnesium salts ↑ peristalsis causing diarrhea, hypermagnesemia.

Nursing Care

- Many antacids contain Na, which should be avoided on low Na diets.
- Shake suspensions well; give 60 mL water to ↑ passage to stomach.
- Encourage foods high in calcium and iron; avoid foods that ↑ GI distress.
- Caution about overuse, which may cause alkalosis, rebound hyperacidity.
- Assess for extent and relief of epigastric and abdominal pain.
- Assess emesis and stool for frank and occult blood.
- Teach to report S&S if they do not resolve in 2 wk.
- Monitor serum calcium and phosphate levels with chronic use.

Antidiarrheals: Decrease Diarrhea and Promote Formed Stool

Mechanism of Action	Examples	Nontherapeutic Effects
Motility Suppressants ↓ peristalsis so water is absorbed by large intestine.	diphenoxylate (Lomotil) loperamide (Imodium)	Tachycardia, respiratory depression, ileus, urinary retention, sedation, dry mouth.
Enteric Bacteria Replacements ↓ pathogenic bacterial growth.	*lactobacillus acidophilus* (Bacid)	Abdominal cramps, ↑ flatulence.

Nursing Care

- Assess bowel movements for frequency, characteristics; assess bowel sounds for ↓ in hyperactivity.
- Assess for F&E imbalances, particularly dehydration.

Antibiotics and Anti-infectives: Destroy or Decrease Growth of Susceptible Microorganisms

Mechanism of Action	Examples	Nontherapeutic Effects
Aminoglycosides ↓ protein synthesis.	gentamicin neomycin	N&V, hypersensitivity reactions such as rash and anaphylaxis.
Cephalosporins Bind to cell wall, causing cell death.	cefazolin (Ancef) ceftriaxone (Rocephin) cephalexin (Keflex)	
Fluoroquinolones ↓ DNA synthesis.	levofloxacin (Levaquin) ciprofloxacin (Cipro)	
Macrolides ↓ protein synthesis.	azithromycin (Zithromax) clarithromycin (Biaxin)	
Penicillins Bind to cell wall → cell death.	amoxicillin penicillin V	
Sulfonamides ↓ protein synthesis.	doxycycline tetracycline	
Anti-infectives ↓ protein and DNA synthesis; bactericidal, trichomonacidal, amebicidal.	chloroquine phosphate clindamycin (Cleocin) metronidazole (Flagyl)	

Nursing Care

- Ensure C&S test is done before starting med; assess S&S of hepatotoxicity, nephrotoxicity, hyperglycemia, med interactions associated with some fluoroquinolones.
- Assess S&S of infection.
- Assess for superinfection: Furry overgrowth on tongue; vaginal discharge; foul-smelling stools.

- Give evenly spaced doses to maintain blood levels.
- Teach that regimen should be completed to prevent resistance.
- Do not crush or chew extended-release tablets.
- Obtain blood specimen 1–3 hr after a dose (depending on med) to measure highest blood level **(peak)** and 30–60 min before next dose to measure lowest blood level **(trough)**.

Anticoagulants: Interfere With Normal Coagulation to Decrease Thrombus Formation or Extension

Mechanism of Action	Examples	Nontherapeutic Effects
Thrombin Inhibitors ↓ conversion of prothrombin to thrombin, thus ↓ conversion of fibrinogen to fibrin.	heparin	• Excessive bleeding such as bruising, melena, hematuria, epistaxis, bleeding gums. • ↓ Hb and ↓ Hct, anemia, thrombocytopenia.
Low Molecular Weight Heparins Block coagulation factor Xa.	dalteparin (Fragmin) edoxaban (Savaysa) enoxaparin (Lovenox) rivaroxaban (Xarelto)	
Clotting Factor Inhibitors Interfere with hepatic synthesis of vitamin K and dependent clotting factors.	warfarin (Coumadin)	
Platelet Inhibitors ↓ platelet aggregation.	acetylsalicylic acid (aspirin) apixaban (Eliquis) clopidogrel (Plavix) ticlopidine (Ticlid)	
Direct Thrombin Inhibitors Attach to thrombin ↓ its ability to clot.	dabigatran (Pradaxa)	• Same as above. • Dyspepsia, esophagitis. • Hypersensitivity reactions.

Nursing Care

- Discontinue anticoagulants before invasive procedures; report if bleeding occurs; prepare to give antidote (protamine sulfate for heparin, vitamin K for warfarin); encourage use of medical alert card or jewelry.
- Assess for bleeding; monitor coagulation studies, platelet count; teach to use electric razor, soft toothbrush; teach to avoid OTC meds, especially aspirin and NSAIDs.
- Teach to avoid alcohol and foods high in vitamin K—they ↓ med effectiveness.
- *Thrombin inhibitors:* Monitor PTT (therapeutic level is 1.5–2.5 times control); half-life of heparin is 1–2 hr.
- *Low molecular weight heparins:* Do not use with another heparin product; if bruising occurs, ice cube massage site before injection.
- *Clotting factor inhibitors:* Monitor PT (therapeutic level is 1.3–2.0 times control) or INR (therapeutic level is 2–4.5 times control).

Antiemetics: Decrease N&V and Prevent and Decrease Motion Sickness

Mechanism of Action	Examples	Nontherapeutic Effects
Phenothiazines ↓ chemoreceptor trigger zone in CNS.	prochlorperazine promethazine	Confusion, sedation, photosensitivity, dry mouth, constipation, extrapyramidal reactions.
5 HT_3 Antagonists Block serotonin at receptor sites in vagal nerve terminals and chemoreceptor trigger zone in CNS.	ondansetron (Zofran)	Headache, dizziness, constipation, diarrhea.
Anticholinergics Correct imbalance of acetylcholine and norepinephrine in CNS that causes motion sickness.	scopolamine (Transderm Scop) trimethobenzamide (Tigan)	• Drowsiness. • *Scopolamine:* Urinary hesitancy, blurred vision, dry mouth, tachycardia. • *Tigan suppository:* ↓ BP, local irritation.

Mechanism of Action	Examples	Nontherapeutic Effects
Nonphenothiazines Block chemoreceptor trigger zone in CNS; ↑ GI motility and ↑ gastric emptying.	metoclopramide (Reglan)	Extrapyramidal reactions, restlessness, drowsiness, anxiety, depression.

Nursing Care

- Give 30–60 min before chemotherapy or activity that causes motion sickness.
- Assess VS; extent and relief of N&V; abdominal distention.
- Ensure safety because of CNS depression; avoid alcohol and other CNS depressants.
- *Assess for extrapyramidal reactions:* Involuntary movements, grimacing, rigidity, shuffling gait, trembling.
- *Phenothiazines:* Encourage sunscreen and protective clothing; assess for **neuroleptic malignant syndrome**: Hyperthermia, diaphoresis, unstable BP, dyspnea, stupor, muscle rigidity, urinary incontinence.

Antifungals: Decrease Fungal Growth

Mechanism of Action	Examples	Nontherapeutic Effects
Systemic Antifungals Impair fungal plasma membrane.	clotrimazole (Mycelex) fluconazole (Diflucan) isavuconazonium (Cresemba) nystatin (Mycostatin)	• Teratogenic, F&E imbalance, N&V, diarrhea, rash, fever. • Nephrotoxicity, ototoxicity, and hepatotoxicity.
Topical Antifungals Disrupt fungal cell wall and metabolism.	amphotericin B (Fungizone) clotrimazole ketoconazole nystatin	Burning, irritation.

Nursing Care

- *Systemic:* Assess for nephrotoxicity, hepatotoxicity, ototoxicity.
- Encourage to complete entire regimen; prevent pregnancy; assess for hypoglycemia in client with DM.
- *Topical:* Assess for irritation; clean skin with tepid water before application.
- Teach difference between *swish and swallow* and *swish and spit.*
- Teach how to administer a vaginal med and to abstain from intercourse until infection clears.

Antiparasitics: Cause Parasite Death

Mechanism of Action	Examples	Nontherapeutic Effects
Parasiticidal Directly absorbed into parasites and eggs (scabies, lice).	lindane	CNS toxicity, seizures.
	permethrin (Nix)	Pruritus, tingling.
Anthelmintic Prevents pinworm growth and reproduction.	mebendazole	• Hypersensitivity such as rash, anaphylaxis. • Abdominal pain.

Nursing Care

- Maintain standard and transmission-based precautions as indicated.
- Teach to wash bedding, clothes, etc., in hot water and dryer; vacuum carpets and furniture; seal nonwashables in plastic bags for 2 wk; teach hand hygiene before meals and after toileting; ensure prescription treats all family members.
- *Pediculosis/scabies:* Use contact precautions and hair cap with direct care; scrub body with soap and water, dry, apply med while avoiding wounds, mucous membranes, face, eyes.
- *Pinworms:* Collect specimen with cellophane tape test in a.m.; assess perianal area.
- *Head lice:* Use medicated shampoo for 5 min; use fine-tooth comb to remove eggs (nits); repeat as prescribed.

Analgesics, Antipyretics, and NSAIDs: Decrease Pain, Fever, and Inflammation

Mechanism of Action	Examples	Nontherapeutic Effects
Analgesic Only Inhibit prostaglandins involved in pain or fever.	acetaminophen (Tylenol)	Hepatic toxicity.
Nonsalicylate NSAIDs Inhibit prostaglandins involved in fever, inflammation, pain.	ibuprofen (Advil, Motrin) meloxicam (Mobic) naproxen (Aleve)	Rash, tinnitus, flulike syndrome.
Salicylate NSAIDs Inhibit prostaglandins involved in inflammation, pain, fever.	acetylsalicylic acid (aspirin)	• Agitation, hyperventilation, lethargy, confusion, diarrhea. • *Toxicity:* Diaphoresis, tinnitus (8th cranial nerve damage).

Nursing Care

- Do not exceed recommended 24-hr dose; withhold 1 wk before invasive procedures because of ↓ platelet aggregation and risk of bleeding; salicylates contraindicated in pregnancy, lactation, children <2 yr of age (associated with Reye syndrome).
- Give with 8 oz water, sit up 15–30 min after ingestion; give with food except for naproxen and ibuprofen; assess for GI bleeding (anemia, melena).
- Avoid alcohol and OTC meds with analgesic or antipyretic properties.
- Discontinue med if serious side effects and report to primary health-care provider.
- *Acetaminophen:* Do not exceed >4 g per 24-hr period to ↓ risk of hepatotoxicity.
- *Salicylates:* Monitor serum salicylate levels.
- *NSAIDs:* Assess for headache, drowsiness, dizziness, photosensitivity.

Antihistamines: Decrease Clinical Indicators of Allergies and Motion Sickness

Mechanism of Action	Examples	Nontherapeutic Effects
Block histamine, which ↓ allergic response and motion sickness.	diphenhydramine (Benadryl) loratadine (Claritin)	Dry eyes and mouth, constipation, blurred vision, sedation.

Nursing Care

- Contraindicated with narrow-angle glaucoma; use caution with opioids because it may cause paradoxical effect.
- May be used to promote sleep; assess older adults for risk of falls.
- Exerts antiemetic, anticholinergic, CNS depressant effects; assess older adults for confusion.
- Give with food and fluid to ↓ GI irritation.
- Caution client to avoid hazardous activities; assess level of sedation.
- Give 1 hr before activity for motion sickness prophylaxis.
- Suggest use of gum and hard candy to ↑ salivation and ↓ dry mouth.
- Teach to wear long sleeves and pants and sunscreen to ↓ effects of photosensitivity.

Antihypertensives: Decrease Blood Pressure (also see Diuretics, p. 256)

Mechanism of Action	Examples	Nontherapeutic Effects
Angiotensin Antagonists (ACE Inhibitors) ↓ release of aldosterone causing ↑ excretion of Na and water.	captopril (Capoten) enalapril (Vasotec) fosinopril (Monopril) lisinopril (Zestril) ramipril (Altace)	Teratogenic, cough, taste disturbances, proteinuria, agranulocytosis, angioedema, neutropenia.

Mechanism of Action	Examples	Nontherapeutic Effects
Calcium Channel Blockers ↑ relaxation and dilation of vascular smooth muscle of coronary arteries and arterioles.	amlodipine (Norvasc) diltiazem (Cardizem) nifedipine (Procardia) verapamil (Calan)	• Flushing, peripheral edema. • *Cardizem, Calan:* Bradycardia.
Angiotensin II Receptor Antagonists ↓ vasoconstriction and ↓ release of aldosterone.	irbesartan (Avapro) losartan (Cozaar) olmesartan (Benicar) valsartan (Diovan)	• Teratogenic, nephrotoxic. • May cause angioedema such as dyspnea, facial swelling.
Beta Blockers (Selective) Block stimulation of $beta_1$ (myocardial) adrenergic receptors.	metoprolol (Lopressor)	• Fatigue, weakness, impotence, bradycardia, pulmonary edema. • May ↑ blood glucose of clients with DM.
Beta Blockers (Nonselective) Block stimulation of $beta_1$ (myocardial) and $beta_2$ (pulmonary, vascular, uterine) adrenergic receptors.	carvedilol (Coreg) labetalol propranolol (Inderal)	• Fatigue, weakness, pulmonary edema, bradycardia. • May cause impotence.
Centrally Acting Antiadrenergics Stimulate CNS $alpha_2$ adrenergic receptors to ↓ sympathetic outflow.	clonidine (Catapres) methyldopa (Aldomet)	• Dizziness, weakness, dry mouth, constipation. • May cause impotence.

Nursing Care

- Abrupt withdrawal may cause life-threatening ↑ BP or dysrhythmias; report to primary health-care provider any dyspnea, severe dizziness, persistent headache, ↑ or ↓ BP, ↑ or ↓ P, or irregular pulse rate.
- Assess BP and pulse for rate, rhythm, and volume before administration and routinely; teach to assess pulse daily and BP twice weekly; hold med if pulse is below preset parameter such as 50 bpm.

- Assess for ↑ fluid volume: ↑ BP, intake more than output, ↑ weight, edema, breath sounds for crackles, bounding pulse, distended neck veins.
- IV route: Assess VS every 5–15 min, ECG.
- Teach to take at same time of day; do not crush, break, or chew extended-release tabs.
- Avoid OTC meds, particularly cold remedies.
- Ensure safety related to orthostatic hypotension, avoidance of hazardous activities.
- Encourage actions to ↓ BP such as ↓ weight, ↓ Na diet, ↑ exercise, ↓ alcohol intake, smoking cessation, stress management.
- Assess for headache, hypotension, dizziness, nausea, dysrhythmias, ↑ sensitivity to cold, impotence.
- *Calcium channel blockers:* Avoid use of calcium-containing antacids or calcium supplements.

Antilipidemics (Lipid Lowering): Decrease Serum LDL, Triglycerides, and Total Cholesterol Levels and Increase HDL Levels

Mechanism of Action	Examples	Nontherapeutic Effects
HMG-CoA Reductase Inhibitors (Statins) Inhibit HMG-CoA—a catalyst in the synthesis of cholesterol.	atorvastatin (Lipitor) rosuvastatin (Crestor) simvastatin (Zocor)	• N&V, abdominal cramps, diarrhea, constipation, muscle soreness, hepatotoxicity, ↓ absorption of fat-soluble vitamins. • *Atorvastatin, rosuvastatin, simvastatin, fenofibrate:* S&S of rhabdomyolysis such as arthralgia, arthritis, myalgia, myositis. • *Ezetimibe:* Angioedema.
Bile Acid Sequestrants Bind cholesterol in GI tract.	cholestyramine	
Fibrates Inhibit peripheral lipolysis; ↓ triglyceride production and synthesis.	fenofibrate (Tricor) gemfibrozil (Lopid)	

Mechanism of Action	Examples	Nontherapeutic Effects
Cholesterol Absorption Inhibitors Inhibit absorption of cholesterol in small intestine.	ezetimibe (Zetia)	
Water-Soluble Vitamins Inhibit release of free fatty acids from adipose tissue; ↓ hepatic lipoprotein synthesis.	niacin	

Nursing Care

- Report occurrence of muscle pain, tenderness, or weakness with fever or malaise; fibrates may ↑ effect of warfarin.
- Encourage ↓ cholesterol, ↓ fat, ↑ fiber; fish high in omega-3 fatty acids 2–3 times a wk in diet.
- Monitor serum cholesterol, triglycerides, Hb, RBC, liver function studies.
- Exchange vegetable oils with polyunsaturated fatty acids (PUFA) to those with monounsaturated fatty acids (MUFA).
- *HMG-CoA reductase inhibitors:* Take at hr of sleep; avoid grapefruit, which ↑ risk of toxicity.
- *Bile acid sequestrants:* Take before meals with 8 oz of water; contraindicated for clients with phenylketonuria.
- *Cholesterol absorption inhibitors:* Explain to avoid these meds during pregnancy and lactation.
- *Water-soluble vitamins:* Explain that transient sensation of warmth may occur; ensure safety if orthostatic hypotension occurs.

Antineoplastics and Related Medications: Destroy or Decrease Growth of Neoplastic Cells to Cure, Control, and/or Palliate

Mechanism of Action	Examples	Nontherapeutic Effects
Alkylating Agents ↓ DNA synthesis preventing replication.	carboplatin cisplatin cyclophosphamide	• S&S of myelosuppression such as ↓ WBC, ↓ platelets. • Skin problems, second malignancies, hypersensitivity, nephrotoxicity, hepatotoxicity. • *Cisplatin:* Ototoxicity, neuropathies, vesicant. • *Cyclophosphamide:* Hemorrhagic cystitis.
Antiandrogens Block testosterone effect at cellular level.	bicalutamide (Casodex) flutamide	Hot flashes, gynecomastia, ↓ libido.
Antiangiogenic Agents ↓ new blood vessel formation in tumors.	bevacizumab (Avastin)	Hypersensitivity, GI perforation, HTN, bleeding, ↓ wound healing, arterial thromboembolic events.
Antiestrogens Compete for estrogen-binding sites in tissue; ↓ aromatase, which ↓ estrogen level.	**Estrogen-binding agents** tamoxifen citrate **Aromatase inhibitors** anastrozole (Arimidex) letrozole (Femara)	• *Estrogen-binding agents:* Hot flashes, N&V, ↓ libido, vaginal bleeding. • *Aromatase inhibitors:* Headache, weakness, hot flashes, musculoskeletal pain.

Mechanism of Action	Examples	Nontherapeutic Effects
Antimetabolites ↓ DNA synthesis and metabolism; cell-cycle S-phase specific.	capecitabine (Xeloda) fluorouracil gemcitabine (Gemzar) hydroxyurea (Hydrea) methotrexate	Myelosuppression, GI and skin problems, alopecia.
Antitumor Antibiotics ↓ DNA synthesis; doxorubicin is cell-cycle S-phase specific.	bleomycin doxorubicin mitomycin	• Myelosuppression, alopecia, skin and GI problems, organ toxicity. • *Bleomycin:* Pulmonary toxicity. • *Doxorubicin:* Red urine, cardiotoxicity.
Cytokines—Hematopoietic Growth Factors ↑ proliferation and function of hematopoietic cells.	**Increase RBC** epoetin alfa (Procrit, Epogen) **Increase WBC** filgrastim (Neupogen) pegfilgrastim (Neulasta)	Bone and injection site pain, N&V.
Cytokines—Immune Stimulants Suppress cell proliferation.	interferon alpha-2a (Roferon-A) interferon alpha-2b (Intron-A)	Flulike symptoms, myelosuppression.
Monoclonal Antibodies Bind to specific receptor sites to ↓ cell proliferation.	cetuximab (Erbitux) rituximab (Rituxan) trastuzumab (Herceptin)	• Fever, N&V, headache, hypersensitivity. • *Cetuximab:* Rash, interstitial lung disease. • *Rituximab:* Tumor lysis syndrome, myelosuppression. • *Trastuzumab:* Diarrhea, cardiotoxicity.
Plant Alkaloids ↓ cell replication, cell-cycle specific.	docetaxel (Taxotere) paclitaxel (Taxol) topotecan (Hycamtin) vinblastine vincristine	Alopecia, diarrhea, N&V, myelosuppression, hypersensitivity, neurotoxicity, vesicant.

Continued

Mechanism of Action	Examples	Nontherapeutic Effects
Tyrosine Kinase Inhibitors (Biological Response Modifiers) ↓ tumor growth; ↑ cell death.	erlotinib (Tarceva)	N&V, photosensitivity, rash.
Combination Therapy Concurrent use of multiple meds to destroy rapidly proliferating cells at different stages of replication; lower doses of each med ↓ toxicity and tumor cell resistance.	**CMF**: cyclophosphamide, methotrexate, fluorouracil. **CHOP**: cyclophosphamide, doxorubicin, vincristine, prednisone **ABVD**: doxorubicin, bleomycin, vinblastine, dacarbazine	See individual meds for nontherapeutic effects.
Nursing care: See Nursing Care for Clients With Cancer or Experiencing Nontherapeutic Effects of Antineoplastic Therapies in Med Surg Tab, p. 172.		

Antituberculars: Decrease Cough, Sputum, Fever, Night Sweats and Produce Negative Culture for *M. tuberculosis*

Mechanism of Action	Nontherapeutic Effects
Isoniazid (INH) ↓ mycobacterial cell wall synthesis, interferes with metabolism.	• Peripheral neuropathy: Numbness, tingling, paresthesia. • Hepatotoxicity: Jaundice, N&V, anorexia, amber urine, weakness, fatigue.
Rifampin ↓ mycobacterial RNA synthesis.	• Thrombocytopenia, hepatotoxicity, red/orange urine and other body fluids. • N&V, abdominal pain, flatulence, diarrhea. • Teratogenic; ↓ effectiveness of oral contraceptives.
Ethambutol ↓ mycobacterial RNA synthesis.	• Optic neuritis: ↓ visual acuity, temporary loss of vision, constriction of visual field, red/green color blindness, photophobia, and eye pain. • Rash.

Mechanism of Action	Nontherapeutic Effects
Pyrazinamide (PZA) Causes cellular destruction.	• Hyperuricemia: Pain in great toe and other joints. • Hepatotoxicity, skin rash, anorexia, N&V.
Rifapentine (Priftin) Inhibits DNA-dependent RNA polymerase.	• Dizziness, headache, hypertension, anorexia, diarrhea.
Badaquiline (Sirturo) Interferes with bacterial energy metabolism and replication.	• N&V, joint pain, headache, ↓ appetite, abdominal pain, dark urine, jaundice.
Combination meds: INH/rifampin (Rifamate); INH/rifampin/PZA (Rifater). **Nontherapeutic effects:** See individual meds for nontherapeutic effects.	

Nursing Care

- Assess VS, breath sounds, amount and characteristics of sputum.
- Monitor liver and renal labs, CBC, serum uric acid, visual tests.
- Obtain specimens for mycobacterial tests to detect possible resistance.
- Encourage avoidance of alcohol to ↓ hepatotoxicity.
- *Isoniazid (INH):* Avoid aluminum-containing antacids within 1 hr of INH; give pyridoxine (vitamin B_6) if prescribed to ↓ neuropathy.
- *Rifampin:* Take on empty stomach.
- *Ethambutol:* Take with food; do not breastfeed; eye exams monthly.
- *Pyrazinamide (PZA):* ↑ fluid to 2–3 L daily.

Antiretrovirals: Treat HIV and AIDS and Prevent or Decrease Severity of Viral Infections

Mechanism of Action	Examples
Nucleoside Reverse Transcriptase Inhibitors (NRTIs) Damage HIV's DNA interfering with ability to control host DNA.	abacavir (Ziagen) emtricitabine (Emtriva) lamivudine (Epivir-HBV) zidovudine (AZT, Retrovir)

Continued

Mechanism of Action	Examples
Non-Nucleoside Reverse Transcriptase Inhibitors (NNRTIs) Prevent conversion of HIV RNA into HIV DNA.	efavirenz (Sustiva) etravirine (Intelence) nevirapine (Viramune)
Protease Inhibitors Inhibit HIV protease, preventing virus maturation.	atazanavir (Reyataz) darunavir (Prezista) fosamprenavir (Lexiva)
Fusion Inhibitors Attach to gp41 protein on surface of HIV cells blocking HIV from entering into CD4 cells.	efuvirtide (Fuzeon) maraviroc (Selzentry)
Integrase Inhibitors Prevent HIV DNA from entering healthy cell DNA.	elvitegravir (Vitekta) raltegravir (Isentress)
Multiple Med Regimens Highly active antiretroviral therapy (HAART).	Atripla Combivir Complera Stribild Triumeq Truvada

Nontherapeutic Effects

- Anorexia, N&V, diarrhea, headache, dizziness, vaginitis, moniliasis.
- *Additional effects depending on med:* Confusion, skin eruptions, allergic response, neuropathies, nephrotoxicity, blood dyscrasias, hepatotoxicity, CNS depression.

Nursing Care

- Explain that GI discomfort and insomnia resolve after 3–4 wk.
- Refer to manufacturer's insert about need to take with or without food and what to do if a dose is missed.
- Take meds exactly as prescribed; avoid OTC meds; compliance of 95% necessary to prevent resistance.
- Assess for S&S of opportunistic infections, nephrotoxicity, hepatotoxicity, blood dyscrasia, and other specific med side effects.
- Encourage routine medical supervision; blood studies every 2 mo.
- Encourage sexual abstinence or use of safer sex practices.

Antivirals: Prevent or Decrease Severity of Viral Infections but Do Not Cure

Mechanism of Action	Examples	Nontherapeutic Effects
↓ entry of virus into host to ↓ effect of influenza type A.	oseltamivir (Tamiflu)	• Anorexia, N&V, diarrhea, headache, dizziness, vaginitis, moniliasis. • *Depending on med:* Skin eruptions, allergic response, neuropathies, nephrotoxicity, CNS depression, blood dyscrasias, confusion, hepatotoxicity.
↓ viral DNA synthesis to prevent or limit episodes of herpes simplex, genitalis, zoster, and varicella.	acyclovir valacyclovir (Valtrex)	
↓ viral DNA synthesis to prevent or limit cytomegalovirus, blood dyscrasias.	ganciclovir (Cytovene)	

Nursing Care

- Obtain C&S before starting therapy.
- Take meds exactly as prescribed to maintain blood levels; avoid OTC meds.
- Assess for S&S of nephrotoxicity, hepatotoxicity, blood dyscrasias, opportunistic infections.
- *Oseltamivir:* Begin treatment as soon as S&S appear.
- *Acyclovir, valacyclovir:* Take for pain and pruritus, which usually occur before eruptions; ↑ fluids to 3 L/day; herpes genitalis: ↑ risk for cervical cancer, avoid sexual activity during exacerbations.
- *Ganciclovir:* Give with food; assess for neutropenia, thrombocytopenia, photosensitivity, ↓ visual acuity; ensure regular eye exams; avoid pregnancy during and for 90 days after treatment (teratogenic); may cause infertility.

Bronchodilators: Promote Bronchial Expansion, Increase Transfer of Gases, Decrease Wheezing and Dyspnea

Mechanism of Action	Examples	Nontherapeutic Effects
Sympathomimetics (Beta-Adrenergic Agonists) Relax bronchial smooth muscle, ↓ spasms.	albuterol metaproterenol terbutaline	Headache, restlessness, tremor, paradoxical bronchospasm evidenced by wheezing, dyspnea.
Xanthines Relax bronchial smooth muscle, ↓ spasms.	theophylline	↑ P, ↓ BP, palpitations, dysrhythmias, nausea, dizziness, headache, restlessness.
Anticholinergics ↓ action of acetylcholine receptors in bronchial smooth muscle.	ipratropium (Atrovent) tiotropium (Spiriva)	Dizziness, headache, nervousness, ↓ BP, palpitations, blurred vision, urinary retention, dry mouth.
Leukotriene Receptor Antagonists ↓ edema, inflammation.	montelukast (Singulair)	• Bronchoconstriction. • Headache, weakness, N&V.
Inhaled and Nasal Route Steroids ↓ local inflammatory response and edema, ↑ airway diameter.	budesonide (Pulmicort) fluticasone (Flovent)	• Headache, oropharyngeal fungal infections, dysphonia, hoarseness. • *Budesonide:* Flulike syndrome.

Nursing Care

- Wait 1–5 min between inhaled meds; use bronchodilator first.
- Use spacer with metered-dose inhaler (MDI) to limit large droplets; rinse mouth and MDI after use.
- Obtain return demonstration of use of peak expiratory flow rate meter, inhaler, nebulizer.
- Assess breath sounds, extent of wheezing, amount and characteristics of sputum.
- Assess respiration rate, depth, characteristics; check heart for ↑ rate and dysrhythmias; ↓ or ↑ BP.
- Encourage use of all prescribed meds because of variety of purposes.
- Teach to avoid second-hand smoke and other respiratory irritants; smoking cessation.
- Encourage intake of 2–3 L of fluid daily to help liquefy respiratory secretions.

- Report if SOB is not ↓ or is accompanied by diaphoresis, dizziness, palpitations, chest pain.
- *Xanthines*: Use cautiously for clients with cardiac problems because it may ↑ P; give with food; monitor serum theophylline level (therapeutic: 10–20 mcg/mL).
- *Anticholinergics:* Ensure client does not have glaucoma because it ↑ intraocular pressure; encourage voiding before taking to ↓ urinary retention; suggest lozenges to ↓ dry mouth.
- *Leukotriene receptor antagonists:* Give on empty stomach.
- *Sympathomimetics:* Use cautiously for clients with cardiac problems; avoid use with tricyclic antidepressants or MAO inhibitors because it may cause hypertensive crisis or dysrhythmias.

Antisecretory Agents: Decrease Gastric Acidity and Epigastric Pain

Mechanism of Action	Examples	Nontherapeutic Effects
H_2 Antagonists ↓ histamine at H_2 receptors in parietal cells promotes ↓ gastric secretions.	famotidine (Pepcid) ranitidine (Zantac)	• Blood dyscrasias such as ↓ RBC, ↓ WBC, ↓ platelets. • CNS disturbances such as confusion, dizziness, drowsiness, headache. • Dysrhythmias, nephrotoxicity, hypersensitivity reactions. • Osteoporosis with long-term use.
Proton Pump Inhibitors ↓ entry of hydrogen ions into gastric lumen.	dexlansoprazole (Dexiante) esomeprazole (Nexium) lansoprazole (Prevacid) omeprazole (Prilosec) pantoprazole (Protonix)	

Nursing Care

- May ↑ anticoagulant effect of warfarin; CNS disturbances often occur in older adults.
- Give 1–2 hr before or after antacids; give oral meds with meals.
- Assess heart rate and rhythm, emesis and stool for frank or occult blood, CBC for blood dyscrasias.
- *H_2 antagonists:* Teach that smoking interferes with med action, may cause diarrhea.
- *Proton pump inhibitors:* Advise not to crush or chew capsule.

Diuretics: Increase Urine Output and Decrease Hypervolemia, BP, Peripheral Edema, ICP, Intraocular Pressure, and Seizures

Mechanism of Action	Examples	Nontherapeutic Effects
Thiazides and Thiazide-Like ↓ sodium (Na) and chloride resorption in distal convoluted tubule and ↓ chloride resorption in ascending loop of Henle.	**Thiazide** hydrochlorothiazide (HCTZ) **Thiazide-like** metolazone (Zaroxolyn)	• Dehydration, orthostatic hypotension, F&E imbalances. • ↓ potassium. • ↓ Na, ↓ chloride, ↓ magnesium, ↑ calcium. • Pain in great toe and other joints.
Loop ↓ Na and chloride resorption in ascending loop of Henle and distal renal tubule.	bumetanide (Bumex) furosemide (Lasix)	
Potassium-Sparing *Spironolactone:* Acts in distal tubule; ↓ action of aldosterone, ↑ Na, and ↓ potassium excretion. *Triamterene:* ↑ excretion of Na, blocks potassium loss.	spironolactone (Aldactone) triamterene (Dyrenium)	• CNS complications such as dizziness, drowsiness, lethargy, weakness, hearing loss. • N&V, photosensitivity, pulmonary edema, ↑ serum glucose. • *Potassium-sparing meds:* ↑ potassium.
Carbonic Anhydrase Inhibitors Diuretic Effect ↓ carbonic anhydrase in proximal renal tubule, thereby ↑ excretion of Na, potassium, bicarbonate, and water. *Ophthalmic effect:* ↓ aqueous humor, which ↓ intraocular pressure. *Anticonvulsant effect:* ↓ abnormal paroxysmal discharge in CNS neurons.	acetazolamide (Diamox)	

Nursing Care

- Assess VS before administration; give in a.m. to ↓ disruption in sleep.
- Assess for F&E imbalances, particularly hypo- and hyperkalemia, which can cause dysrhythmias.

- Assess for S&S of hypervolemia such as ↑ BP, bounding pulse, intake exceeds output, ↑ weight, pitting edema, crackles in lungs.
- Assess for S&S of hypovolemia such as ↓ BP, thready pulse, tenting of skin, dry sticky mucous membranes.
- Change position slowly to ↓ orthostatic hypotension.
- Avoid sun to ↓ photosensitivity; suggest use of sunscreen, protective clothing.
- Take meds even if feeling better because meds control, not cure, HTN.
- Encourage other interventions to ↓ BP such as ↓ weight, low Na diet, smoking cessation, ↑ exercise and stress management.

Thrombolytic Agents: Dissolve Clots in Blood Vessels or Venous and Arterial Catheters

Mechanism of Action	Examples	Nontherapeutic Effects
Activate conversion of plasminogen to plasmin, which breaks down clots.	alteplase (Activase) reteplase (Retavase) streptokinase	• Bleeding: GI, genitourinary, retroperitoneal, CNS; ecchymoses. • Reperfusion dysrhythmias, rash, dyspnea, anaphylaxis.

Nursing Care

- Give prescribed agent within 6 hr of event, preferably 3 hr for a coronary artery thrombus; also give for PE, acute ischemic brain attack, DVT, arterial thromboembolism, occluded central venous access devices.
- *Identify clients at ↑ risk of bleeding:* >75 yr; ≤10 days postpartum; or receiving warfarin, aspirin, NSAIDs, heparin, heparin-like agents.
- *Identify clients with conditions that contraindicate therapy:* History of brain attack, recent surgery or trauma, uncontrolled HTN, bleeding tendencies, intracranial neoplasm, atriovenous malformation.
- Follow manufacturer's directions for solution and med compatibility and infusion rate; use IV infusion pump.
- Assess VS and for bleeding every 15 min 1st hr, every 15–30 min next 8 hr, and then every 4 hr; assess for coffee-ground emesis, tarry stool, occult blood, hematuria, epistaxis; ↓ neurological status, sudden severe headache, indicating cranial bleeding; joint pain, back and leg pain, indicating retroperitoneal bleeding; abdominal pain, T 104°F, indicating internal bleeding; hold med and call primary health-care provider immediately.
- Monitor Hb, Hct, platelets, activated partial thromboplastin time, prothrombin time, thrombin time, INR, and bleeding time.
- Have blood and antidote aminocaproic acid (Amicar) available to treat hemorrhage.

Hypoglycemics: Control Blood Glucose in Type 2 Diabetes

Mechanism of Action	Examples	Nontherapeutic Effects
Sulfonylureas Stimulate beta cells to release insulin.	glimepiride (Amaryl) glipizide (Glucotrol) glyburide	Hypoglycemia.
Biguanides ↑ sensitivity to insulin, ↑ binding of insulin to its receptor.	metformin (Glucophage)	• Lactic acidosis: Drowsiness, hyperventilation, myalgia, malaise. • Hypoglycemia.
Meglitinides ↑ release of insulin in pancreas.	repaglinide (Prandin)	Hypoglycemia.
Thiazolidinediones ↑ insulin action in muscle and fat, ↓ gluconeogenesis.	pioglitazone (Actos) rosiglitazone (Avandia)	• Upper respiratory tract infection. • Hypoglycemia does not occur.
Incretin Mimetics Mimic effects of GLP-1, an intestinal hormone, that ↑ secretion of insulin, ↓ glucose absorption from the gut, ↓ action of glucagon.	dulaglutide (Trulicity) liraglutide (Victoza)	• N&V, diarrhea, abdominal pain, ↓ appetite, indigestion, fatigue.
Dipeptidyl Peptidase-4 Inhibitors Prevent GLP-1 and GIP activation, ↑ the secretion of insulin, ↓ the release of glucagon.	sitagliptin (Januvia)	• N&V, common cold-like S&S, photosensitivity.
Glifozin Inhibits renal glucose reabsorption.	canagliflozin (Invokana, Sulisent)	• Dizziness, ↑ urination, pain or burning on urination, allergic reaction, genital discharge, hyperkalemia, ketoacidosis.

Nursing Care

- *Identify clients with conditions that contraindicate therapy:* Uncontrolled infection; pregnancy; breastfeeding; serious burns; trauma; renal, hepatic, or endocrine disease.
- Assess for hypoglycemia, hyperglycemia, and hyperosmolar nonketotic coma.
- Perform finger stick for serum glucose; ketones in urine if blood glucose is ≥300.
- Teach to avoid alcohol because it may produce severe N&V (Antabuse-like reaction).
- Teach to not crush sustained-release tablets; take 30 min before meal or follow prescription exactly.
- *Dulaglutide and liraglutide:* Injectable forms are given Sub-Q.
- *Thiazolidinediones:* Monitor liver function.
- For hyper- and hypoglycemia and related nursing care, see Alterations in Blood Glucose Associated With DM, Nursing Care, in Med Surg Tab, p. 188.

Insulins: Time-Action Profiles

Insulin Type	Examples	Onset	Peak	Duration
Rapid Acting	aspart (NovoLog)	10–20 min	1–3 hr	3–5 hr
	glulisine (Apidra)	15–30 min	30 min–1.5 hr	3–4 hr
	lispro (Humalog)	15–30 min	30 min–1.5 hr	3–4 hr
Short Acting	regular (Humulin R)	30–60 min	1–5 hr	6–10 hr
	regular (Novolin R)	30–60 min	2–5 hr	5–8 hr
Intermediate Acting	Humulin N Novolin N NPH (N)	1.5–4 hr	4–12 hr	18–24 hr

Continued

Insulin Type	Examples	Onset	Peak	Duration
Long Acting	detemir (Levemir)	50 min–2 hr	Unknown	24 hr
	glargine (Lantus)	1–1.5 hr	Steadily delivered, no peak action	20–24 hr
Premixed	Humalog 75/25	15 min	30 min–2.5 hr	16–20 hr
	Humulin 50/50	30 min	2–5 hr	18–24 hr
	Humulin 70/30	30 min	2–4 hr	14–24 hr
	Novolin 70/30	30 min	2–12 hr	24 hr
	NovoLog Mix 70/30	10–20 min	1–4 hr	24 hr

Nursing Care

- Generally, only regular insulin can be given IV; however, rapid-insulin analogs such as aspart and glulisine may be given IV in selective situations with medical supervision.
- Roll, do not shake, vials of insulin; avoids bubbles in solution.
- Use calibrated insulin syringe to ensure accurate dose.
- Give prescribed dose of insulin based on blood glucose levels; usually before meals and before bedtime.
- **Procedure for mixing insulins**
  Proper technique prevents NPH insulin from ↓ purity of solution in the short-acting regular insulin vial.
    1. Use insulin syringe calibrated in units (0.3, 0.5, 1 mL; 1/2-, 5/8-, 1-inch needle).
    2. Draw up air equal to combined volume of both insulins.
    3. Inject NPH vial with amount of air equal to prescribed amount of NPH without dipping needle into solution while keeping vial right-side up.
    4. Inject remaining air into regular insulin vial without dipping needle into solution while keeping vial right-side up.

5. Invert vial, and draw up the prescribed amount of regular insulin.
6. Reinsert needle into NPH vial, invert vial, and withdraw prescribed amount.
7. Administer within 5 min of preparation or insulins will bind, decreasing their action.

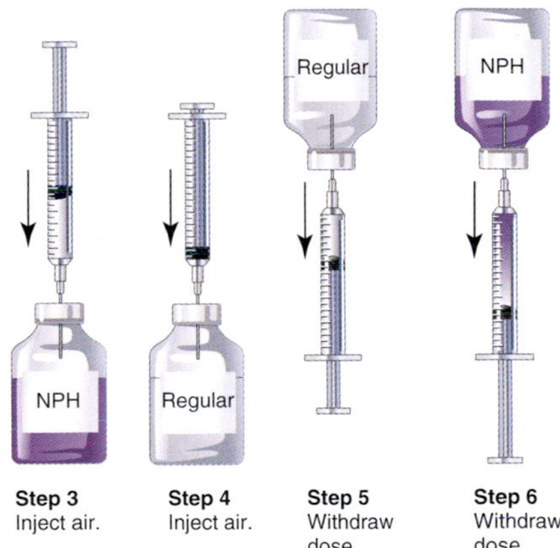

Laxatives and Cathartics: Decrease Constipation and Promote Evacuation of Bowel

Mechanism of Action	Examples	Nontherapeutic Effects
Bulk-Forming Laxatives and Cathartics ↑ bulk stimulates peristalsis.	methylcellulose (Citrucel) psyllium (Metamucil)	Cramps, F&E imbalances, dependence.
Stool Softeners Cause water and fat to enter feces to soften and ↓ drying of stool.	docusate sodium (Colace)	
Stimulants and Irritants Irritate mucosa, causing rapid propulsion of contents.	bisacodyl (Dulcolax) senna (Senokot)	
Lubricants Soften feces.	mineral oil	
Saline Osmotics Draw water into intestinal lumen, distending bowel and stimulating peristalsis.	magnesium salts (Milk of Magnesia)	

Nursing Care

- Identify clients for whom the med is contraindicated: N&V, abdominal pain, or S&S of acute abdomen because these may indicate bowel obstruction; do not use sodium osmotic with older adults or children because it may cause F&E imbalances.
- Give at bedtime.
- Encourage ↑ fluid intake, activity, dietary fiber; assess stool frequency, consistency.
- *Bulk-forming:* Teach to mix in 8 oz of fluid and follow with 8 oz fluid; may take ≥12 hr to act.
- *Stool softeners:* Inform that results may take several days to act.
- *Stimulants/irritants:* Inform that results occur quickly; fluid may be passed with feces.
- *Lubricants:* Inform that absorption of fat-soluble vitamins may decrease.
- *Saline osmotics:* Inform that results occur quickly; monitor for S&S of dehydration, hypernatremia, ↓ absorption of fat-soluble vitamins.

Opioid (Narcotic) Antagonists: Reverse Opioid-Induced CNS Depression and Decreased Respiratory Function

Mechanism of Action	Examples	Nontherapeutic Effects
Displace opioid at receptor sites via competitive antagonism.	naloxone	N&V, ↓ or ↑ BP, ventricular fibrillation.
	naltrexone	N&V, abdominal cramps, muscle and joint pain, insomnia, anxiety, headache, hepatotoxicity; may cause early fetal loss.

Nursing Care

- Assess VS, particularly respiratory rate and BP.
- Assess for S&S of opioid withdrawal such as restlessness, ↑ BP, ↑ T, abdominal cramps, and N&V.

Opioid (Narcotic) Analgesics: Decrease Transmission of Pain Impulses, Coughing, and GI Motility

Mechanism of Action	Examples	Nontherapeutic Effects
Combine with opioid receptors in CNS.	codeine fentanyl (Duragesic-72-hr transdermal patch) hydrocodone (Hycodan) hydromorphone (Dilaudid) methadone (Dolophine) morphine (MS Contin) oxycodone (OxyContin) *Atypical opioid:* tramadol (Ultram)	• ↓ R, sedation, constipation, nausea, drowsiness, pruritus. • *Fentanyl:* Dry mouth, diaphoresis, weakness.

Opioid and Nonopioid Analgesic Combinations: Provide More Effective Pain Relief Due to Synergistic Effect

- Codeine phosphate and acetaminophen (Tylenol with codeine 1, 2, 3, or 4).
- Hydrocodone and acetaminophen (Vicodin).
- Oxycodone and acetaminophen (Percocet).
- Oxycodone and aspirin (Percodan).

Nursing Care

- Assess for respiratory depression; if respiratory rate is ≤10 breaths per min, hold dose and call primary health-care provider.
- Keep opioid antagonist available, such as naloxone or naltrexone, for toxicity or overdose.
- Assess pain, VS, ↓ BP, drowsiness, confusion, constipation, N&V, tolerance and dependence.
- Give before pain is severe because regularly scheduled doses maintain therapeutic blood levels and ↑ effectiveness.
- Give additional prescribed med for breakthrough pain; common with continuous infusion, sustained-release med, or intractable pain.
- Give cautiously because combinations ↑ effectiveness **(synergistic effect)** and may ↑ risk of toxicity.
- Decrease slowly after chronic use to ↓ S&S of withdrawal.
- Encourage coughing and deep breathing every 2 hr.
- Increase fluids, fiber, and activity to limit constipation; give prescribed stool softeners and laxatives.
- Provide for safety; encourage avoidance of hazardous activities; change position slowly.
- Use cautiously with ↑ ICP because it can mask S&S of ICP.
- Teach how to self-administer meds such as IM, Sub-Q, sublingual, transdermal.

Skeletal Muscle Relaxants: Limit Muscle Spasms

Mechanism of Action	Examples	Nontherapeutic Effects
Central Acting ↓ muscle activity at the level of the brain stem.	carisoprodol (Soma) cyclobenzaprine (Flexeril) diazepam (Valium) metaxalone (Skelaxin)	• Drowsiness, dizziness, fatigue, weakness, constipation. • *Metaxalone and dantrolene:* GI upset, vomiting, diarrhea. • *Botox:* Effects depend on site of injection.
Direct Acting ↓ release of calcium within skeletal muscles, preventing contraction and suppressing hyperactive reflexes.	botulinum toxin (Botox) dantrolene (Dantrium)	

Nursing Care

- Assess pain, muscle stiffness, area around injection site, ROM.
- Give with food to ↓ GI irritation; avoid alcohol and CNS depressants.
- Avoid hazardous activity until sedative effect is known.
- ↑ fluids and fiber to ↓ constipation; give prescribed stool softeners.

Antiseizure Agents: Decrease Occurrence, Frequency, and/or Severity of Seizures

Mechanism of Action	Examples	Nontherapeutic Effects
Action depends on med classification. Choice of med depends on seizure type.	acetazolamide (Diamox) carbamazepine (Tegretol) gabapentin (Neurontin) lamotrigine (Lamictal) levetiracetam (Keppra) pregabalin (Lyrica) topiramate (Topamax) valproic acid (Depakene) *Status epilepticus:* diazepam (Valium) lorazepam (Ativan)	• Drowsiness, dizziness, N&V, rash, headache. • ↓ BP, respiratory depression. • Blood dyscrasias such as ↓ WBC, ↓ RBC, ↓ platelets. • Hepatotoxicity.

Nursing Care

- Increase gradually as prescribed until seizure control is achieved; may require two antiseizure meds.
- Shake suspensions before administration; give with food to ↓ GI irritation.
- Teach that med may be continued indefinitely; withdrawal may be attempted after 3 yr of being seizure free.
- Advise med may ↓ effectiveness of oral contraceptives; advise to consult primary health-care provider when planning pregnancy or lactation.
- Withdraw med over 6–12 wk; seizures occur with abrupt withdrawal.
- *Status epilepticus:* Give prescribed IV diazepam or lorazepam; keep resuscitative equipment available.

Bone Resorption Inhibitors: Decrease Bone Resorption and Potential for Fractures and Increase Bone Density

Mechanism of Action	Examples	Nontherapeutic Effects
Bisphosphonates ↓ osteoclast activity, ↓ bone resorption.	alendronate (Fosamax) ibandronate (Boniva) pamidronate (Aredia) risedronate (Actonel) zoledronic acid (Reclast, Zometa)	• N&V, diarrhea, bone pain, abdominal pain, flushing. • May cause osteonecrosis of jaw.
Hormonal Agents *Calcitonin salmon:* ↓ rate of bone turnover and lowers serum calcium. *Teriparatide:* ↑ osteoblastic activity and bone mineral density.	calcitonin salmon (Miacalcin) teriparatide (Forteo)	• Transient N&V, diarrhea. • Flushing and/or warmth 1 hr after IM or Sub-Q. • *Calcitonin salmon:* Nasal irritation with nasal route.

Nursing Care

- Teach that effect takes >1 mo.
- Assess for hypocalcemia such as ↓ BP, muscle spasms, paresthesias, laryngospasm, positive Chvostek and/or Trousseau signs.
- Teach to discuss plans for pregnancy or lactation with primary health-care provider.
- Encourage intake of calcium foods and prescribed calcium and vitamin D supplements.
- Encourage weight-bearing exercise; avoid smoking, alcohol, and cola, which ↑ osteoporosis; ensure baseline bone density test.

- *Bisphosphonates:* Teach to take oral dose in a.m. with water on empty stomach.
- *Calcitonin salmon:* Perform intradermal allergy test first because med may cause anaphylaxis; alternate nostrils daily with intranasal calcitonin.

Erectile Dysfunction Agents

- **Sildenafil (Viagra), tadalafil (Cialis), alprostadil (Muse)**
  - *Action:* ↑ strength and duration of erections.
  - *Nontherapeutic effects:* HTN, UTI, headache, insomnia, constipation, dry mouth, erection lasting ≥4 hr.
  - *Nursing care:* Assess for S&S of cardiac distress, med interactions; call primary health-care provider if erection lasts ≥4 hr; avoid concurrent use with a nitrate because of risk of fatal brain attack, MI.

Contraceptive Agents

- **Oral monophasic, biphasic, triphasic formulations (combined estrogen and progestin in different doses and cycles):** ↓ ovulation; suppresses follicular-stimulating hormone and luteinizing hormone. *Nontherapeutic effect:* Uterine bleeding, nausea, vaginal candidiasis, ↑ BP, fluid retention, pigmentation of face, thromboembolism.
- **Medroxyprogesterone (Depo-Provera), etonogestrel implant (Implanon):** ↓ sperm and ovum transport, ↓ ovum implantation. *Nontherapeutic effect:* Uterine bleeding, thromboembolism; etonogestrel implant - ↑ BP, headache.
- **Emergency contraception: levonorgestrel/ethinylestradiol, levonorgestrel:** ↓ implantation; 75% effective. *Nontherapeutic effect:* Thromboembolism, nausea, abdominal pain, fatigue, headache, menstrual changes.
- **Contraindications for all types:** ≥35-yr-old smoker, history of thromboembolism.
- **Nursing care**
  - Teach ↑ pregnancy risk with use of antibiotics, phenobarbital, phenytoin, and rifampin.
  - Instruct to have regular Pap smears, physicals, mammograms, stop smoking.
  - *Oral formulations:* Assess for ectopic pregnancy, avoid breastfeeding.
  - *Medroxyprogesterone:* Administer injection 4 times a yr.
  - *Etonogestrel implant:* Assess implant site (upper arm); teach to replace within 3 yr because effectiveness ↓.
  - *Emergency contraception:* Teach to begin within 72 hr after intercourse; refer to contraception counseling.

Medications for Degenerative Diseases of the Nervous System

Parkinson Disease Medications: Restore Dopamine and Acetylcholine Balance; Decrease Motor S&S Such as Stooped Posture, Nonintention Tremors, Rigidity, Impaired Coordination

Mechanism of Action	Examples	Nontherapeutic Effects
Dopamine Agonists Stimulate dopamine receptors	amantadine apomorphine (Apokyn) bromocriptine (Parlodel) carbidopa-levodopa (Sinemet) pramipexole (Mirapex) ropinirole (Requip)	• ↓ BP, ↑ P, fatigue, anorexia, N&V, dry mouth, tremors, constipation, dizziness, weakness. • Sleepiness, compulsive behaviors, hallucinations. • *Toxicity:* Muscle twitching, mood changes. • *Carbidopa-levodopa:* Urine and sweat may darken in color.
Anticholinergics ↓ excess cholinergic activity in brain.	benztropine (Cogentin)	Dry mouth, blurred vision, ↑ P, constipation, urinary retention.
COMT Inhibitors Inhibit the enzyme COMT, prevent levodopa breakdown.	entacapone (Comtan) tolcapone (Tasmar)	• Brownish/orange urine, dyskinesia, N&V, ↓ BP. • *Entacapone:* Disintegration of muscle **(rhabdomyolysis)**, neuroleptic malignant syndrome.
Monoamine Oxidase (MAO) Type B Inhibitor Inactivates MAO thereby ↑ dopamine.	selegiline (Eldepryl)	CNS stimulation or depression, confusion, dizziness, nausea.

Nursing Care

- Teach that effect may take several mo; therapy is palliative.
- Give exactly as prescribed and slowly because of dysphagia.
- Encourage eating after taking to use advantage of ↓ dysphagia and to ↓ GI irritation.
- Assess VS; change position slowly; avoid hazardous activity.
- Do not discontinue abruptly because parkinsonian crisis may occur.
- *Dopamine Agonists:* Teach to avoid food such as veal, lamb, pork, egg yolks, and potatoes that are high in pyridoxine (B_6) because they ↓ effectiveness.
- *Sinemet:* Ensure not given with narrow-angle glaucoma and MAO inhibitors.
- *Anticholinergics:* Provide frequent oral care; encourage use of gum or hard candy to ↑ salivation; give prescribed stool softeners; catheterize for urinary retention if prescribed.
- *MAO inhibitors:* Avoid concurrent use with an opioid, SSRI, or tricyclic because it may cause a fatal interaction.

Medications for Neurocognitive Disorders Particularly Alzheimer Disease: Slow Progressive Deterioration of Cognition and Behavior

Mechanism of Action	Examples	Nontherapeutic Effects
Acetylcholinesterase (AchE) Inhibitors ↑ acetylcholine levels in cerebral cortex.	donepezil (Aricept) galantamine (Razadyne) rivastigmine (Exelon)	• Anorexia, N&V, diarrhea, ↓ BP, headache, dizziness, insomnia. • *Overdose:* Severe N&V, diaphoresis, salivation, ↓ P, seizures, ↑ muscle weakness, including respiratory muscles.
***N*-methyl D-aspartate Receptor (NMDAR) Antagonists** ↓ action of NMDAR.	memantine (Namenda)	Dizziness, confusion, headache, vomiting, constipation.

Nursing Care

- Use with caution in clients with COPD or asthma.
- Teach that therapy is palliative and lifelong, not a cure.
- Ensure med is prescribed in form client can swallow.
- Monitor VS, respiratory status, Hb, Hct, stool for melena, weekly weight.
- Protect from injury.

Myasthenia Gravis Medications: Increase Strength of Skeletal Muscle Contractions

Mechanism of Action	Examples	Nontherapeutic Effects
Anticholinesterase Muscle Stimulants ↓ cholinesterase, thus ↑ acetylcholine.	neostigmine pyridostigmine (Mestinon)	*Cholinergic S&S:* ↑ salivation, ↑ lacrimation, N&V, diarrhea, intestinal cramping, ↓ P, pupillary constriction.
Immunosuppressants Inhibit immune cells such as T and B cells.	azathioprine (Imuran) cyclosporine (Sandimmune) mycophenolate mofetil (CellCept) prednisone tacrolimus (Prograf)	N&V, GI upset, infection, nephrotoxicity, hepatotoxicity.

Nursing Care

- Assess for myasthenic crisis due to insufficient meds: Dyspnea, dysphagia, dysarthria, respiratory arrest.
- Assess for cholinergic crisis due to overdose of anticholinergics: Ptosis; weakness; difficulty chewing, swallowing, breathing; keep IV atropine sulfate available as antidote for anticholinesterase muscle stimulants.
- Administer edrophonium **(Tensilon Test)** as prescribed to distinguish between myasthenic crisis (S&S will ↓) from cholinergic crisis (S&S will ↑).
- Give meds carefully due to dysphagia; give with food or milk to ↓ GI irritation.
- Give meds exactly as scheduled; usually before meals to ↑ chewing and swallowing.
- Have tracheostomy set and resuscitative equipment available.
- Evaluate response as dosage is adjusted accordingly.
- Balance activity and rest; plan activities when strength is greatest.

Medications for Cardiac Problems

Antidysrhythmics: Decrease Abnormal Electrical Conduction Through Heart

Mechanism of Action	Examples	Nontherapeutic Effects
Calcium Ion Antagonists Slow conduction; local anesthetic; used for ventricular dysrhythmias.	flecainide (Tambocor) lidocaine procainamide	Heart failure, new dysrhythmias, ↓ BP, GI distress, blood dyscrasias, anticholinergic effects, diarrhea, neurotoxicity.
β-adrenergic Blockers ↓ cardiac excitability, output, and workload; ↓ heart rate and ↓ BP; used for angina, HTN, and dysrhythmias.	atenolol (Tenormin) metoprolol (Lopressor) nadolol (Corgard) nebivolol (Bystolic) propranolol (Inderal)	
Potassium Channel Blockers Slow heart rate and conduction; used for ventricular and supraventricular dysrhythmias.	amiodarone (Cordarone) dofetilide (Tikosyn) ibutilide (Corvert) sotalol (Betapace)	
Calcium Channel Blockers ↓ entry of calcium into myocardial and vascular smooth muscle cells; ↓ SA and AV node conduction; used for atrial fibrillation and supraventricular tachycardia.	clevidipine butyrate (Cleviprex) diltiazem (Cardizem) felodipine (Plendil) nifedipine (Procardia) verapamil (Calan)	
Selective Sinus Node Inhibitor ↑ ventricular filling and coronary perfusion.	ivabradine (Corlandor)	↓ P, temporary visual disturbances (flashes of light, blurred vision), HTN.

Nursing Care

- Keep resuscitative equipment available.
- Use infusion pump for IV; assess VS, BP, and ECG until stable.
- Obtain heart rate before administration; withhold med based on preset parameters.
- Monitor therapeutic blood levels.
- Assess for S&S of ↑ fluid volume such as crackles, edema, weight gain.
- Maintain safety; change position slowly to ↓ risk of hypotension.
- Teach about med regimen; need to ↓ Na intake; report side effects; identify irregular beats or ↑ or ↓ heart rate; need for continued medical supervision.
- Counsel females of childbearing age about teratogenic risk of specific meds.

Cardiac Glycosides: Increase Force of Cardiac Contraction and Cardiac Output and Decrease Heart Rate

Mechanism of Action	Example	Nontherapeutic Effects
Cardiac Glycoside ↑ force of cardiac contractions. ↓ rate of cardiac contractions. ↓ conduction velocity.	digoxin (Lanoxin)	• ↓ P, headache, drowsiness, fatigue, weakness. • *Toxicity:* N&V; anorexia; visual disturbances such as blurred, yellow vision; premature ventricular complexes; diarrhea.

Nursing Care

- Initiate digoxin therapy as prescribed **(digitalization)**.
  - *Slow method:* Dose gradually increased; used in less acute situations.
  - *Fast method:* Dose rapidly increased; used in acute heart failure.
- Teach to take own pulse; hold med and notify primary health-care provider if less than preset parameters such as <50–60 bpm.
- Teach S&S of toxicity; report if they occur.
- Monitor therapeutic blood level (0.8–2 ng/mL); has narrow therapeutic window.
- Monitor potassium levels; notify primary health-care provider if below 3.5 mEq/L because it may precipitate digoxin toxicity.
- Assess for hyperkalemia if on potassium-sparing diuretic.
- Encourage foods high in potassium unless taking potassium-sparing med.

Cardiac Stimulants: Increase Heart Rate

Mechanism of Action	Examples	Nontherapeutic Effects
Cardiac Stimulants Stimulate alpha and beta receptors in the heart to ↑ heart rate, contractility.	atropine sulfate dobutamine dopamine epinephrine norepinephrine (Levophed)	• Dysrhythmias, ↑ P, headache, angina. • *Atropine sulfate:* Anticholinergic effects such as dry mouth, blurred vision, urinary retention.

Nursing Care

- Assess VS frequently during administration.
- Monitor ECG continuously when given IV.
- Ensure ongoing follow-up care and ECGs.

Coronary Vasodilators: Dilate Arteries and Decrease Preload, Afterload, and Myocardial Oxygen Consumption

Mechanism of Action	Examples	Nontherapeutic Effects
Coronary Vasodilators Mechanism varies by med; blocks calcium channels or relaxes smooth muscle to treat angina, mild hypertension.	amlodipine (Norvasc) clonidine (Catapres) hydralazine (Apresoline) isosorbide dinitrate (Isordil, Sorbitrate) nifedipine (Procardia) nitroglycerin (Nitro-Dur, Sublingual Nitrostat) terazosin (Hytrin)	Orthostatic hypotension, ↑ P, headache, dizziness, N&V, flushing, confusion.

Nursing Care

- Assess BP; hold at set parameters.
- Teach to take prescribed acetaminophen for headache.
- *Nitroglycerin (transdermal):* See Med Administration, Transdermal Route p. 290.
- *Nitroglycerin (sublingual)*
  - Teach to take sip of water; put tablet under tongue; expect slight tingling as tablet dissolves.
  - Take 1 pill every 5 min up to 3 times for chest pain; if pain continues, get emergency help such as dial 911.
  - Store tablets in dark, tightly closed bottle; meds expire in 6 mo.

Psychotropic Medications

Anxiolytics, Sedatives, and Hypnotics: Decrease Anxiety, Induce Sleep, Ease Alcohol Withdrawal

Mechanism of Action	Examples	Nontherapeutic Effects
Benzodiazepines ↑ action of gamma-aminobutyric acid (GABA) inhibitory neurotransmitter.	**Short Acting** alprazolam (Xanax) midazolam (Versed) **Medium Acting** lorazepam (Ativan) **Long Acting** chlordiazepoxide (Librium) clonazepam (Klonopin) diazepam (Valium)	• ↓ mental alertness, ↓ BP, drowsiness, dizziness, headache. • Paradoxical reactions such as euphoria, excitement.
Nonbenzodiazepines All have CNS-depressant effect, variable action, depending on med.	buspirone (BuSpar) diphenhydramine (Benadryl) eszopiclone (Lunesta) hydroxyzine (Vistaril) zaleplon (Sonata) zolpidem (Ambien) zopiclone (Zimovane)	

Nursing Care

- Avoid alcohol because it ↑ effects; avoid caffeine because it ↓ effects.
- Avoid hazardous activities until tolerance develops.
- Avoid concurrent use with herbal products such as St. John's wort, kava, ginseng.
- Hold med if systolic BP falls <20 mm Hg on standing.
- Discontinue gradually to prevent S&S of withdrawal; use more than 2 wk may cause dependence.
- *Buspirone:* Teach that effect takes 3–6 wk, which is longer than other anxiolytics.
- Administer flumazenil (Romazicon) for reversal of benzodiazepines.

Antidepressants: Lift Depressed Mood, Minimize Panic Response and Narcolepsy

Mechanism of Action	Examples	Nontherapeutic Effects
Tricyclics (TCAs) ↓ reuptake of norepinephrine and serotonin into presynaptic nerve terminals.	amitriptyline doxepin (Silenor) imipramine (Tofranil) nortriptyline (Pamelor)	Anticholinergic effects, ↓ BP, CNS stimulation effects.
Selective Serotonin Reuptake Inhibitors (SSRIs) ↓ reuptake of serotonin into presynaptic nerve terminals.	citalopram (Celexa) duloxetine (Cymbalta) escitalopram (Lexapro) fluoxetine (Prozac) paroxetine (Paxil) sertraline (Zoloft) trazodone (Oleptro)	• Sexual dysfunction. • ↑ appetite, ↑ weight. • Anticholinergic and CNS stimulation or depression. • Hepatotoxicity, photosensitivity.
Monoamine Oxidase Inhibitors (MAOIs) ↓ breakdown of dopamine, norepinephrine, and serotonin in CNS neurons.	phenelzine (Nardil) selegiline (Eldepryl) tranylcypromine (Parnate)	• Sexual dysfunction, rash, anticholinergic effects. • CNS stimulation or depression.
Atypical New-Generation Meds ↑ effects of dopamine serotonin and/or norepinephrine at neural membranes.	bupropion (Wellbutrin) mirtazapine (Remeron) venlafaxine (Effexor)	Drowsiness, dizziness, headache, insomnia, N&V, anticholinergic effects.

Nursing Care

- Assess for suicidal potential; especially as mood lifts and physical and psychic energy increase.
- Ensure minimum of 2–6 wk between concurrent use of TCAs, MAOIs, or SSRIs to avoid serotonin syndrome; do not discontinue med abruptly.
- Assess for anticholinergic and CNS effects.
- Avoid prescription, OTC, or herbal products without supervision.
- Take at hr of sleep if sedation occurs or in a.m. if insomnia occurs.
- Avoid hazardous activities until sedative effect is known.
- Change positions slowly to ↓ orthostatic hypotension.

Tricyclics

- Avoid giving with narrow-angle glaucoma or cardiac condition.
- Teach that effect may take 2–6 wk.

SSRIs

- Teach that effect may take 5 wk.
- Obtain baseline weight, assess regularly.
- Teach to ↑ exercise and ↓ caloric intake to ↓ weight gain.
- Teach to wear protective clothing and sunscreen outdoors.

MAOIs

- Prevent hypertensive crisis by eliminating foods containing tyramine such as aged cheese, beer, wine, chocolate, caffeine, licorice, bananas, raisins, pepperoni, salami, bologna, liver, sour cream, yogurt.
- Assess BP when given with antihypertensive because hypotension may occur.
- Teach that effect may take 4–8 wk.

Atypical New-Generation Medications

- Give with food to ↓ GI irritation; teach to not chew or crush sustained-release capsules.
- Teach to avoid alcohol during therapy because of potentiation.
- Assess VS routinely for ↑ BP and ↑ P; ↑ or ↓ weight.
- Institute seizure precautions; assess for S&S of seizure.
- Instruct to notify primary health-care provider if pregnancy is planned.

Antipsychotic Agents: Decrease Agitated Behavior, Disorganized Thinking, and Positive and Negative Psychotic Signs and Symptoms

Mechanism of Action	Examples	Nontherapeutic Effects
Typical Antipsychotics Specific action depends on med. ↓ *positive symptoms:* Delusions, hallucinations, agitation, catatonia, disorganized speech and behavior.	chlorpromazine haloperidol (Haldol) prochlorperazine	• Sedation, ↓ BP, anorexia, sexual dysfunction, anticholinergic effects, photosensitivity. • Signs of cardiotoxicity, hepatotoxicity, agranulocytosis.
Atypical Antipsychotics Specific action depends on med. ↓ *negative symptoms:* Blunt affect, passivity, apathy, withdrawal, lack of pleasure, inability to decide and speak.	aripiprazole (Abilify) brexpiprazole (Rexulti) clozapine (Clozaril) olanzapine (Zyprexa) paliperidone palmetate (Invega Sustenna) quetiapine (Seroquel) risperidone (Risperdal) ziprasidone (Geodon)	**Extrapyramidal tract side effects** Dystonia (early in therapy); akathisia (most common); parkinsonism, tardive dyskinesia (prolonged use); may be reversible if dose is ↓ or withdrawn but some may be permanent. **Neuroleptic malignant syndrome** ↑ temp (cardinal sign), muscular rigidity, tremors, impaired ventilation, unstable BP, autonomic hyperactivity, muteness, altered LOC.

Nursing Care

- Teach that effect may take 1–2 wk; sedation may occur immediately; avoid hazardous activities; avoid coffee, tea, cola, antacids that ↓ med effectiveness.
- Obtain BP before each dose; hold med based on systolic and diastolic parameters.
- Assess for ↓ anticholinergic effects; ↑ fluids, ↑ fiber diet, suggest use of hard candy.

- Monitor CBC and liver function studies routinely.
- Assess weight to evaluate response to anorexia and energy expenditure related to extrapyramidal side effects.
- Assess for S&S of cardiotoxicity, particularly during initiation of therapy.
- Teach to limit exposure to sun; wear clothing, sunblock, sunglasses.
- Give prescribed med to ↓ extrapyramidal side effects: benztropine, clonazepam.
- Give prescribed meds to ↓ neuroleptic malignant syndrome: amantadine, bromocriptine, dantrolene.

Antimanic and Mood-Stabilizing Agents: Minimize Extreme Shifts in Emotions Between Mania and Depression

Mechanism of Action	Examples	Nontherapeutic Effects
Lithium Affects neurotransmitters dopamine, serotonin, norepinephrine, acetylcholine, and GABA.	lithium carbonate	• Headache, fatigue, recent memory loss, anorexia, N&V, diarrhea, muscle weakness, ↓ BP, dizziness. • Teratogenic effect during 1st trimester. • *Toxicity:* Slurred speech, ataxia, tremors, disorientation, confusion, severe thirst, cogwheel rigidity, dilute urine, tinnitus, respiratory depression, and coma.
CNS Agents, Antiseizure Agents Action varies depending on med.	carbamazepine (Tegretol) divaproex (Depakote) lamotrigine (Lamictal) topiramate (Topamax) valproic acid (Depakene)	• Drowsiness, fatigue, headache, nausea, blurred vision, psychomotor slowing. • May cause ↓ WBC and ↓ platelets.

Nursing Care

- **Lithium**
  - Teach that effect may take 1–2 wk, take with meals to ↓ GI irritation, not to crush or chew med.
  - Maintain fluid and Na intake because dehydration and hyponatremia may cause toxicity.
  - Assess therapeutic blood levels (0.15–1.5 mEq/L) weekly and then every 2–3 mo; has narrow therapeutic window.
- **CNS and antiseizure agents**
  - Teach that tablets and sustained-release tablets are swallowed whole, chewable tablets are chewed, and carbonated beverages are not used to dilute elixir.
  - Teach to avoid hazardous activities; protect from injury.
  - Monitor CBC and platelet counts routinely.

Medications for Attention Deficit Hyperactivity: Decrease Hyperactivity and Distractibility; Increase Alertness and Ability to Focus

Mechanism of Action	Examples	Nontherapeutic Effects
CNS Stimulants ↑ dopamine and norepinephrine in brain.	amphetamine/ dextroamphetamine (Adderall) lisdexamfetamine (Vyvanse) methamphexamine (Desoxyn) methylphenidate (Concerta, Ritalin)	• Anorexia, insomnia, hypersensitivity, tachycardia, palpitations, HTN, restlessness, weight loss, growth suppression. • May cause paradoxical hyperactivity.
Nonstimulant Norepinephrine Reuptake Inhibitors Inhibit norepinephrine uptake and transport.	atomoxetine (Strattera)	Headache, insomnia, anorexia, vomiting, abdominal pain, cough, irritability, aggression, impotence.

Nursing Care

- Give 30–45 min before meals to ↑ food intake before anorexia occurs.
- Give 6 hr before sleep to ↓ sleep disturbances.
- Obtain baseline and periodic weight because dose is based on weight.
- Assess for S&S of depression or aggression; may require stopping med.
- Inform school nurse and teacher of med regimen.
- Teach that a med holiday may be prescribed to assess progress and ↓ dependence.
- Withdraw gradually with medical supervision.
- *CNS stimulants*
  - Teach that duration is 3–6 hr; 8 hr for sustained-release forms.
  - Teach to not chew or crush sustained-release tablets.
- *Strattera*
  - Teach that duration is 12–24 hr.

Nontherapeutic Effects of Psychotropic Medications

Agranulocytosis

- S&S of infection: Fever, sore throat, cough.
- Urinary frequency, urgency due to UTI.

Anticholinergic Effects

- Dry mouth, urinary retention, constipation, blurred vision, ↑ P.

Cardiac Toxicity

- S&S of heart failure: ↓ BP, dysrhythmias, SOB, fatigue, ↑ weight, edema.

CNS Depression

- Drowsiness, sedation, orthostatic hypotension.

Peripheral CNS Stimulation (Sympathomimetic)

- ↑ P, ↑ BP, tremor, dysrhythmias.
- Restlessness, nightmares, insomnia, confusion.

Extrapyramidal Side Effects (EPS)

- *Akathisia:* Motor agitation, inability to rest or relax, pacing, restless legs, compulsive movements.
- *Dystonia:* Severe muscle spasms of back, neck, face, tongue.
- *Parkinsonism:* Tremor, muscle rigidity, bradykinesia, masklike facies, stooped posture, shuffling gait **(cogwheel gait)**, drooling, restlessness.
- *Tardive dyskinesia:* Involuntary movements of tongue and face such as rolling or protrusion of tongue, lip smacking, teeth grinding, chewing motions, tics; movements disappear during sleep.

Hepatotoxicity

- Altered liver function studies, jaundice.

Hypersensitivity

- Rash, fever, arthralgia, urticaria.

Hypertensive Crisis

- Caused by high-dose antipsychotic meds or med interactions.
- Headache, palpitations, stiff neck, photophobia, nausea, flushing, diaphoresis, dysrhythmias, death.

Hyponatremia

- N&V, diarrhea, fasciculations, stupor, seizures.

Neuroleptic Malignant Syndrome

- Caused by dopamine blockade in hypothalamus due to ↑ or prolonged dose of antipsychotic meds.
- ↑ temp (cardinal sign), diaphoresis, muscle rigidity, drowsiness, unstable BP, ↓ ventilation, dysrhythmias.

Serotonin Syndrome

- Caused by high dose of antidepressants; can be fatal.
- Confusion, anxiety, hyperpyrexia, ataxia, restlessness, tremors, hypertension, sweating.

Sexual Dysfunction

- ↓ libido, ↓ ability to reach orgasm, delayed ejaculation, impotence, cessation of menses or ovulation.

Herb-Drug Interactions

Herb/Use	Interactions
Echinacea Anti-infective, antipyretic.	↑ hepatotoxicity with amiodarone, anabolic steroids, ketoconazole, and methotrexate.
Feverfew Migraine headache.	↑ bleeding potential with aspirin, heparin, NSAIDs, and warfarin (Coumadin).
Garlic Lipid-lowering agent.	↑ bleeding potential with aspirin, NSAIDs, and warfarin. ↑ hypoglycemic effect of insulin and oral hypoglycemics.

Continued

Herb/Use	Interactions
Ginger Antiemetic.	↑ bleeding potential with aspirin, heparin, NSAIDs, and warfarin.
Ginkgo Antiplatelet agent, CNS stimulant.	↑ bleeding potential with aspirin, heparin, NSAIDs, and warfarin. ↓ effect of anticonvulsants, tricyclic antidepressants.
Ginseng ↑ stamina, ↑ immune response, ↑ appetite, antidepressant.	↓ anticoagulant effect of warfarin and ↓ effect of diuretics. ↑ hypoglycemic effect of insulin and oral hypoglycemics. ↑ digoxin toxicity and ↑ effect of CNS depressants.
Kava Kava Antianxiety agent, sedative, hypnotic.	↑ sedation with barbiturates, CNS depressants, and benzodiazepines. ↑ dystonia with phenothiazines.
Melatonin Promotes sleep, ↑ immune response.	↑ risk of bleeding with aspirin and anticoagulants. ↓ effectiveness of immunosuppressants and antihypertensives. ↑ level of melatonin in body when taken with birth control pills.
St. John's Wort Antidepressant.	↑ sedation with CNS depressants. ↓ effect of cyclosporine, reserpine, and theophylline. ↓ anticoagulant effect of warfarin and dabigatran. ↓ antiretroviral effect of protease inhibitors. ↑ risk for serotonin syndrome with tricyclics and SSRIs. ↑ risk for hypertensive crisis with MAO inhibitors.
Valerian Antianxiety agent, sedative, hypnotic.	↑ sedation with barbiturates, benzodiazepines, and CNS depressants.

Medication Administration: Key Points

Five Rights of Medication Administration	Client Rights
• Right **client** (check armband; date of birth; follow agency policy). • Right **medication**. • Right **dose**. • Right **route**. • Right **time**.	• Right to refuse medication. • Right to be educated. • Right to administration by knowledgeable, licensed person. • Right to be assessed before administration and evaluated after administration. • Right to have appropriate documentation.

Triple-Check Before Administration

- *First:* Check label when removing from storage.
- *Second:* Compare med label to med administration record (MAR).
- *Third:* Check again after med preparation, before administration.

Client Teaching

- Assess client attitude and ability for self-administration.
- Provide clear oral and written instructions; use understandable language.
- Include family members when appropriate.
- Evaluate learning; obtain return demonstration.
- Teach significant information
  - Generic and trade name, purpose, therapeutic effect.
  - Dose, route, frequency, and when to take prn meds.
  - Nontherapeutic effects and what to do if S&S occur.
  - How to store meds, to take with or without food; pre- and postadministration assessments; and what to do if a dose is missed.

Safe Medication Administration

Preadministration Activities

- Check clinical record for known allergies.
- Obtain history of prescription and OTC meds.
- Confirm written prescription; repeat back with a witness for verbal or phone prescriptions.
- Be informed; check sources when unfamiliar with med.
- Investigate compatibilities and interactions.
- Question overdose, subtherapeutic dose, med duplication, extended use, med prescription without indication.

Administration Activities

- Verify prescription against MAR.
- Calculate med dosage; double-check your calculation.
- Follow rights of med administration and triple-check procedure.
- Do not rush client; ensure oral meds are ingested.
- Record meds given; document reasons for nonadministered meds.
- Identify therapeutic and nontherapeutic responses.
- Notify primary health-care provider of concerns or if client vomits within 10 min of ingestion.

Safety and Legal Issues

- Do not borrow meds from another client.
- Give only meds personally prepared.
- Do not leave meds at bedside.
- Double-lock controlled meds; have wasted controlled meds witnessed.
- Use filtered needle when drawing meds from an ampule.
- Crush meds and mix with smallest amount of applesauce to facilitate ingestion of entire dose; do not crush enteric or time-release meds.
- Document after, not before, med is given; document and report med errors.

Factors Affecting Medication Therapy

- **Development level**
    - *Infants:* Immaturity of liver and kidneys require ↓ dose.
    - *Older adults:* ↓ liver and kidney function → accumulation; ↓ circulation and gastric function → ↓ med absorption; many meds **(polypharmacy)** ↑ interactions.
    - *Pregnancy:* May cause abnormal fetal development **(teratogenic)**.
- **Diet:** Nutrients can ↑ or ↓ absorption or action of med.
- **Gender:** Distribution of body fat, fluid, and hormones may affect med action.

- **Environment**: Cold temperature can ↑ peripheral vasoconstriction; warm temperature can ↑ vasodilation; noise can ↓ effect of sedatives and analgesics.
- **Pathology**: ↓ liver or kidney function can cause ↑ med accumulation; ↓ gastric or ↓ circulatory function can cause ↓ med absorption.
- **Time of administration**: ↑ absorption on empty stomach; given with food to ↓ GI distress; circadian and sleep cycles can affect response.
- **Body weight**: Dose calculated by client's weight or body surface area.
- **Genetic/ethnic/culture**: Usual dose may be toxic; herbal agents may ↑ or ↓ med action; Asian clients may need ↓ dose of antipsychotic and antianxiety meds due to slower metabolism of these meds; African American clients may need ↑ dose of antihypertensives.
- **Psychological**: Client's positive or negative expectations can ↑ or ↓ response.

Effects of Medications

- **Adverse effect**: Severe side effect or toxicity.
- **Allergic reaction**: Immunological reaction.
- **Anaphylactic reaction**: Hypersensitive, life-threatening reaction.
- **Cumulative effect**: Excessive level of med in body when intake is higher than metabolism or excretion.
- **Drug misuse**: Inappropriate intake of a med.
- **Drug dependence**: State that results from repeated substance use that causes S&S of withdrawal upon stopping the substance.
- **Drug habituation**: Degree of psychological, rather than psychological, dependence on continued use of a med to maintain a sense of well-being.
- **Drug interaction**: When one med alters the effect of one or more meds.
- **Drug tolerance**: Requiring ↑ dose to achieve therapeutic effect.
- **Drug toxicity**: Dangerous effect due to excessive amount of med.
- **Idiosyncratic effect**: Unexpected or unique response.
- **Inhibiting effect**: One med decreases effect of another med.
- **Potentiating**: One med adds to, prolongs, or ↑ action of another med.
- **Side effect**: Predictable nontherapeutic effect that is tolerable.
- **Synergistic effect**: Combined effect of two meds is greater than when effect of each are added together.
- **Therapeutic effect**: Reason med is prescribed; desired effect.

Medication Administration Routes

Route	Advantages (Pro) and Disadvantages (Con)	Nursing Care
Buccal Tablet or troche held between cheek and gum until dissolved. Local or systemic effect, depending on med. Absorbed within min.	**Pro**: Rapid relief. **Con**: Remains until dissolved; can be swallowed, chewed, or aspirated accidentally.	• Use standard precautions. • Alternate cheeks to avoid mucosal irritation. • Warn not to chew or swallow tablet or sleep until dissolved to ↓ risk of aspiration.
Nasogastric Tube, Gastrostomy Tube Instillation of med via a tube into stomach.	**Pro**: Used for ↓ gag reflex and unconscious clients. **Con**: Risk for aspiration; requires enteral tube and special equipment.	• Use standard precautions. • ↑ HOB; ensure placement of tube in stomach by aspirating gastric contents; clear tube with 30 mL of water; insert med through tube; clear tube with 30 mL of water after. • Assess for aspiration.
Inhalation Medications Dispersed through aerosolized solution or powder that penetrates airways, rapidly promoting absorption. MDI—metered-dose inhaler. NPA—nonpressurized aerosol nebulizer. DPI—dry powdered inhaler.	**Pro**: Rapid effect; can be given to unconscious client. Use of spacer/extender with MDI ↓ particle size, promoting ↑ absorption and less droplets on tongue. **Con**: Can cause undesired systemic effects. Equipment must be cleaned and stored.	**MDI** • Shake canister before each depression. • Exhale through pursed lips. • Hold 2 cm from mouth or insert mouthpiece beyond teeth with lips around mouthpiece (may use spacer).

Route	Advantages (Pro) and Disadvantages (Con)	Nursing Care
	Client with ↓ cognition, infants, or children may be unable to follow directions. MDI: Requires coordination with inhalation and device compression.	• Depress device while inhaling slowly and deeply; hold breath 5–10 sec. • Exhale slowly via pursed lips; wait 1–2 min between inhalations. • Rinse mouth and clean MDI afterward. **NPA** • Insert dose in chamber. • Breathe in and out with lips closed around mouthpiece. • Take deep breath every 5 breaths. • Repeat until no misting. • Rinse mouth and clean equipment afterward. **DPI** • Prepare inhaler for use. • Close mouth around mouthpiece. • Take deep breath; dose in chamber is aerosolized when inhaled. • Hold breath 5–15 sec. • Rinse mouth and clean DPI afterward.

Continued

Route	Advantages (Pro) and Disadvantages (Con)	Nursing Care
Intradermal (ID) Solution injected into dermis just under epidermis. Slow absorption. Volume 0.1–0.3 mL.	**Pro:** Used for allergy testing. **Con:** Pierces skin.	• Use sterile technique to prepare syringe. • Wear clean gloves to administer. • Assess for allergic or anaphylactic reaction when used for allergy testing.
Intramuscular (IM) Solution injected into muscle. Onset 3–5 min. Volume 1–3 mL.	**Pro:** Used when oral route is contraindicated; more rapidly absorbed than oral, topical, or Sub-Q. **Con:** Pierces skin; more tissue damage than Sub-Q. Requires adequate peripheral circulation. Can cause anxiety.	• Use sterile technique to prepare syringe. • Wear clean gloves to administer. • Position client to access injection site. • Landmark sites. • Rotate sites.
Intravenous (IV) Solution Injected into intravascular compartment via a vein. Immediate onset.	**Pro:** Immediate therapeutic effect. **Con:** More costly than oral; can cause anxiety.	• Use sterile technique to prepare infusion. • Wear gloves to administer infusion. • Administer IV push, intermittent, continuous titrated drips as prescribed. • Change tubing every 24–72 hr and site 3–7 days as per agency policy.

Route	Advantages (Pro) and Disadvantages (Con)	Nursing Care
Oral (PO) Taken by mouth in tablet, capsule, or liquid form. Absorbed in GI tract. Onset 30–45 min.	**Pro:** Convenient, does not invade skin, economical; less psychological stress than other routes. **Con:** May irritate gastric mucosa, have bad taste or odor, discolor or erode teeth, cause aspiration. **Contraindications:** Vomiting, dysphagia, unconsciousness, continuous NG suction.	• ↑ HOB to ensure safe swallowing. • Pace intake to ↓ aspiration. • Crush meds and mix with food if client has dysphagia; do not crush extended-release and enteric-coated meds; obtain liquid form if available. • Obtain prescription for alternate route if contraindication exists.
Rectal (PR) Suppository or solution inserted into anus. Slow absorption; local or systemic effect.	**Pro:** Used if oral route is contraindicated. **Con:** Client embarrassment; absorption unpredictable. **Contraindications:** Rectal surgery or rectal bleeding.	• Use standard precautions. • Position client in lateral or Sims position for insertion.
Subcutaneous (Sub-Q) Solution inserted into tissue just below skin. Onset 3–20 min. Volume ≤1 mL.	**Pro:** Faster than oral. **Con:** Pierces skin; can be irritating to tissue.	• Use sterile technique to prepare syringe. • Wear clean gloves to administer. • Landmark sites. • Rotate injection sites.
Sublingual (SL) Under tongue. Rapid absorption.	**Pro:** Immediate therapeutic response. **Con:** Can be swallowed, chewed, or aspirated accidentally.	• Use standard precautions. • Instruct to keep liquid or tablet under tongue. • Warn not to chew or swallow tablet or sleep until it is absorbed.

Continued

Route	Advantages (Pro) and Disadvantages (Con)	Nursing Care
Swish and Spit Solution dispersed throughout oral cavity and expelled from mouth. **Swish and Swallow** Solution dispersed throughout oral cavity and swallowed.	**Pro**: Easy and inexpensive to implement; provides local effect. **Con**: Some clients may not be able to follow directions to swish solution; may swallow the solution meant for a swish and spit; may be accidentally aspirated.	• Instruct to keep lips closed and by puffing cheeks in and out move solution around entire oral cavity and then: • *Swish and spit:* Expel solution from mouth. • *Swish and swallow:* Swallow solution.
Transdermal Via the skin (percutaneous). Prolonged absorption.	**Pro**: Prolonged systemic effect; limited side effects; avoids GI irritation. **Con**: Residue may irritate skin or soil clothes.	• Wear gloves to prevent self-contamination. • Use site indicated by manufacturer such as chest, upper arms, anterior thighs. • Rotate sites. • Avoid impaired skin; use hairless area to ensure patch contact. • Wash site after removing patch.
Vaginal Inserted into vaginal vault.	**Pro**: Local effect. **Con**: Limited use; client embarrassment.	• Use standard precautions. • Clean perineum before and after insertion. • Position in dorsal recumbent or Sims position. • Lubricate applicator or finger with water-soluble gel.

Route	Advantages (Pro) and Disadvantages (Con)	Nursing Care
		• Insert applicator into vagina to depth recommended by manufacturer and depress plunger; insert suppository full length of index finger. • Instruct to remain supine for 15 min. • Wash and dry applicator.

Intradermal (ID), Subcutaneous (Sub-Q), and Intramuscular (IM)

	ID	Sub-Q	IM
Site	Inner forearm, chest, and back.	Outer upper arm, anterior thigh, upper and lower back, "love handles," abdomen.	Gluteus, vastus lateralis, deltoid muscles.
Gauge	27–30	25–28	22–23
Length	1/4–3/8 inch	5/16, 1/2, 5/8 inch	1–1½ inch
Angle	10–15°	90° 45° for very thin clients.	90°
Volume	0.1–0.2 mL	0.5–1 mL	Up to 3 mL; small muscles (deltoid) no more than 1 mL.

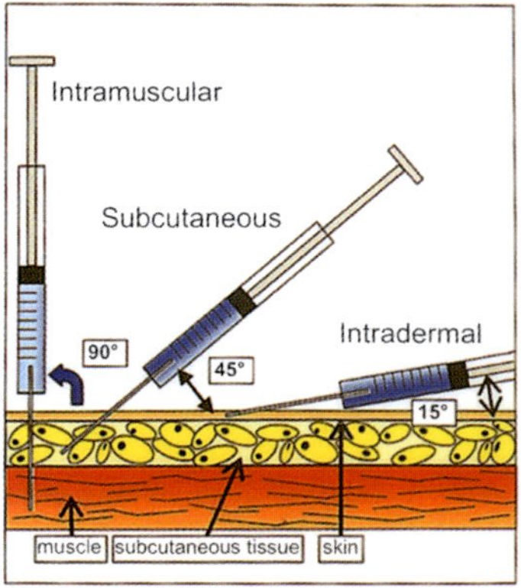

Sub-Q Heparin and Low Molecular Weight Anticoagulant Injections

Site	Gauge and Angle	Aspirate	Massage Site
Abdomen, posterior upper arm, low back, thigh, and upper back.	25–26 gauge, 1/2–5/8 inch. 90° angle (45° if client is underweight).	No	No

Injection Techniques

Commonalities of Injection Techniques

- Use sterile technique to prepare syringe.
- Wear clean gloves for administration.
- Provide privacy.
- Landmark injection site.
- Wipe insertion site with alcohol.
- Inject solution slowly to ↓ discomfort.
- Withdraw needle via same needle track after administration.
- Activate needle guard.
- Discard syringe in sharps container.

Subcutaneous Injection Sites

	Specific Injection Techniques
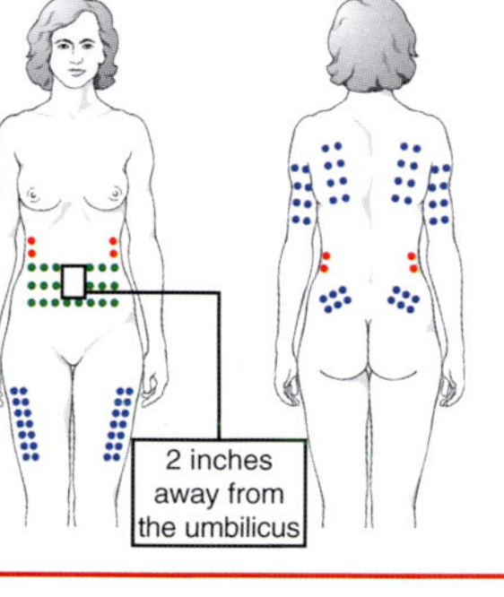	• See Commonalities of Injection Techniques, p. 293. • Landmark sites: Abdomen—green dots; extremities, scapular area, upper buttocks—blue dots; love handles—red dots. • Pinch or spread skin. • Insert 1-inch needle at 45° angle and ≤1-inch needle at 90° angle. • Follow agency policy regarding whether to aspirate syringe or not; never aspirate an anticoagulant or insulin.

Intramuscular Injection Sites

Specific Injection Techniques

- See Commonalities of Injection Techniques, p. 293.
- Spread skin, insert needle at 90° angle.
- Insert needle to hub in dartlike, steady motion.
- Aspirate to ensure no blood return; follow agency policy if different.
- Massage site; do not massage site when using Z track.

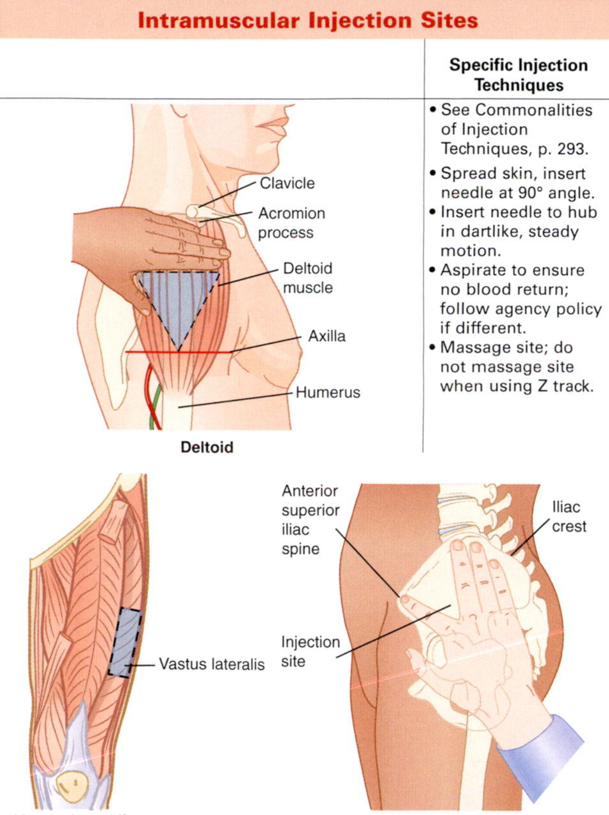

Z-Track Method for Giving IM Injections

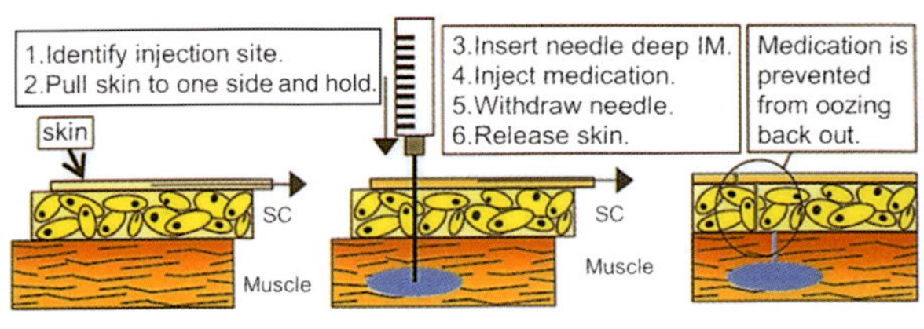

IV Piggyback (IVPB) Setup

- Assess integrity of primary IV site such as no S&S of infiltration or inflammation; ensure primary set is patent and not expired.
- Ensure compatibility of primary solution and med in IVPB.
- Attach secondary tubing to IVPB bag; flush tubing without wasting any solution; clamp tubing.
- Hang IVPB bag higher than primary IV bag; primary IV bag may need a hook to extend bag lower.
- Connect secondary tubing to primary set using port most distal from client.
- Open IVPB tubing clamp, set rate via primary set roller clamp.

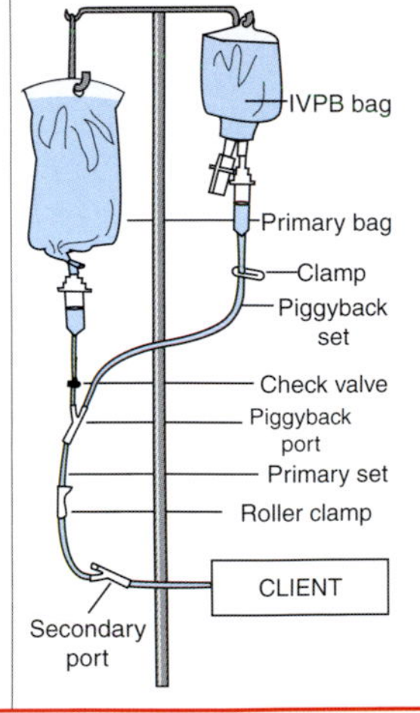

Complications of IV Therapy

Complication	Nursing Assessment	Nursing Care
Infiltration IV fluid escapes into subcutaneous tissue; ↓ or no fluids infusing.	Assess site for swelling, pale, cool to touch. No blood return when IV bag is held lower than insertion site.	• Discontinue IV; apply prescribed warm compress as per policy; restart in new site. • *Prevention:* Discourage movement of limb with IV.
Phlebitis Inflammation of vein. **Thrombus** Blood clot.	*Phlebitis:* Assess for red line or burning pain along course of vein, heat, and swelling. *Thrombus:* IV flow may stop due to obstruction.	• Discontinue IV; apply prescribed warm compress as per policy; do not massage or rub affected area; restart in new site; notify primary health-care provider. • *Prevention:* Discourage movement of limb with IV; flush as per policy; rotate sites as per policy (generally every 72 hr).
Fluid Overload Client cannot tolerate rate of infusion; rate is faster than prescribed.	Assess for hypervolemia: Bounding, ↑ P; ↑ BP; ↑ R; lung base crackles; dyspnea; distended neck veins.	• ↓ IV rate and notify primary health-care provider. • If experiencing respiratory complications: ↑ HOB; provide O_2 at 2 L/min. • *Prevention:* Assess response during 1st 15 min frequently after hanging new solution; assess rate regularly; use time tape and volume control device.

Continued

Complication	Nursing Assessment	Nursing Care
Incorrect Solution Solution other than what was prescribed is infusing.	Check IV prescription with hanging IV fluid.	• ↓ IV rate to maintain patency; immediately hang correct solution; notify primary health-care provider; complete incident report. • *Prevention:* Verify solution with prescription 3 times before hanging IV solution.
IV Rate Is Too Slow Volume absorbed is ↓ than volume prescribed.	Inspect factors affecting flow such as kinks, lying on tubing, dependent loops; IV bag too low; arm position that impairs flow rate.	• Remove tubing from under client; coil tubing on bed; reposition arm; maintain at prescribed rate (do not increase rate faster than prescribed rate because it may precipitate fluid overload). • Change IV site if infiltrated. • *Prevention:* Assess flow rate routinely, use time tape and volume control device, position bag 3 feet above IV site, coil tubing on bed surface, discourage movement of limb with IV.
Air Embolus Air in intravascular compartment.	Assess for respiratory distress, ↑ P, cyanosis, ↓ BP, ↓ LOC.	• Secure system to prevent entry of air; place client on left side in modified Trendelenburg position; continue to assess VS, O_2 sat. • Notify primary health-care provider. • *Prevention:* Flush IV lines of air before use; assess integrity of system frequently.

Medication Calculation Formulas

IV Drop Rate Formula

- Drop factor equals number of drops per mL delivered by IV tubing.

$$\text{Drops per minute} = \frac{\overset{\text{(total volume in drops)}}{\text{total mL X drop factor}}}{\underset{\text{(total time in minutes)}}{\text{1 hour X 60 minutes}}}$$

Conversion of Pounds to Kilograms (kg)

- Solve for X by cross multiplying.
- Divide both sides of resulting equation by the number in front of the X.
- Reduce to lowest terms to achieve child's weight in kg.

$$\frac{\text{child's weight in lb}}{\text{2.2 lb}} = \frac{\text{x kg}}{\text{1 kg}}$$

Ratio and Proportion Formulas

- Prescribed dose and dose on hand must be in same unit of measure.
- **Formulas 1 and 2:** Solve for X by cross multiplying.
- **Formula 3:** Solve for X by multiplying the means and the extremes.
- Divide both sides of all resulting equations by the number in front of the X.
- Reduce to lowest terms to achieve the quantity of dose.

#1 $$\frac{\text{desired}}{\text{have}} = \frac{\text{prescribed dose}}{\text{dose on hand}} = \frac{\text{X quantity desired}}{\text{quantity on hand}}$$

#2 $$\frac{\text{quantity on hand}}{\text{dose on hand}} = \frac{\text{X quantity desired}}{\text{prescribed dose}}$$

#3 dose on hand : quantity on hand :: prescribed dose : X quantity desired
(extreme) **(means)** **(means)** **(extreme)**

Pediatric Dosage Calculations

Body Surface Area (BSA) Method

- Estimate the child's BSA in square meters (m^2) by using a BSA chart (nomogram).*
- The BSA chart consists of three columns. The left column is height, the middle column is body surface area, and the right column is weight. These numbers increase from the bottom to the top of each column.
- Draw a straight line from the child's height in the left column to the child's weight in the right column. The number found where the line crosses the middle column is the child's estimated BSA.
- The BSA should be used in the formula for the body surface area method to calculate a pediatric dose.

$$\text{Pediatric dose in mg} = \frac{\text{child's BSA in square meters } (m^2) \times \text{adult dose in mg}}{1.73\ m^2}$$

Young's Rule: Age-Based (1–12 Yr) Method

$$\text{Child's dose} = \frac{\text{child's age (in yr)}}{\text{child's age (in yr + 12)}} \times \text{average adult dose}$$

*Vallerand and Sanoski, with Deglin; *Davis's Drug Guide for Nurses*, 14th Ed., 2015; F.A. Davis Co., Philadelphia; Appendix F, Body Surface Area Nomograms, p.1402.

Test Analysis Tools

- This tab includes tips and analysis tools that will help you pass the NCLEX-RN®. Seven tools are included to help you analyze your test performance:
  1. Performance Trends
  2. Information Processing Errors
  3. Knowledge Deficits: Universal Information
  4. Knowledge Deficits: Medical-Surgical Nursing
  5. Knowledge Deficits: Pediatric Nursing
  6. Knowledge Deficits: Childbearing Nursing
  7. Knowledge Deficits: Mental Health and Psychiatric Nursing
- Performance trends and information-processing errors focus on the process of test taking, and corrective-action plans are presented to address your identified deficits.
- Knowledge deficits: Basic information focuses on content common to all disciplines in nursing practice.
- Four tools concerning knowledge deficits (medical-surgical, pediatric, childbearing, and mental health/psychiatric nursing) focus on discipline-specific content.

Instructions for Performance Trends

- Answer the following questions to identify opportunities to improve your test-taking skills:

Performance Trends	
• I am able to focus with little distraction.	Yes ( ) No ( )
• I feel calm and in control.	Yes ( ) No ( )
• I effectively use test-taking techniques to reduce options.	Yes ( ) No ( )
• I change answers from wrong to right.	Yes ( ) No ( )
• I have no error clusters: beginning, middle, or end of exam.	Yes ( ) No ( )

- If you answered **No** to any of these questions, see the tool **Corrective Action Plan**.

Instructions for Information-Processing Errors and Knowledge-Deficit Tools

- First look over each tool. After taking and scoring your test, use the tools to help you identify your area of weakness.
- Complete all tools in the same way:
  1. Identify the **processing error** or **knowledge category** associated with a question you got wrong.
  2. Insert the number of the question you got wrong in the box in the column to the right of the processing error or knowledge category you identified.
  3. Complete the first 2 steps for all the questions you got wrong.
  4. Tally the total number of questions you got wrong for each row in the last column on the right; after you identify clusters of deficits, see the tool **Corrective Action Plan** and follow the suggestions addressing your specific deficit.

Information-Processing Errors

Knowledge Category	Question Numbers							
Stem								
• Missed negative polarity								
• Missed word that set priority								
• Missed important clues								
• Misinterpreted information								
• Missed central point, theme								
• Read into the question								
• Missed step in nursing process								
• Incompletely analyzed stem								
• Did not understand question								
• Did not know the content								

Information-Processing Errors—cont'd

Knowledge Category	Question Numbers							
Options								
• Selected the answer too quickly								
• Misidentified the priority								
• Misinterpreted information								
• Read into options								
• Did not know the content								
• Misapplied concepts, principles								
• Transcribed incorrectly								

Knowledge Deficits: Basic Information

Knowledge Category	Question Numbers							
• A&P and pathophysiology								
• Basic care (including pain)								
• Community care								
• Complementary, alternative care								
• Death/dying/loss/grief								
• Emergency care								
• Fluid and electrolyte balance								
• Growth and development								
• Inflammation/infection								
• Leadership and management								
• Legal and ethical issues								

Continued

Knowledge Deficits: Basic Information—cont'd

Knowledge Category	Question Numbers							
• Perioperative								
• Pharmacology								
• Psychosociocultural/spirituality/ communication								
• Safety (physical/ microbiological)								
• Teaching and learning								

Knowledge Deficits: Medical-Surgical Nursing

Knowledge Category	Question Numbers								
• Cardiac									
• Endocrine									
• GI, accessory organs of digestion (gallbladder, liver, pancreas)									
• GI, upper (mouth, esophagus, stomach)									
• GI, lower (small and large intestines)									
• Hematological, immunological, lymphatic									
• Integumentary									
• Musculoskeletal									
• Neoplastic									
• Neurological									
• Peripheral vascular									
• Reproductive (female)									

Knowledge Deficits: Medical-Surgical Nursing—cont'd

Knowledge Category	Question Numbers								
• Reproductive (male)									
• Respiratory									
• Urinary									
• Other									

Knowledge Deficits: Pediatric Nursing

Knowledge Category	Question Numbers								
• Cardiac disease (congenital, acquired)									
• Endocrine									
• GI, accessory organs of digestion (gallbladder, liver, pancreas)									
• GI, upper (mouth, esophagus, stomach)									
• GI, lower (small and large intestines)									
• Genitourinary									
• Growth and development									
• Health promotion and immunization									
• Hematological, immunological, lymphatic									

Continued

Knowledge Deficits: Pediatric Nursing—cont'd

Knowledge Category	Question Numbers								
• Integumentary									
• Musculoskeletal									
• Neoplastic									
• Neurological									
• Peripheral vascular									
• Respiratory									
• Other									

Knowledge Deficits: Childbearing Nursing

Knowledge Category	Question Numbers								
• Family									
• Diagnostic testing									
• Nutrition: Maternal, infant (breast/formula)									
• Prenatal care									
• Intrapartal care (labor/birth)									
• High-risk pregnancy									
• Obstetric emergencies									
• Postpartum care									
• Healthy newborn									
• High-risk newborn									
• Other									

Knowledge Deficits: Mental Health Nursing

Knowledge Category	Question Numbers								
• Defense mechanisms									
• Domestic violence									
• Legal and ethical issues									
• Mental health assessment									
• Therapeutic communication									
• Therapeutic modalities									
• Other									
Disorders									
• Anxiety, panic, PTSD									
• Bipolar and depressive disorders									
• Dissociative disorders									
• Eating disorders (anorexia, bulimia)									
• Gender dysphoria and paraphilic disorders									
• Neurocognitive disorders (dementia, Alzheimer)									
• Neurodevelopmental disorders (autism, ADHD, intellectual disability)									
• Obsessive-compulsive and related disorders									
• Personality disorders									
• Schizophrenia									
• Somatic symptom and related disorders									
• Substance use disorders									
• Other									

Corrective Action Plan

Performance Trends

- Implement recommendations if you scored **No** on the Performance Trends tool.
  1. Be comfortable, rested, sit in area free of distractions; wear earplugs.
  2. Develop a positive mental attitude (challenge negative thoughts, use positive self-talk: "I can do this!").
     - Regain control (use deep breathing, imagery, muscle relaxation).
     - Desensitize yourself to fear response (practice test taking).
     - Establish control on day of exam (manage routine, travel, environment, supplies).
     - Stop exam, take a break, and regain control; do not get bogged down on answering questions on content you do not know—move on; overprepare for the exam.
  3. Practice test-taking tips presented on Davis*Plus*.
  4. If you change more answers from right to wrong on practice tests, **do not** change your first answer unless you are absolutely certain that the new answer is correct.
  5. Use anxiety-reducing techniques during the exam at times when error clusters appeared in practice; if due to fatigue, stop exam and take a short break; work at practice tests longer to increase stamina.

Information-Processing Errors

- Practice test-taking tips presented on Davis*Plus*.
- For more detail see Nugent, *Test Success: Test-Taking Techniques for Beginning Nursing Students,* F. A. Davis, Philadelphia.

Knowledge Deficits: All Areas

- Focus study on clustered gaps in knowledge.
- Review notes, text, computer-assisted instruction, videos, and practice test questions with rationales; use study workbooks and computer programs.
- Do not waste time studying areas you know.
- Explore the F. A. Davis Notes series and Davis Essential Nursing Content + Practice Questions Series for additional resources when preparing for the NCLEX exam.

Illustration Credits

Tab 2: ©1983 Wong-Baker FACES Foundation. www.WongBakerFACES.org. Used with permission. Originally published in *Whaley & Wong's Nursing Care of Infants and Children.* © Elsevier Inc.

Tab 4: The Centers for Disease Control and Prevention.

Tab 7: Wilkinson J. M., and Treas L. S. *Fundamentals of Nursing Theory, Concepts, and Applications,* 3rd ed. F. A. Davis, Philadelphia, 2015.

Index